Chapman & Hall/CRC Biostatistics Series

Statistical Methods for Drug Safety

Robert D. Gibbons

University of Chicago

Illinois, USA

Anup K. Amatya

New Mexico State University

Las Cruces, USA

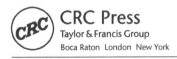

CRC Press

Taylor & Francis Group

Boca Raton London New York

CRC Press is an imprint of the
Taylor & Francis Group, an **informa** business

A CHAPMAN & HALL BOOK

Chapman & Hall/CRC Biostatistics Series

Published Titles

Chapman & Hall/CRC Biostatistics Series

Statistical Methods for Drug Safety

Robert D. Gibbons

University of Chicago

Illinois, USA

Anup K. Amatya

New Mexico State University

Las Cruces, USA

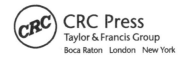

CRC Press

Taylor & Francis Group

Boca Raton   London   New York

CRC Press is an imprint of the
Taylor & Francis Group, an **informa** business

A CHAPMAN & HALL BOOK

CRC Press
Taylor & Francis Group
6000 Broken Sound Parkway NW, Suite 300
Boca Raton, FL 33487-2742

First issued in paperback 2022

ISBN 13: 978-1-03-247729-9 (pbk)
ISBN 13: 978-1-4665-6184-7 (hbk)

DOI: 10.1201/b18698

**Visit the Taylor & Francis Web site at
http://www.taylorandfrancis.com**

**and the CRC Press Web site at
http://www.crcpress.com**

To Carol, Julie, Jason and Michael and the memory of Donna and Sid
R.D.G.

To my family and friends
A.K.A.

Contents

Preface

"It is a capital mistake to theorize before one has data. Insensibly one begins to twist facts to suit theories, instead of theories to suit facts."
(Sir Arthur Conan Doyle, Sherlock Holmes)

My (RDG) first encounter with statistical issues related to drug safety came on the heels of then President George Bush senior taking the drug Halcion and throwing up on the Japanese ambassador. Sidney Wolfe of Public Citizen immediately filed suit against the U.S. FDA and the Upjohn Company for a myriad of adverse effects of the drug. The FDA turned to the Institute of Medicine (IOM) of the National Academy of Sciences to review the matter. I received a call from Dr. Andy Pope of the IOM asking if I would be willing and interested in being a member of the IOM committee that was to opine on this question. I told him that I would think about it and get back to him. I then called Dr. Joe Flaherty, Dean of the School of Medicine, and asked him if the IOM (which I had never really heard of) was some kind of right-wing religious organization. He told me that it was, but that I should do whatever they asked. I agreed to be a member of the committee, and it led to a series of different committees which have been among the most interesting, challenging, and rewarding scientific experiences of my career.

In terms of the safety and efficacy of the drug Halcion, during the first IOM committee meeting, I sat quietly and listened while the group of distinguished scientists discussed the evidence base and voiced their opinions. The late Bill Brown from Stanford and I were the two statisticians on the committee and at the end of the meeting we said, this all sounds great, but why don't we just get the data and find out what is really going on. This turned out to be a really bad idea because a truck pulled up to my office with a room full of paper supplied by Upjohn, and Don Hedeker (now at the University of Chicago) and I spent about a month digging through it. We ultimately found the appropriate measures of safety and efficacy for each study which we were able to synthesize across the 25 or so randomized clinical trials (RCTs) and show that the drug was indeed efficacious at its currently labeled dosages and that it had a similar safety profile to the other drugs in its class. Most importantly we found no evidence that the drug would increase one's level of nausea in the presence of foreign dignitaries beyond the already elevated base rate when in the company of politicians.

The IOM report was published in 1997 (IOM, 1997) and reports in the medical (Bunney et al. 1999) and statistical literatures (Gibbons et al. 1999) followed. This early experience led to two more IOM studies that involved drug safety issues, the IOM Study on the Prevention of Suicide (Goldsmith et al. 2002) and the IOM Study on the Future of Drug Safety (Burke et al. 2006). It was clear to me at this time that there were several singular statistical features of interest in the analysis of pharmacoepidemiologic data that had yet to be explored. The issue of whether drugs, in particular antidepressants, increased the risk of suicide, a condition they were at least in part designed to treat, was one of the more interesting problems that I had encountered, and because of my service to the IOM committee on the prevention of suicide, I was asked to be on the FDA Scientific Advisory Committee which ultimately placed a black box warning on all antidepressants with regards to suicidal thoughts and behavior in children, adolescents and young adults. My former student now colleague and co-author of this book, Anup Amatya, and I have spent many years studying both this question and the impact of the black box warning on the treatment of depression in youth and on its relationship to suicidal events. Statistically it is a very challenging area because suicidal thoughts and behavior may lead to antidepressant treatment, but the question is can we disentangle these selection effects from the possible causal effect of antidepressant treatment on suicidal thoughts, behavior, and completion. The public health importance of this question is enormous given the large number of patients with depression and related mental health disorders and the frequency with which they receive antidepressant treatment. As such, many of the illustrations of statistical methods presented in this book are drawn from this area. If you can solve this problem, you can solve most other pharmacoepidemiologic problems, because most other drug safety problems are far less complicated.

I tell my students that applied statistics is a lot like dating; you should hang around wealthy people and marry for love. The same is true in applied statistics; it takes just as much effort to provide a rigorous statistical solution to an unimportant problem as it does to solve important problems that can change the world and improve our public health. Drug safety is certainly one of the most important problems in this era. What I don't tell them is that working at the interface between public policy and statistics is not for the faint of heart. For every person that admires your work, there is one, and often far more, that are not at all pleased with the conclusions that you or others draw from your statistical work. These individuals can be quite vocal about their dissatisfaction. My favorite blogger comment is "Dr. Gibbons should stick to his statistical knitting, he doesn't know his front end from his rear end when it comes to clinical judgment." These are generally not waters where statisticians have experience treading.

This book covers a wide variety of statistical approaches to pharmacoepidemiologic data, some of which are commonly used (e.g., proportional reporting ratios for analysis of spontaneous adverse event reports) and others which are quite new to the field (e.g., use of marginal structural models for controlling dynamic selection bias in analysis of large-scale longitudinal observational data). Readers of this book will learn about linear and non-linear mixed-effects models, discrete-time survival models, new approaches to the meta-analysis of rare binary adverse events and when the traditional approaches can get you into trouble, research synthesis involving reanalysis of complete longitudinal patient records from RCTs (not to be confused with meta-analysis which attempts to synthesize effect sizes), causal inference models such as propensity score matching, marginal structural models, differential effects; mixed-effects Poisson regression models for the analysis of ecological data such as county-level adverse event rates, and a wide variety of other methods useful for analysis of within-subject and between-subject variation in adverse events abstracted from large scale medical claims databases, electronic health records, and other observational data streams. We hope that this book provides a useful resource for a wide variety of statistical methods that are useful to pharmacoepidemiologists in their work and motivation for statistical scientists to work in this exciting area and develop new methods that go far beyond the foundation provided here.

Acknowledgments

We are thankful to Fan Yang and Don Hedeker of the University of Chicago, and Arvid Sjolander of the Karolinska Institute for their helpful review and suggestions. Hendricks Brown (Northwestern) was instrumental in conceiving of many of the original examples related to suicide and antidepressants and Kwan Hur (Veterans Administration and the University of Chicago) helped greatly in the preparation of the illustrations. The book would not have been possible without financial support of the National Institute of Mental Health R01 MH8012201 (Gibbons and Brown Principal Investigators) and the Center for Education and Research on Therapeutics (CERT) grant U19HS021093 funded by the Agency for Healthcare Research and Quality (Bruce Lambert (Northwestern) Principal Investigator) [1]. And of course, to my (RDG) teacher, R. Darrell Bock, Professor Emeritus at the University of Chicago, who taught me (and in turn all of my students) how to think as a statistician and ignited my passion for the development of new statistical methodologies for interesting applied problems. I (RDG) have been an expert witness on various legal cases involving problems in drug safety for the U.S. Department of Justice, Wyeth, Pfizer, GlaxoSmithKline, and Merck pharmaceutical companies

---

[1] This project was supported by grant number U19HS021093 from the Agency for Healthcare Research and Quality. The content is solely the responsibility of the authors and does not necessarily represent the official views of the Agency for Healthcare Research and Quality.

1

Introduction

"All drugs are poisons, the benefit depends on the dosage."
(Philippus Theophrastrus Bombast that of Aureolus Paracelsus - 1493-1541)

As noted in the Institute of Medicine report on the Future of Drug Safety (Burke et al. 2006):

"Every day the Food and Drug Administration (FDA) works to balance expeditious access to drugs with concerns for safety, consonant with its mission to protect and advance the public health. The task is all the more complex given the vast diversity of patients and how they respond to drugs, the conditions being treated, and the range of pharmaceutical products and supplements patients use. Reviewers in the Center for Drug Evaluation and Research (CDER) at the FDA must weigh the information available about a drug's risk and benefit, make decisions in the context of scientific uncertainty, and integrate emerging information bearing on a drug's risk-benefit profile throughout the lifecycle of a drug, from drug discovery to the end of its useful life. These processes may have life-or-death consequences for individual patients, and for drugs that are widely used, they may also affect entire segments of the population. The distinction between individual and population is important because it reflects complex determinations that FDA must make when a drug that is life-saving for a specific patient may pose substantial risk when viewed from a population health perspective. In a physicians office, the patient and the provider make decisions about the risk and benefits of a given drug for that patient, whereas FDA has to assess risks and benefits with a view toward their effects on the population. The agency has made great efforts to balance the need for expeditious approvals with great attention to safety, as reflected in its mission to protect and advance the health of the public."

Although pre-marketing clinical trials are required for all new drugs before they are approved for marketing, with the use of any medication comes the possibility of adverse drug reactions (ADRs) that may not be detected in the highly selected populations recruited into randomized clinical trials. A primary aim in pharmacovigilance is the timely detection of either new ADRs or a relevant change in the frequency of ADRs that are already known to be associated with a certain drug that may only be detected in more typical clinical populations with their greater range of illness severity and more co-morbid illness and use of other medications (Egberts 2005). Moreover, less common ADRs will require larger populations to be detected, than are typically available in RCTs. Historically, pharmacovigilance relied upon case studies such as the "yellow card" system in Britain, and case control studies (Rawlins 1984). The Uppsala Monitoring Center paper and classic Venning publications also highlighted the importance of individual case reports for signal detection (Venning 1983). More recently, pharmacovigilance has relied upon large-scale spontaneous reporting systems in which adverse events experienced within a population (the entire United States or the Veterans Administration) are the focus of analytic work. Such data are useful for the detection of rare adverse events which are unlikely to occur for natural causes, such as youthful death, but are questionable for adverse events which occur commonly in the population for a myriad of possible reasons. While there are many reasons that a person may feel blue, whether they are or are not exposed to a pharmaceutical, there are far fewer alternative explanations for patients turning blue following a drug exposure. The purpose of this book is to provide the applied statistician and pharmacoepidemiologist with a detailed statistical overview of the various tools that are available for the analysis of possible ADRs. To various degrees, these tools will fill in the gap between identification of ADRs like feeling blue and turning blue.

1.1   Randomized Clinical Trials

Drawing inferences from pharmacoepidemiologic data is complicated for many reasons. While randomized clinical trials generally insulate one from bias in that the process by which patients are selected for the treatment that they receive is governed by the laws of probability, they invariably suffer from lack of generalizability to the population that is truly of interest. This is because the patients who are either recruited for such trials or are willing to subject themselves to the experience may have little resemblance to those people who ultimately will receive the treatment in routine practice. As an example, most pediatric antidepressant medication trials excluded children with evidence of suicidal ideation or behavior. These trials formed the basis for FDA analysis of a possible link between antidepressant treatment and suicidality (i.e., a rather poor term that is intended to encompass suicidal thoughts, behavior and completion), for which it can and has been argued that this exclusion criterion rendered the results of the analysis of little value in terms of our ability to draw inferences to "real world" drug exposures. Pharmacoepidemiology is also one of the few areas where randomization itself does not insure the absence of biased conclusions. Comparison of patients receiving an active medication versus those receiving placebo can lead to ascertainment bias in which patients receiving active medication will experience more side-effects in general than patients randomized to placebo, leading to increased contact with medical study staff and greater likelihood of the spontaneous reporting of an adverse event of interest, regardless of whether or not there is any real causal link between the drug and the adverse event. Returning to the pediatric suicide example, a variety of ascertainment biases seem likely. Depressed children often have suicidal thoughts and increased physician contact due to increased risk of gastrointestinal side effects from modern antidepressant medications such as selective serotonergic reuptake inhibitors (SSRIs) can lead to increased frequency of reports of suicidal thoughts among children randomized to active SSRI treatment. Equally threatening to our ability to draw unbiased conclusions in this area is related to suicide attempts that are made by children (or adults) in antidepressant RCTs. A suicide attempt made by taking an overdose of study medication will have serious consequence and high likelihood of detection if the patient was randomized to active medication, but little likelihood of detection for a patient who attempts suicide by overdosing on placebo. The net result is an apparent association between active treatment and a very serious adverse event that may not be causal in nature despite the unquestionable benefits of randomization.

Of course, there are many adverse events that are simply too rare to even be studied in the context of an RCT. As an example suicide has an annual rate of 11 per 100,000 in the United States and 5-10 times that rate among depressed patients. Even then, there are no studies large enough to have the statistical power to examine the effects of a medication on suicide. Even in FDA's (2006) meta-analysis of 372 RCTs consisting of almost 100,000 patients, there were only 8 completed suicides which were seen in equal distribution among patients randomized to placebo and antidepressant medication (Thomas 2006). As will be discussed, while meta-analysis is useful for synthesizing information across a large number of similarly designed RCTs, meta-analysis is itself an observational study of studies and insulation from bias provided by randomization in an individual study is not always guaranteed when studies are combined. For example, studies may recruit subjects with different indications for treatment (e.g., antiepileptic drugs are used for the treatment of epilepsy, chronic pain, and bipolar disorder), the different drugs have different mechanisms of action, and the different studies have different randomization schedules (1:1, 2:1, and 3:1). Differences in the base-rate of an adverse event that may be confounded with randomization schedule can lead to the appearance of an association between the drug exposure and the adverse event where none exists, depending on the statistical method used for combining the data across studies. Furthermore, as will be described, when the adverse event is rare, many traditional and widely used statistical methods for meta-analysis can yield results that are biased in the direction of finding a significant ADR when none exists.

1.2　Observational Studies

In contrast to RCTs, observational studies can be (1) much larger in size making evaluation of even rare ADRs possible, (2) are generally more representative of routine clinical practice than RCTs, and (3) are capable of identifying drug interactions which may explain heterogeneity of drug safety profiles in the population. However, the price paid for this generalizability is that observational studies are highly prone to selection bias. Stated simply, characteristics of the individual can lead patients and/or their physicians to select different treatments and those characteristics become confounded with the treatment effects. This is sometimes referred to as "confounding by indication." A classic example relates back to the suicide example in which the likelihood of suicide and related thoughts and behavior are elevated in patients with depression and those are the same patients who receive antidepressants; therefore, antidepressants will invariably be found to be associated with increased rates of suicidality in the general population. However, even if we were to select a cohort that was restricted to patients with depression, confounding by indication may still be in operation because among depressed patients, the most severely ill will have the highest likelihood of receiving antidepressant treatment and reporting suicidal thoughts and/or behavior. To make matters worse, these confounds are not static, but rather dynamic throughout the treatment process. The choice of switching from drug A to drug B may be due to lack of treatment response on drug A; hence, more treatment resistant patients will receive drug B, and in some cases the presence of the adverse event may be due to this treatment resistance and not the drug itself.

Insulation from bias when analyzing observational data is no simple task. The statistical field of causal inference is relevant, because it is based on methods that under certain assumptions are capable of supporting causal inferences from observational studies. The general idea is to extract something similar to a randomized controlled trial out of a larger observational dataset. This can be done in a variety of different ways based on matching (e.g., propensity score matching), weighting (e.g., marginal structural models), or identifying an appropriate instrumental variable. An instrument is a variable which in and of itself is not an explanatory variable for the adverse effect, but is related to the probability that the patient will receive the treatment and is uncorrelated with the error terms of the ADR prediction equation. As an example, Davies et al. (2013) used prior prescription of an SSRI vs. tricyclic antidepressant (TCA) by the treating physician as a surrogate instrument for the actual prescription the next patient received. Prior prescriptions were strongly related to new prescriptions; however, they were far less correlated with other measured confounders relative to actual prescriptions. These findings suggest that there is considerable treatment selection bias for actual prescribed treatment, but use of prior prescriptions as an instrument may eliminate this selection bias for both observed and unobserved potential confounders.

RCTs and observational studies are in fact quite complimentary. RCTs are generally (although not always) free from bias, but they may not be generalizable to the ultimate population who will use the drug. RCTs are small by comparison to large scale observational studies, so the types of endpoints considered may be more distal to the actual outcome of interest (e.g., suicidal thoughts versus suicide attempts and/or completion). However, the coherence of findings from RCTs and large scale observational studies helps to provide evidence of an ADR which is both unbiased and generalizable. It is through the synthesis of both lines of evidence that strong causal inferences can be derived.

1.3 The Problem of Multiple Comparisons

In the demonstration of efficacy, great care is taken in carefully defining one or a small number of endpoints by which to judge the success of the study and the efficacy of the intervention. This is done because of the concern that in exploring a large number of possible endpoints, some may be statistically significant by chance alone. If we ignore the effect of performing multiple comparisons on the overall experiment-wise Type I error rate (i.e., false positive rate), then we may incorrectly conclude that there is a true effect of the drug when none exists. If we adjust for the number of endpoints actually examined, then the study may not have sufficient statistical power to detect one of the many endpoints considered, even if it is a real treatment related effect of the drug.

While great care in dealing with multiple comparisons is taken in determining efficacy of pharmaceuticals (particularly by the FDA), little or no attention is paid to considering multiple comparisons as they relate to safety. This is not an oversight; from a public health perspective, the danger of a false negative result far outweighs that of a false positive. However, in our litigious society, there is now a substantial cost associated with false positive results as well. In the context of RCTs designed to look at efficacy, pharmaceutical companies routinely look at large numbers of safety endpoints, without any adjustment for multiple comparisons. The net result is that at least for commonly observed adverse events (e.g., 10% or more), they will invariably find at least some statistically significant findings. For example, for a Type I error rate of 5%, the probability of at least 1 of the next 50 adverse event comparisons being statistically significant by chance alone is $1 - (1 - .05)^{50} = 0.92$ or a 92% chance of at least one statistically significant finding. This is not a good bet. Conversely, for rare events, the likelihood of detecting a significant ADR is quite low, and looking at multiple rare events does little to amplify any potential signal to the level of statistical significance. There is of course no good answer. We must evaluate all potential drug safety signals and use coherence across multiple studies using different methodologies (both RCTs and observational studies following approval) to determine if the signal is real. Only the most obvious ADRs would be identifiable from a single study that was not specifically designed to look at that particular adverse event.

1.4   The Evolution of Available Data Streams

We live in a world in which "big data" are becoming increasingly available. Historically, safety decisions were based largely on case reports. With the advent of RCTs, safety was evaluated study by study by analyzing spontaneously reported adverse events during the course of each study. Needing larger populations to assess rare ADRs, pharmacoepidemiology turned to nationwide spontaneous reporting systems. While these reporting systems provide access to the experiences of millions of potential users, they are limited due to lack of information regarding the population at risk, incomplete reporting, stimulated reporting based on media attention, and very limited information regarding the characteristics of the patients exposed, the nature of the exposure and concomitant medications. The IOM report on the Future of Drug Safety led to the establishment of new legislation (Kennedy-Enzi bill), and FDA initiatives (FDA Sentinel Network) to provide new large scale ADR screening systems. These systems are based on integrated medical claims data from a variety of sources including private health insurance companies, and government agencies such as the Veterans Administration and Medicaid/Medicare. The advantage of these new data streams is that they are longitudinal, person-level, the population at risk is generally well characterized, and considerable information regarding filled prescriptions, concomitant medications, and co-morbid conditions are generally available. However, they are limited because they are based on insurance reimbursement codes (e.g., ICD-9/ICD-10 codes) for medical claims, and the claims may not always reflect the nature of the condition for which treatment was received. As an example, many physicians may be reluctant to file claims for suicide attempt and may simply list it for depression treatment or an accidental injury unrelated to self-harm. Obtaining information on cause of death is also complicated by the fact that these databases are generally not linked to the National Death Index.

The availability of large integrated medical practice networks (e.g. DART-Net), using common treatment protocols and prospective measurement systems will help fill gaps in the existing claims-based data structures. Furthermore, the availability of the electronic health record (EHR) and new tools to mine it may also increase the precision of measuring potential ADRs in populations of a size, and at a level of detail not previously considered.

1.5   The Hierarchy of Scientific Evidence

In the hierarchy of scientific evidence, we must place randomized placebo-controlled RCTs at the highest position. RCTs permit researchers to compare the incidence, or risk, of specific outcomes, including suicidal or violent behavior, between patients who are exposed to the medication and similar patients who are administered an identical-looking but chemically inactive sugar pill (placebo). The unparalleled advantage of the RCT is that the omission of important variables in the design will increase measurement error, but it will not produce bias. This is because each subject's treatment assignment (active treatment of interest versus placebo or an active comparator) is based on a random process with predetermined sampling proportion (e.g., 1:1, 2:1, or 3:1). This advantage does not hold true for observational studies, where patients or their physicians select the treatment, often on the basis of personal characteristics. In this case, omitted variables of importance cannot only increase measurement error (i.e., variability in the response of interest), but they can also produce biased estimates of the treatment effect of interest. However, as previously noted, well conducted observational studies also have an important advantage over RCTs, in that RCTs often exclude the patients that are at the highest risk for the event of interest. For example, some patients at serious risk for suicide have been excluded from RCTs based on study entrance criteria. This exclusion criterion can limit generalizability to representative populations of people who take these drugs. In contrast, observational studies (e.g., pharmacoepidemiologic studies) are based on "real-world" data streams, the results of which are typically generalizable to the routine practice. Again, it is for this reason that coherence between RCTs and observational studies is so important for drawing inferences that are both unbiased and generalizable to every-day life.

At this point it is important to draw a distinction between large-scale pharmacoepidemiologic studies that are based on person-level data, often include a relevant control group, and have clear knowledge regarding the characteristics of the population at risk (including the number of patients exposed), versus pharmacovigilance studies in which spontaneous reports of adverse events (AEs) are tallied for particular drugs, without a clear description of the population at risk or even the number of patients taking the drug. Person-level data describe the experiences (drugs taken, diagnoses received, and adverse events experienced) of each individual subject in a cohort from a well defined population. As such, for any potential adverse drug reaction, we know the number of patients at risk, for example, the exact number of patients who did or did not take a drug and the corresponding frequency of the AE of interest in these two groups. By contrast, for spontaneous reports from pharmacovigilance studies, we have reports for only a small subset of those patients who took a drug and experienced the AE. We do not know the number of patients who took the drug and did not experience the AE, and we do not know the frequency with which patients who did not take the drug experienced the AE. Indeed, a drug can have spontaneous reports of an AE and actually be protective (i.e., reduce risk) if the base-rate of the AE in patients with the same condition who did not take the drug is higher than for those who took the drug. While "pseudo-denominators" can be obtained (Gibbons et al. 2008), based on number of prescriptions filled during a specific time-frame, this is no real substitute for knowing the exact number of patients taking the drug and the period of time during which the drug was consumed (or prescription filled). In most cases, no attempt at all is made to even adjust the raw number of AEs for the population at risk.

Pharmacovigilance data based on spontaneous reports are hypothesis generating and cannot and should not be relied upon to yield causal inferences regarding a drug-AE relationship. Causal inferences can be drawn from RCTs, and the generalizability of those inferences can be demonstrated using observational (pharmacoepidemiologic) studies.

A note about meta-analysis. The objective of meta-analysis is to synthesize evidence across a series of studies and to draw an overall conclusion. Even if the individual studies are RCTs, meta-analysis is an observational study of studies. Differences between the studies and their characteristics, can lead to a biased overall conclusion. While this does not mean that meta-analysis is not useful, it would be wrong to draw a causal inference from such studies. Similar to other observational studies, meta-analysis can be quite useful in demonstrating generalizability of a treatment-related effect across a wider variety of patient populations.

1.6   Statistical Significance

A fundamental premise of the scientific method is the formulation and testing of hypotheses. In pharmacoepidemiology, the null hypothesis is that there is no effect of the drug exposure on the adverse event of interest. To test this hypothesis, we collect data, for example on the rate of heart attacks in patients treated with a drug versus those not treated or between two different active medications, and statistically compare the rate of the events between the two treatment arms (i.e., conditions) of the study. We use statistical methods and corresponding probabilities to determine the plausibility of the null hypothesis. Traditionally, if the probability associated with the null hypothesis of no difference between treated and control conditions is less than 0.05 (i.e., 5%), we reject the null hypothesis in favor of the alternative hypothesis that states that the difference between treated and control conditions is beyond what we would expect by chance. If the probability is 0.05 or greater, we fail to reject the null hypothesis and depending on many factors which include our degree of uncertainty, the sample size, the rarity of the event, we either conclude that there is no difference between treated and control conditions in terms of the outcome of interest or that further data are necessary. Note that we can never definitively prove the null hypothesis.

An alternative yet in many ways complementary and potentially more informative approach to determining the effect of a drug on an adverse event is to compute an odds ratio (OR) or a relative risk (RR) and corresponding confidence interval (e.g., 95% confidence interval) for the treatment effect. If the confidence interval contains the value of 1.0 then the result is deemed non-significant, similar to what was previously described for a p-value being greater than or equal to 0.05. The difference, however, is that the width of the confidence interval describes the plausible values of the parameter of interest. The confidence interval indicates that if the statistical model is correct and the study was unbiased, then in say 95% of replications of the study, the true value for the parameter (e.g., RR or OR) will be included within the computed confidence interval. This does not mean that we can have 95% certainty that the true population value is within the computed confidence interval from this particular instance of the study. In some cases, the confidence interval is quite large, indicating that either due to the sample size or the rarity of the event or both, we have too much uncertainty to provide a meaningful inference. In such cases assuming either no effect or a harmful effect (assuming the OR or RR is greater or less than 1.0) is inappropriate.

The RR is the ratio of risk of the event of interest in treated versus control conditions. For example, if the rate is 4% in treated and 2% in control, the RR is 4/2=2. This is intuitively what we think of in terms of the effect of a drug on the risk of an event. The OR is the ratio of the probability of the event in treated and control conditions. With respect to studies examining rare adverse events, the RR and OR are virtually identical.

If there is no association between an exposure and a disease, the RR or OR will be 1.0. Note that even if there is no effect, half of the time the RR or OR will be greater than 1.0. As such it is quite dangerous to conclude that any RR or OR that is greater than 1.0 provides evidence of risk. This is why we test the null hypothesis of no effect using statistical tests and also report the confidence interval to better understand the range of possible effects that are consistent with the observed data. An OR or RR below 1.0 means that those people exposed are less likely to develop the outcome. In an RCT, this is referred to as a protective effect and in an observational study an exposure that is associated with reduced risk. Again, hypothesis testing and confidence interval estimation are critical for interpretation of both increases and decreases in risk, since by chance alone half of the studies will produce point estimates of the RR or OR that are above 1.0 and half will produce point estimates of the RR or OR that are below 1.0 when the true value of RR=OR=1.0 (i.e., no true effect of the drug exposure on the adverse event of concern).

It has unfortunately become the practice of many epidemiologists to infer risk to any OR or RR greater than 1.0 ignoring statistical significance. Perhaps of even greater concern is the practice of attributing increased risk to a drug exposure with upper confidence limit greater than 1.0, even if the point estimate is less than 1.0. This practice leads us to only conclude that a drug is not harmful if it is significantly protective. Since most drugs do not prevent adverse events, one can only conclude from this practice that all drugs cause all adverse events, since for any finite sample under the null hypothesis of no drug effect, the upper confidence limit for the RR or OR will exceed 1.0.

Interestingly, there is evidence of this movement almost 30 years ago (Fleiss 1986). As noted by Fleiss:

> "There is no doubt that significance tests have been abused in epidemiology and in other disciplines: statistically significant associations or differences have, in error, been automatically equated to substantively important ones, and statistically nonsignificant associations or differences have, in error, been automatically equated to ones that are zero. The proper inference from a statistically significant result is that a nonzero association or difference has been established; it is not necessarily strong, sizable or important, just different from zero. Likewise, the proper conclusion from a statistically nonsignificant result is that the data have failed to establish the reality of the effect under investigation. Only if the study had adequate power would the conclusion be valid that no practically important effect exists. Otherwise, the cautious "not proven" is as far as one ought to go."

However, Fleiss goes on to note that:

> "In part as a reaction to abuses due to misinterpretation, a movement is under way in epidemiology to cleanse its literature of significance tests and p-values. A movement that aimed at improving the interpretation of tests of significance would meet with the approbation of most of my statistical colleagues, but something more disturbing is involved. The author of one submission to a journal that publishes articles on epidemiology was asked by an editor that "*all* (emphasis mine) references to statistical hypothesis testing and statistical significance be removed from the paper." The author of another submission to that journal was told, "We are trying to discourage use of the concept of 'statistical significance,' which is, in our view, outmoded and potentially misleading. Thus, I would ask that you delete references to p-values and statistical significance."

As noted by Rothman et al. (2008), the confusion arises because statistics can be viewed as having a number of roles in epidemiology; "data description is one role and statistical inference is another." They point out that hypothesis testing uses statistics to make decisions "such as whether an association is present in a source population of "super-population" from which the data are drawn." They suggest that this view has been declining because "estimation, not decision making, is the proper role for statistical inference in science."

We believe that there are valid roles for both hypothesis testing and interval estimation in pharmacoepidemiology. It is through better understanding of the meaning and interpretation of these statistical concepts that statistical practice will improve.

1.7   Summary

Statistical practice in pharmacoepidemiology has borrowed heavily from traditional epidemiology. This has in some ways limited advances because many of the problems encountered in pharmacoepidemiology are unique from mainstream epidemiology in particular and the medical research in general. In the following chapters we provide an overview of both basic and more advanced statistical concepts which lay the foundation for new discoveries in the field of pharmacoepidemiology. Some of these advancements are straightforward applications of statistical methodologies developed in related fields whereas some appear unique to problems encountered in drug safety. The interplay between statistics and practice is critical for further advances in the field.

2

Basic Statistical Concepts

*"If we doctors threw all our medicines into the sea, it would be that much
better for our patients and that much worse for the fishes."*
(Supreme Court Justice Oliver Wendel Holmes, MD)

2.1 Introduction

Analyses in drug safety studies involve simple to rather complex statistical
methods. Often they involve categorical outcomes, such as whether a certain adverse event occurred or not. The risk factors of interest are also often
categorical, such as whether a patient was on a certain medication or not.
Therefore, knowledge regarding analysis of 2×2 contingency tables is fundamental. Analyses involving multiple risk factors require stratification or
covariate adjustment. These studies sometimes involve millions of data points
and hundreds of covariates. Bayesian methods are particularly useful in modeling such high dimensional data. In this chapter, we discuss some measures of
effect, basic modeling techniques and parameter estimation methods in both
frequentist and Bayesian domains. It is assumed that readers are familiar with
basic statistical concepts including measures of central tendency, measures of
dispersion and sampling variability.

2.2 Relative Risk

Risk of experiencing an ADR is measured by comparing estimates of probabilities of an ADR in exposed or drug treated patients versus untreated patients
or patients taking an active comparator drug. The relative risk (or risk ratio)
is the ratio of the observed proportions r_t/r_c, where r_t and r_c are the proportion of ADRs in patients who are treated with a particular drug or class of
drugs versus untreated patients. If the data are summarized as in Table 2.1,
the relative risk (RR) is estimated by the expression in (2.1).

13

TABLE 2.1: Contingency table of a drug-adverse event pair.

	ADR	
	yes	no
Treatment	a	b
Placebo	c	d

$$\widehat{RR} = \frac{\frac{a}{a+b}}{\frac{c}{c+d}} \tag{2.1}$$

The standard error of $ln(\widehat{RR})$ is

$$SE[ln(RR)] = \sqrt{\frac{1}{a} + \frac{1}{c} - \frac{1}{a+b} - \frac{1}{c+d}}. \tag{2.2}$$

The sampling variability in the point estimate is reflected in the interval estimate which provides a range within which the true value of the parameter will be contained a certain percentage of the time (e.g., 95%). The confidence level of the interval determines the percentage of time the confidence interval will contain the true value of the estimated parameter. For example, the 95% confidence interval for the RR is

$$95\% \text{ CI for RR} = \left(\frac{\widehat{RR}}{e^{(1.96 \times SE[ln(\widehat{RR})])}}, \widehat{RR} \times e^{(1.96 \times SE[ln(\widehat{RR})])} \right), \tag{2.3}$$

which indicates that under repeated sampling, 95% of the CIs constructed as in (2.3) will contain the true RR.

In dealing with rare ADRs, the high RR does not necessarily mean that the treatment is harmful, because even when the absolute risk difference is low, the RR can be relatively high. For example, assume that 4 out of 10000 exposed patients experience an adverse event (AE), whereas only 2 out of 10000 unexposed patients experience the AE. The RR of 2 suggests incidence of the AE is 2 times as high for drug users. Although it is a correct statement, the adverse event rate of 0.0004 and 0.0002 are so close that the absolute risk increase is only 0.0002. Because the absolute risk increase is so small, the ADR is marginal. Another issue with using RR is that it's calculation requires a true denominator, i.e., population at risk. Such a denominator is typically unavailable in classical drug safety studies which are based on passive surveillance data where the total number of people exposed is typically unavailable.

Example

In the Hypertension Optimal Treatment Study, 9399 patients were randomized to receive soluble aspirin 75 mg daily and 9391 patents were randomized to receive placebo in addition to treatment with felodipine to establish the relation between achieved blood pressure and cardiovascular events. Aspirin is suspected to cause serious gastrointestinal (GI) bleeding. In the aspirin group 77 patients had major GI bleeding and in the placebo group 37 patients had GI bleeding. Data are summarized in Table 2.2. The relative risk and 95% CI of GI bleeding is found by evaluating equations (2.1)-(2.3).

TABLE 2.2: Contingency table of an aspirin and major GI bleeding.

	ADR	
	yes	no
Aspirin	77	9322
Placebo	37	9354

$$\widehat{RR} = \frac{\frac{a}{a+b}}{\frac{c}{c+d}} = \frac{\frac{77}{9399}}{\frac{37}{9391}} = 2.08$$

$$SE[ln(\widehat{RR})] = \sqrt{\frac{1}{77} + \frac{1}{37} - \frac{1}{9399} - \frac{1}{9391}} = 0.12$$

$$95\% \text{ CI for RR} = \left(\frac{\widehat{RR}}{e^{(1.96 \times SE[ln(\widehat{RR})])}}, \widehat{RR} \times e^{(1.96 \times SE[ln(\widehat{RR})])} \right)$$

$$= (1.41, 3.07).$$

The risk of GI bleeding for patients on aspirin is 2.08 times higher than for patients on placebo. The 95% CI is $(1.41, 3.07)$ and does not include the value 1.0 (the null hypothesis value) suggesting that the increase in the risk of GI bleeding for aspirin users is statistically significant.

2.3 Odds Ratio

Another simple way to measure the likelihood of an ADR is to compare the odds of such events for patients using active drug with the odds for placebo or no drug. The odds in favor of a certain event E is defined as the ratio $P(E)/[1 - P(E)]$. The odds ratio is the ratio of odds in favor of the event in the treatment group and in the control group. Odds ratios greater than 1.0 suggest greater likelihood of events in the treatment group. The odds ratio is an appropriate measure of effect magnitude in retrospective studies. It closely approximates the RR when the event is rare. For the general data in Table 2.1, the odds ratio is found by evaluating the following expression.

$$\widehat{OR} = \frac{ad}{bc} \tag{2.4}$$

The standard error of $ln(\widehat{OR})$ is

$$SE[ln(OR)] = \sqrt{\frac{1}{a} + \frac{1}{b} + \frac{1}{c} + \frac{1}{d}}. \tag{2.5}$$

The 95% confidence interval for OR is

$$95\% \text{ CI for OR} = \left(\frac{\widehat{OR}}{e^{(1.96 \times SE[ln(\widehat{OR})])}}, \widehat{OR} \times e^{(1.96 \times SE[ln(\widehat{OR})])}\right). \tag{2.6}$$

Example

Consider the data in Table 2.2. A likelihood of GI bleeding in the aspirin users compared to placebo is found by evaluating equations (2.4)-(2.6).

$$\widehat{OR} = \frac{ad}{bc} = \frac{77 \times 9354}{37 \times 9322} = 2.09$$

$$SE[ln(OR)] = \sqrt{\frac{1}{77} + \frac{1}{9322} + \frac{1}{37} + \frac{1}{9354}} = 0.2$$

$$95\% \text{ CI for OR} = \left(\frac{2.09}{e^{(1.96 \times 0.2)}}, 2.09 \times e^{(1.96 \times 0.2)}\right) = (1.41, 3.09).$$

The likelihood of GI bleeding for patients on aspirin is 2.09 times higher than for patients on placebo. The 95% CI is $(1.41, 3.09)$ and does not include the value 1.0 (the null hypothesis value) suggesting that the increased likelihood of GI bleeding for aspirin users is statistically significant.

2.4 Statistical Power

Hypothesis testing is a decision making process where the null hypothesis is either rejected or retained. Note that failure to reject the null hypothesis does not prove that the null hypothesis is true. The decision can be correct - retaining a true null hypothesis or rejecting a false null hypothesis; or it can be incorrect - rejecting a true null hypothesis or retaining a false null hypothesis. The incorrect decision of the first type is called *type I error* (α) and of the second type is called *type II error* (β). Statistical power is the probability of not making a *type II error*. It depends on the significance level of the test, sample size, effect size, and whether the test is one- or two-tail. Let T and c be the test statistic and critical value respectively, and H_1 be the alternative hypothesis. Then the probabilistic expression for power is as follows:

$$P(|T| > |c| \,|H_1) = 1 - P(|T| \leq |c| \,|H_1) \tag{2.7}$$
$$= 1 - \beta. \tag{2.8}$$

Example

Consider hypothesis testing of a one sample proportion. Let X be the Bernoulli random variable and $\hat{p}$ be the point estimate of the true proportion of successes in n trials. The null hypothesis of the right-sided test is $H_0 : p \leq p_0$ and alternative hypothesis is $H_1 : p > p_0 (= p_1)$. An asymptotic test of H_0 against H_1 is the following z-test:

$$
\begin{aligned}
z^* &= \frac{\hat{p} - p_0}{\sqrt{\frac{p_0 q_0}{n}}} \\
P(z^* > c | H_0) &= \alpha \\
\Rightarrow c &= \Phi^{-1}(1 - \alpha) = z_{1-\alpha} \\
Power &= P(z^* > c | H_1) \\
&= P\left(\frac{\hat{p} - p_0}{\sqrt{\frac{p_0 q_0}{n}}} > c \,\middle|\, H_1 \right) \\
&= P\left(\frac{\hat{p} - p_1}{\sqrt{\frac{p_1 q_1}{n}}} > c \sqrt{\frac{p_0 q_0}{p_1 q_1}} - \frac{\sqrt{n}(p_1 - p_0)}{\sqrt{p_1 q_1}} \,\middle|\, H_1 \right) \\
&= P\left(z > c \sqrt{\frac{p_0 q_0}{p_1 q_1}} - \frac{\sqrt{n}(p_1 - p_0)}{\sqrt{p_1 q_1}} \right) \\
&= 1 - \Phi\left(c \sqrt{\frac{p_0 q_0}{p_1 q_1}} - \frac{\sqrt{n}(p_1 - p_0)}{\sqrt{p_1 q_1}} \right) \\
&= 1 - \Phi\left(\frac{c\sqrt{p_0 q_0} - \sqrt{n}(p_1 - p_0)}{\sqrt{p_1 q_1}} \right) \\
&= 1 - \Phi\left(\frac{z_{1-\alpha}\sigma_0 - \sqrt{n}(p_1 - p_0)}{\sigma_1} \right) \quad (2.9)
\end{aligned}
$$

The power function of (2.9) is plotted in Figure 2.1 for varying alternative hypothesis values and p_0 set at 0.5. Power of the test increases with the increasing value of p_1 and with the increasing sample size (n). A simple manipulation of (2.9) gives the required sample size to achieve a predetermined level of statistical power.

2.5 Maximum Likelihood Estimation

The likelihood function is the basis for deriving estimates of parameters from a given dataset. The likelihood function L is a probability density viewed as a function of parameters given the data; that is, the roles of data and parameters are reversed in the probability density function. In the method of

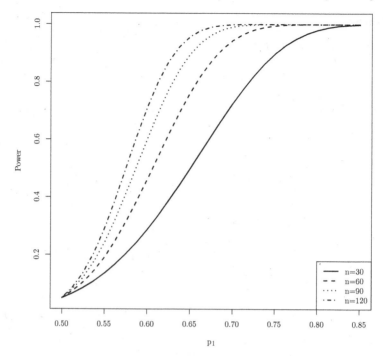

FIGURE 2.1: Power of right sided test as a function of p_1 for $p_0 = 0.5$.

maximum likelihood, the parameter values that maximize L are estimated for a given dataset. The estimated values are called maximum likelihood estimates of the parameters. These are the most likely values of the parameters that are produced by the observed data. Maximum likelihood estimators involve working with first and second derivatives of the likelihood function in the multiplicative scale. Since it is more complicated to compute derivatives in multiplicative scale, $ln(L)$ is used for maximization. As the logarithm function is a monotonic function of L, the maximum values of L and $ln(L)$ occur at the same points. The $ln(L)$ is called the log-likelihood function.

Consider a set of observations x_i from a population with probability density function $f(x_i; \boldsymbol{\theta})$, where $i = 1, \cdots, N$ and $\boldsymbol{\theta}$ is the vector of unknown parameters. Since observations are assumed to be independent, the probability of observing a given set of observations is the product of N $f(x_i; \boldsymbol{\theta})$. Thus the likelihood and log-likelihood functionof the parameters given the observed data are:

$$L(\boldsymbol{\theta}|\boldsymbol{x}) = \prod_{i=1}^{N} f(x_i; \boldsymbol{\theta}) \tag{2.10}$$

$$ln[L(\boldsymbol{\theta}|\boldsymbol{x})] = \sum_{i=1}^{N} f(x_i; \boldsymbol{\theta}). \tag{2.11}$$

The estimating equations of the parameters $\boldsymbol{\theta}$ are:

$$\frac{d \, ln[L(\boldsymbol{\theta}|\boldsymbol{x})]}{d\theta} \Big|_{\boldsymbol{\theta}=\hat{\boldsymbol{\theta}}} = \mathbf{0}; \tag{2.12}$$

where $\hat{\boldsymbol{\theta}}$ is the value of $\boldsymbol{\theta}$ which maximizes the $ln[L(\boldsymbol{\theta}|\boldsymbol{x})]$ function. Variance of $\hat{\boldsymbol{\theta}}$ is estimated by extracting diagonal elements of the inverse of the negative of the expected value of the Hessian matrix, also known as the information matrix, of $ln[L(\boldsymbol{\theta}|\boldsymbol{x})]$ evaluated at $\hat{\boldsymbol{\theta}}$. For the cases where closed form solution of (2.12) do not exist, iterative optimization techniques are used to obtain maximum likelihood estimates (MLE). The MLE has desirable asymptotic properties. It converges in probability to the true parameter, its variance-covariance is the Rao-Cramer lower bound. It has an asymptotic normal distribution and the MLE of a function of a parameter is the same function of the MLE, i.e., MLE of $g(\boldsymbol{\theta})$ is $g(\hat{\boldsymbol{\theta}})$.

2.5.1 Example with a Closed Form Solution

Consider estimating risk of an adverse event in a given population exposed to a particular drug. Let X be the Bernoulli random variable representing incidence or absence of the adverse event. Let p denote the unknown probability of the adverse event. If x_i, $i = 1. \cdots , N$ are the observed outcomes for N patients, then the likelihood function for p is as follows:

$$L(p|\boldsymbol{x}) = \prod_{i=1}^{N} p^{x_i}(1-p)^{1-x_i} = p^{\sum_{i=1}^{N} x_i}(1-p)^{N-\sum_{i=1}^{N} x_i}$$

$$ln[L(p|\boldsymbol{x})] = \sum_{i=1}^{N} x_i ln(p) + (N - \sum_{i=1}^{N} x_i)ln(1-p)$$

$$\frac{d \, ln[L(p|\boldsymbol{x})]}{dp} = \frac{\sum_{i=1}^{N} x_i}{p} - \frac{N - \sum_{i=1}^{N} x_i}{1-p}.$$

The MLE of $\hat{p}$ satisfies the following estimating equations:

$$\frac{\sum_{i=1}^{N} x_i}{\hat{p}} - \frac{N - \sum_{i=1}^{N} x_i}{1 - \hat{p}} = 0$$

$$\Rightarrow \quad \sum_{i=1}^{N} x_i - N\hat{p} = 0$$

$$\Rightarrow \quad \hat{p} = \frac{\sum_{i=1}^{N} x_i}{N}.$$

Thus, $\hat{p}$ is the average, which is the MLE of p. The variance of $\hat{p}$ is found by evaluating inverse of $-E\left(\frac{d^2 \ln[L(p|x)]}{dp^2}\right)|_{p=\hat{p}}$ as follows:

$$\frac{d^2 \ln[L(p|x)]}{dp^2} = \frac{d}{dp}\left[\frac{\sum_{i=1}^{N} x_i}{p} - \frac{N - \sum_{i=1}^{N} x_i}{1 - p}\right]$$

$$E\left(\frac{d^2 \ln[L(p|x)]}{dp^2}\right) = E\left[-\frac{\sum_{i=1}^{N} x_i}{p^2} - \frac{N - \sum_{i=1}^{N} x_i}{(1 - p)^2}\right]_{p=\hat{p}}$$

$$= -\frac{Np}{p^2} - \frac{N - Np}{(1 - p)^2}$$

$$= -\frac{N}{p(1 - p)}.$$

Thus,

$$V(\hat{p}) = \left[-E\left(\frac{d^2 \ln[L(p|x)]}{dp^2}\right)\right]_{p=\hat{p}}^{-1} = \frac{\hat{p}(1 - \hat{p})}{N}.$$

2.5.2 Example without a Closed Form Solution

Consider again a problem of determining risk of adverse events where along with adverse event status Y, patient characteristics X are also available for N patients. Let $\{y_i, x_i\}$ denote a pair of AE status and J risk factors, and p_i be the probability of the AE for the ith patient. Thus, Y is an $N \times 1$ vector, x_i is a $1 \times J + 1$ vector including constant term, and X is an $N \times J + 1$ matrix. Logistic regression is a common choice for modeling the odds of the AE adjusting for known risk factors.

$$\ln\left(\frac{p}{1 - p}\right) = X\beta.$$

Since the ith outcome variable y_i is a Bernoulli variable, the log-likelihood function in terms of parameter vector β is

$$\ln L(\beta) = Y^T X\beta - 1^T \ln\left(1 + e^{X\beta}\right).$$

Let p be a column vector of length N with elements $\frac{e^{x_i^T\beta}}{1+e^{x_i^T\beta}}$ and W be an $N \times N$ diagonal matrix with elements $\frac{e^{x_i^T\beta}}{(1+e^{x_i^T\beta})^2}$. Then the score equation (i.e., first derivatives) and the Hessian matrix is given by the following two sets of equations:

$$\frac{d\ln L(\beta)}{d\beta} = X^T(Y - p)$$

$$\frac{d^2\ln L(\beta)}{d\beta d\beta^T} = -X^TWX.$$

The MLE for β satisfies the following estimating equation:

$$X^T(Y - p) = 0. \tag{2.13}$$

Equation (2.13) is a system of $J+1$ non-linear simultaneous equations without a closed form solution. The Newton-Raphson algorithm is commonly used to solve (2.13). The kth step of Newton-Raphson is as follows:

$$\beta^k = \beta^{k-1} - [X^TWX]^{-1}X^T(Y - p). \tag{2.14}$$

The algorithm starts with the initial value β^0 and iteration continues until convergence. β^0 is the best guess of β. For this example, β^0 can be found by linear regression of Y on X.

2.5.3 Bayesian Statistics

From a Bayesian perspective, the unknown parameter θ is viewed as a random variable, and its probability distribution is used to characterize its uncertainty. Prior knowledge of θ is characterized by the prior distribution $p(\theta)$; the probabilistic mechanism which has generated the observed data D is represented by the probability model $p(D|\theta)$; and the updated distribution, known as posterior density $p(\theta|D)$ of the parameter incorporating information from the observed data is obtained by using Bayes theorem. According to Bayes theorem

$$p(\theta|D) \propto p(D|\theta)p(\theta). \tag{2.15}$$

$p(D|\theta)$ is viewed as a function of θ called a likelihood function. Thus, the posterior is proportional to the likelihood times the prior. In general, $p(\theta|D)$ is more concentrated around the true value of the parameter than $p(\theta)$. Selection of a prior density depends on what is known about the parameter before observing the data. However, prior knowledge about the quantity of interest is not always available. In such cases a non-informative prior – a prior that would have a minimal effect, relative to the data, on the posterior inference – can be used to represent a state of prior ignorance.

The point estimates and the statistical inferences are based on the quantities derived from the posterior distribution. A posterior mode or the posterior expectation (mean) is used as the point estimate of the unknown parameter. Statistical inference may be based on interval estimation known as a *credible interval*. A $(1-\alpha)\%$ credible interval is simply a continuous interval on θ such that the posterior probability mass contained in that interval is $(1-\alpha)$. In other words, the probability that the true value of θ lies within the $(1-\alpha)\%$ credible interval is $(1-\alpha)$.

2.5.4 Example

Consider again a problem of estimating risk of an adverse event in a given population exposed to a particular drug. Let X be the binomial random variable representing number of patients experiencing the adverse event and k be the observed value. Let θ denote the unknown probability of incidence of the adverse event and N denote a total number of patients in the sample. Thus, the binomial likelihood is

$$p(X|\theta, N) = \frac{N!}{k!(N-k)!}\theta^k(1-\theta)^{N-k}. \tag{2.16}$$

A very common choice for prior distribution in this situation is the beta distribution. It has the following form

$$p(\theta|\beta_1, \beta_2) = \frac{\Gamma(\beta_1+\beta_2)}{\Gamma(\beta_1)\Gamma(\beta_2)}\theta^{\beta_1-1}(1-\theta)^{\beta_2-1}, \tag{2.17}$$

where β_1 and β_2 are the two parameters of the beta distribution $B(\beta_1, \beta_2)$, and the gamma function is defined as $\Gamma(c) = \int_0^\infty e^{-u}u^{c-1}du$. Then posterior probability of θ is found by Bayes theorem.

$$
\begin{aligned}
p(\theta|N, k, \beta_1, \beta_2) &\propto p(X|\theta, N)p(\theta|\beta_1, \beta_2) \\
&= \frac{N!}{k!(N-k)!}\theta^k(1-\theta)^{N-k}\frac{\Gamma(\beta_1+\beta_2)}{\Gamma(\beta_1)\Gamma(\beta_2)}\theta^{\beta_1-1}(1-\theta)^{\beta_2-1} \\
&\propto \theta^k(1-\theta)^{N-k}\theta^{\beta_1-1}(1-\theta)^{\beta_2-1} \\
&= \theta^{\beta_1+k-1}(1-\theta)^{\beta_2+N-k-1}.
\end{aligned} \tag{2.18}
$$

This posterior distribution has the same form as the prior distribution. It is a consequence of selecting a special prior called the *conjugate prior* for the binomial likelihood. Priors are called conjugate priors for the likelihood if the posterior distributions are in the same family as the prior probability distributions. They are convenient tools in Bayesian statistics because they make computations analytically tractable. The following (Table 2.3) are some additional examples of conjugate priors.

The posterior distribution (2.18) is a beta distribution with parameters β_1+k and β_2+N-k, i.e., $\theta|N, k, \beta_1, \beta_2 \sim B(\beta_1+k, \beta_2+N-k)$, and posterior

TABLE 2.3: Example of Conjugate Priors

prior	likelihood	posterior
$N(\mu_0, \sigma_0^2)$	$N(\mu, \sigma^2)$	$N\left[\left(\frac{\mu_0}{\sigma_0^2} + \frac{\sum_i^n x_i}{\sigma^2}\right) / \left(\frac{1}{\sigma_0^2} + \frac{n}{\sigma^2}\right), \left(\frac{1}{\sigma_0^2} + \frac{n}{\sigma^2}\right)^{-1}\right]$
$\Gamma(\alpha, \beta)$	$Poisson(\lambda)$	$Gamma(\alpha + \sum_{i=1}^n x_i, \beta + n)$
$Dirichlet(\boldsymbol{\alpha})$	$Multinomial(\boldsymbol{p})$	$Dirichlet(\boldsymbol{\alpha} + \sum_i^n \boldsymbol{x}_i)$

mean $\frac{\beta_1 + k}{\beta_1 + \beta_2 + N}$. Naturally, the posterior distribution depends on the choice of prior. In absence of strong prior information on the rate of the AE for drug users, a *diffuse prior* which assigns equal probabilities to all possibilities is a reasonable choice. For this example, a flat prior a $B(1,1)$ can be used without having undue influence on the posterior distribution. With a $B(1,1)$ prior, the estimated posterior mean $(\tilde{\theta})$ of AE probability for drug users is $\frac{k+1}{N+2}$. The 95% credible interval is given by $(\tilde{\theta}_l \leq \tilde{\theta} \leq \tilde{\theta}_u)$, where $\tilde{\theta}_l$ and $\tilde{\theta}_u$ are the 2.5^{th} and 97.5^{th} percentile points of the posterior distribution, respectively.

2.6 Non-linear Regression Models

Drug safety studies commonly involve categorical or discrete outcomes, such as the presence of an AE, severity of an AE or episodes of AE experience in a period of time. By design or as a consequence of sample selection, subjects in the studies are also exposed to multiple risk factors in addition to the drug in question. Regression is the commonly used technique to analyze the impact of drug exposure on AE, adjusting for extraneous risk factors. Regression analyses of non-linear outcomes are more complex to compute and to interpret. Non-linear regression models most commonly encountered in drug safety studies are: binary and multinomial logistic regression, Poisson regression, and time to event or Cox regression models. Parameters of each of these models can be estimated using the maximum likelihood approach. Alternatively, these models can be viewed as a member of family of the generalized linear models in which case the *quasi-likelihood* method is used for estimating parameters. Most statistical software packages provide a way to fit non-linear regression models.

Example

John Ulicny and his colleague at the Temple Bone Marrow Transplant Program analyzed the number of adverse events experienced by a Hematopoietic Cell Transplant patient in the reporting period under study. Hematopoietic Cell Transplantation (HCT) is performed on patients for a variety of severe illnesses, typically affecting the bone marrow and circulating blood. Adverse reactions including anemia, nausea, diarrhea, and mucositis are common due to high dose chemotherapy and radiation. Six covariates considered for adjustment are: temporal risk index (TRI), in-patient length of stay (LTIP), whether or not a follow up visit has occurred (FLFLAG), an indicator to account for personnel change (OBSERVER), an indicator to account for carcinoma patients who received fludarabine, total body irradiation as a preparative regimen (DREG), and transplant year (BMTYR). Poisson regression was used to obtain adverse event rates adjusted for these covariates. Table 2.4 displays the parameter estimates obtained using the SAS GENMOD procedure which uses the quasi-likelihood method. The resulting regression equation is

$$
\begin{aligned}
ln(\lambda_i) \;=\; & \beta_0 + \beta_1 TRI_i + \beta_2 FLFLAG_i + \beta_3 LTIP_i \\
& + \beta_4 OBSERVER_i + \beta_5 DREG_i + \beta_6 BMTYR_i \\
\;=\; & 305.31 + 0.0868 TRI_i - 0.3898 FLFLAG_i + 0.9468 LTIP_i \\
& + 0.7258 OBSERVER_i + 1.5146 DREG_i - 0.1554 BMTYR_i
\end{aligned}
$$

where λ_i is the mean adverse event rate for the ith individual, and the β's are the regression coefficients.

TABLE 2.4: Analysis of Parameter Estimates

Parameters	Ref.	DF	Estimate	Std Err	Wald 95% CI		χ^2	p-value
Intercept		1	305.31	167.94	-23.85	634.48	3.30	0.0691
TRI		1	0.0868	0.0064	0.0742	0.0994	182.98	< .0001
FLFLAG	0	1	-0.3898	0.1158	-0.6167	-0.1629	11.34	0.0008
FLFLAG	1	0	0	0	0	0	0	.
LTIP		1	0.9468	0.0937	0.7632	1.1304	102.18	< .0001
OBSERVER	0	1	0.7258	0.2263	0.2822	1.1694	10.29	0.0013
OBSERVER	1	0	0	0	0	0	.	.
DREG	1	1	1.5146	0.4789	0.5759	2.4532	10	0.0016
DREG	0		0	0	0	0	0	.
BMTYR		1	-0.1554	0.0839	-0.3198	0.0089	3.44	0.0638
Scale	0		1	0	1	1		

The results in Table 2.4 show that the TRI, LTIP, FLFLAG, OBSERVER, and DREG are significant predictors of the adverse event. The BMT year variable, BMTYR, is only borderline significant. After accounting for the other five risk factors, the adverse event rate increases by a factor of $e^{0.0868} = 1.09$ for a one unit increase in TRI; increases by a factor of 2.57 for a one unit increase in LTIP; increases by a factor of 2.07 if responsibility for assigning toxicity grades did not change from one group of observers to another; increases by a factor of 4.52 for renal cell carcinoma patients who received fludarabine and total body irradiation as a preparative regimen; and it decreases by the factor 0.68 if a follow up visit did not occur in the current reporting period. Each category of categorical covariates is compared with its corresponding reference category.

2.7 Causal Inference

Regulatory actions related to a drug already on the market depend on the causal effect of the drug. Ideally, development or non-development of the outcome (ADRs) would be evaluated on the same patient when exposed, and when not exposed to the treatment (a drug). However, the "fundamental problem of causal inference" is that we can at most observe one of these outcomes (Holland 1986). This problem arises because at any given time a patient can only be either exposed or not exposed to the treatment. Therefore, the common approach to assess the effect of treatment is to compare distinct treated and untreated individuals. If the differences between these individuals (e.g., age) influence the outcome, causal comparison of outcomes by treatment may not be valid. More details on a topic of drawing causal inference from observational data is covered in Chapter 4. This section reviews two fundamental concepts of causal inference (1) counterfactuals, and (2) average treatment effect.

2.7.1 Counterfactuals

Suppose Y_{1i} and Y_{0i} represent the i-th subjects's ADR status if she is exposed to a certain drug and if she is not exposed to the drug, respectively. Y_{1i} and Y_{0i} are called potential outcomes. If both of these potential outcomes were available, the individual treatment effect for subject i can be defined as $Y_{1i} - Y_{0i}$. If $Y_{1i} - Y_{0i} > 0$ then the treatment has an adverse effect on the subject. Let W_i indicate whether individual i is exposed to the drug, such that $W_i = 0$ if individual i is not, and $W_i = 1$ if individual i is, exposed to the drug. The treatment indicator W_i is called the observed treatment. The observed outcome Y_i is defined as

$$Y_i = Y_{1i}W_i + Y_{0i}(1 - W_i),$$

such that, if individual i is exposed to the drug, Y_{1i} will be observed. If, on the other hand, individual i is not exposed to the drug, Y_{0i} will be observed. However, individual i cannot be exposed and unexposed at the same time, and thus only one of the two potential outcomes can be observed. Because we can only observe Y_{1i} or Y_{0i}, but not both, up to 50% of the data are missing. The unobservable missing outcome is called the *counterfactual* outcome. For example, if Y_{1i} is observed, then Y_{0i} is the counterfactual. Due to the missing value problem, it is impossible to identify the individual effect.

2.7.2 Average Treatment Effect

Not only is the individual treatment effect impossible to identify, it is also not very useful from a policy perspective. A more interesting and useful metric of treatment evaluation is the average treatment effect (ATE), which is defined as the expectation of the individual causal effects, $Y_{1i} - Y_{0i}$. The mathematical expression of the ATE is as follows:

$$ATE = E(Y_1 - Y_0).$$

Unlike the individual treatment effect, ATE is estimable. Typically, it is solved by utilizing information contained in the sampling process. However, the missing data problem continues to pose substantial challenges. Several different mechanisms (discussed in Chapter 4) are available to deal with the ATE identification problems arising due to the missing data.

3

Multi-level Models

"Doctors give drugs of which they know little, into bodies, of which they know less, for diseases of which they know nothing at all."
(Voltaire)

3.1 Introduction

In this chapter, we review statistical methods for the analysis of clustered and longitudinal data that are commonly encountered in pharmacoepidemiologic research. Longitudinal data represent a collection of repeated observations within units. The units may represent individual patients or an ecological unit such as a county for which the rate of an adverse event is repeatedly measured over time. By contrast, clustered data represent cross-sectional measurements, typically taken at a single point in time, however the units (e.g., patients) upon which the measurements are made, are nested within a higher order ecological structure such as clinics, medical practices, hospitals, or counties. The endpoints or outcomes of interest can be either continuous (e.g., cholesterol levels or blood pressure) or discrete (e.g., presence or absence of a particular adverse event such as a myocardial infarction). The distributional form of the continuous measurements can be normal, as in linear mixed-effects regression models, or it can take on a skewed distribution such as the gamma distribution. For continuous and normally distributed outcomes we will focus attention on the useful class of linear mixed-models (Laird and Ware 1982, Longford 1995, Verbeke and Molenberghs 2000, Diggle et al. 2002, Raudenbush and Bryk 2002, Singer and Willett 2003, Fitzmaurice et al. 2004, Hedeker and Gibbons 2006, Goldstein 2011), whereas for discrete outcomes such as the presence or absence of an adverse event or the rate of the event within a specific time interval we focus on non-linear mixed-models (e.g., mixed-effects logistic regression for a binary event and mixed-effects Poisson regression for a count of the number of events within a given time interval, see Hedeker and Gibbons (2006) for detailed overview). We note that an important case is when data are both clustered and longitudinal. This is termed a "three-level model," where for example, level 1 represents the measurement occasion, level

2 an individual, and level 3 a clustering unit such as a county. Multi-center longitudinal randomized clinical trials are an example of three-level models, because measurement occasions are nested within individuals and individuals are nested within centers. Note however, that such trials are rarely analyzed in this way, rather, the center to center variability is most frequently ignored and more simplistic statistical models are used. However, these more simplistic approaches are not conservative and can lead to biased and misleading results when there are center-specific effects leading to correlation of responses within centers. By adding random person effects and random center effects we can accommodate the complex correlational structure produced by repeatedly measuring the same people over time and by ecological and practice characteristics which produce correlated outcomes within ecological units. Viewed in this way, meta-analysis is a type of multilevel model in which response rates or adverse event rates under treated and control conditions are nested within studies. Using a mixed-effects logistic regression model, we can allow both the background rate and the effect of treatment on the adverse event to vary from study to study. Again, these more advanced statistical approaches are unfortunately underrepresented in routine statistical practice.

In pharmacoepidemiology, longitudinal data related to safety endpoints are commonly encountered in both randomized clinical trials and in observational studies such as analysis of person-level longitudinal medical claims data. The key ingredient is that the units of interest (e.g., patients) are repeatedly assessed over time. At this point it is important to draw a distinction between time-to-event data and longitudinal data, both of which encompass time in the analysis. In time-to-event data, which are often analyzed using survival analytic methods, a given individual can only experience the event once. As such the times within individuals are conditionally independent and the survival time, in many cases censored at the end of the follow-up period, is the focus of the analysis. Events which are generally fatal are analyzed in this way. By contrast, longitudinal data represent events which can be repeatedly assessed, such as weight, blood pressure, cholesterol, neuropsychiatric events, non-fatal suicidal ideation or behavior, to name a few. In this chapter we focus on longitudinal data, not time-to-event data. Note however, that time-to-event data may be collected within ecological units such as clinics, hospitals and counties within which survival times may be correlated. Mixed-effects models that are appropriate for clustered survival times are described in Chapters 8 and 10 (also see Hedeker and Gibbons, 2006).

Since the pioneering work of Laird and Ware (1982) on the linear mixed-effects regression model, statistical methods for the analysis of longitudinal data have advanced dramatically. Prior to this time, a standard approach to analysis of longitudinal data principally involved using the longitudinal data to impute end-points (e.g., last observation carried forward - LOCF) and then to simply discard the valuable intermediate time-point data, favoring the simplicity of analyses of change scores from baseline to study completion (or the last available measurement treated as if it was what would have been obtained had it been the end of the study). Laird and Ware (1982) showed that mixed-effects regression models could be used to perform a more complete analysis of all of the available longitudinal data under much more general assumptions regarding the missing data (i.e., missing at random - MAR). The net result was a more powerful set of statistical tools for analysis of longitudinal data that led to more powerful statistical hypothesis testshypothesis testing, more precise estimates of rates of change (and differential rates of change between experimental and control groups), and more general assumptions regarding missing data, for example because of study drop-out or differential length of follow-up in a medical claims database.

3.2 Issues Inherent in Longitudinal Data

While longitudinal studies provide far more information than their cross-sectional counterparts, they are not without complexities. In the following sections we review some of the major issues associated with longitudinal data analysis.

3.2.1 Heterogeneity

In pharmacoepidemiology, individual differences are the norm rather than the exception. The overall mean response in a sample drawn from a population tells us little regarding the experience of the individual. In contrast to cross-sectional studies in which it is reasonable to assume that there are independent random fluctuations at each measurement occasion, when the same subjects are repeatedly measured over time, their responses are correlated over time, and their estimated trend line or curve can be expected to deviate systematically from the overall mean trend line. For example, behavioral, biological and genetic patient-level characteristics can increase the likelihood of an adverse event to a particular medication. In many cases, these personal characteristics may be unobservable, leading to unexplained heterogeneity in the population. Modeling this unobserved heterogeneity in terms of variance components that describe subject-level effects is one way to accommodate the correlation of the repeated responses over time and to better describe individual or ecological differences in the statistical characterization of the observed data. These variance components are often termed "random-effects," leading to terms like random-effects or mixed-effects regression models.

3.2.2 Missing Data

Perhaps the most important issue when analyzing data from longitudinal studies is the presence of missing data. Stated quite simply, not all subjects remain in the study for the entire length of the study. Reasons for discontinuing the study may be differentially related to the treatment. For example, some subjects may develop side-effects to an otherwise effective treatment and must discontinue the study. In pharmacoepidemiology interest may be in the very side-effect that leads to study discontinuation. In medical claims data, patients may change their insurance coverage or provider, leading to censoring (i.e., discontinuation) of the medical claims record. Characteristics of patients who are likely to change insurance coverage may in turn be related to their health status and likelihood of experiencing an adverse event of interest. Alternatively, some subjects might achieve the full benefit of treatment early on and discontinue the study because they feel that their continued participation will provide no added benefit. These subjects may then be weighted less than subjects not benefiting as well from treatment and may therefore count more heavily in the analysis because they have a longer measurement period.

The treatment of missing data in longitudinal studies is itself a vast literature, with major contributions by Laird (1988), Little (1995), Rubin (1976), Little and Rubin (2002) to name a few. The basic issue is that even in a randomized and well controlled clinical trial, the subjects who were initially enrolled in the study and randomized to the various treatment conditions may be quite different from those subjects that are available for analysis at the end of the trial. If subjects "drop-out" because they already have derived full benefit from an effective treatment, an analysis that only considers those subjects who completed the trial may fail to show that the treatment was beneficial relative to the control condition. This type of analysis is often termed a completer analysis. To avoid this type of obvious bias, investigators often resort to an analysis in which the last available measurement is carried forward to the end of the study as if the subject had actually completed the study. This type of analysis, often termed an end-point analysis, introduces its own set of problems in that (a) all subjects are treated equally regardless of the actual intensity of their treatment over the course of the study, and (b) the actual responses that would have been observed at the end of the study, if the subject had remained in the study until its conclusion, may in fact, be quite different than the response made at the time of discontinuation. Returning to our example of the study in which subjects discontinue when they feel that they have received full treatment benefit, an end-point analysis might miss the fact that some of these subjects may have had a relapse had they remained on treatment. Many other objections have been raised about these two simple approaches of handling missing data, which have led to more statistically reasoned approaches to the analysis of longitudinal data with missing observations.

3.2.3   Irregularly Spaced Measurement Occasions

It is not at all uncommon in real longitudinal studies either in the context of designed experiments or observational studies, for individuals to vary both in the number of repeated measurements they contribute and even in the time at which the measurements are obtained. This may be due to drop-out or simply due to different subjects having different schedules of availability. While this can be quite problematic for traditional analysis of variance based approaches (leading to highly unbalanced designs which can produce biased parameter estimates and tests of hypotheses), more modern statistical approaches to the analysis of longitudinal data are all but immune to the "unbalancedness" that is produced by having different times of measurement for different subjects. Indeed, this is one of the most useful features of the regression approach to this problem, namely the ability to use all of the available data from each subject, regardless of when the data were specifically obtained.

3.3   Historical Background

Existing methods for the analysis of longitudinal data are an outgrowth of two earlier approaches for repeated measures data. The first approach, the so called "repeated measures ANOVA" was essentially a random intercept model that assumed that subjects could only deviate from the overall mean response pattern by a constant that was equivalent over time. A more reasonable view is that the subject-specific deviation is both in terms of the baseline response (i.e., intercept) and in terms of the rate of change over time (i.e., slope or set of trend parameters). This more general structure could not be accommodated by the repeated measures ANOVA. The random intercept model assumption leads to a compound-symmetric variance-covariance matrix for the repeated measurements in which the variances and covariances of the repeated measurements are constant over time. In general, for continuous outcomes, we often find that variances increase over time and covariances decrease as time-points become more separated in time. Finally, based on the use of least-squares estimation, the repeated measures ANOVA breaks down for unbalanced designs, such as those in which the sample size decreases over time due to subject discontinuation. Based on these limitations, the repeated measures ANOVA and related approaches are rarely used for the analysis of longitudinal data.

The second early approach for analysis of repeated measures data was a multivariate growth curve, or MANOVA model (Potthoff and Roy 1964, Bock 1975). The primary advantage of the MANOVA approach versus the ANOVA approach is that the MANOVA assumes a general form for the correlation of repeated measurements over time, whereas the ANOVA assumes the much more restrictive compound-symmetric form. The disadvantage of the MANOVA model is that it requires complete data. Subjects with incomplete data are removed from the analysis, leading to potential bias. In addition, both MANOVA and ANOVA models focus on comparison of group means and provide no information regarding subject-specific growth curves. Finally, both ANOVA and MANOVA models require that the time points are fixed across subjects (either evenly or unevenly spaced) and are treated as a classification variable in the ANOVA or MANOVA model. This precludes analysis of unbalanced designs in which different subjects are measured on different occasions. Finally, software for the MANOVA approach often makes it difficult to include time-varying covariates, which are often essential to modeling dynamic relationships between predictors and outcomes, for example concomitant medications which are added or deleted to naturalistic treatment regimens in observational studies.

3.4   Statistical Models for the Analysis of Longitudinal and/or Clustered Data

In an attempt to provide a more general treatment of longitudinal/clustered data, with more realistic assumptions and associated missing data mechanisms, statistical researchers have developed a wide variety of more rigorous approaches to the analysis of longitudinal and clustered data. Among these, the most widely used include mixed-effects regression models (Laird and Ware, 1982), and generalized estimating equations (GEE) models (Zeger and Liang 1986). Variations of these models have been developed for both discrete and continuous outcomes and for a variety of missing data mechanisms. The primary distinction between the two general approaches is that mixed-effects models are "full-likelihood" methods and GEE models are "partial-likelihood" methods. The advantage of statistical models based on partial-likelihood is that (a) they are computationally easier than full-likelihood methods, and (b) they easily generalize to a wide variety of outcome measures with quite different distributional forms. The price of this flexibility, however, is that partial likelihood methods are more restrictive in their assumptions regarding missing data than their full-likelihood counterparts. In addition, full-likelihood methods provide estimates of person-specific effects (e.g., person-specific trend lines) that are quite useful in understanding inter-individual variability in the longitudinal response process and in predicting future responses for a given subject or set of subjects from a particular subgroup (e.g., a clinic, hospital, or county). In the following sections we will focus our attention on full-likelihood methods and only briefly discuss partial-likelihood methods.

3.4.1   Mixed-effects Regression Models

Mixed-effects regression models (MRMs) are now widely used for the analysis of longitudinal and clustered data (Hedeker and Gibbons 2006). Variants of MRMs have been developed under a variety of names: random-effects models (Laird and Ware, 1982), variance component models (Dempster et al. 1981) multilevel models (Goldstein 2011), two-stage models (Bock 1989), random coefficient models (De Leeuw and Kreft 1986), mixed-models (Longford 1987, Wolfinger 1993), empirical Bayes models (Hui and Berger 1983, Strenio et al. 1983), hierarchical linear models (Bryk and Raudenbush 1992, Raudenbush and Bryk 2002) and random regression models (Bock 1983a,b, Hedeker et al. 1988). A basic characteristic of these models is the inclusion of random-effects into regression models in order to account for the correlation produced by the clustering of data within experimental units (subjects, clinics, hospitals, counties). These random subject effects thus describe each unit's deviation from the overall population mean. For example, in the case of a longitudinal data they can describe how an individual subject's rate of change in cholesterol level deviates from the overall population mean. In clustered data, the random-effect may describe how the rate of suicide for a particular county deviates from the overall national average.

There are several features that make MRMs especially useful for analysis of longitudinal data. First, subjects are not assumed to be measured the same number of times, thus, subjects with incomplete data across time are included in the analysis. The ability to include subjects with incomplete data is an important advantage relative to procedures that require complete data across time because (a) by including all data, the analysis has increased statistical power, and (b) complete-case analysis may suffer from biases to the extent that subjects with complete data may not be representative of the larger population of subjects. Because time can be treated as a continuous variable in MRMs, subjects do not have to be measured at the same time-points. This is useful for analysis of longitudinal studies where follow-up times are not uniform across all subjects. Both time-invariant and time-varying covariates can be easily included in the model. Thus, changes in the outcome variable may be due to both stable characteristics of the subject (e.g., their gender or race) as well as characteristics that change across time (e.g., concomitant medications and comorbid conditions).

To help fix ideas, we consider the following simple linear regression model for the measurement y of individual i ($i = 1, 2, \ldots, N$ subjects) on occasion j ($j = 1, 2, \ldots n_i$ occasions):

$$y_{ij} = \beta_0 + \beta_1 t_{ij} + \beta_2(t_{ij} \times Trt_i) + \varepsilon_{ij}. \tag{3.1}$$

Ignoring subscripts, this model represents the regression of the outcome variable y on the independent variable time (denoted t). The subscripts keep track of the particulars of the data, namely whose observation it is (subscript i) and when the observation was made (the subscript j). The independent variable t gives a value to the level of time, and may represent time in weeks, months, etc. Since y and t carry both i and j subscripts, both the outcome variable and the time variable are allowed to vary by individuals and occasions. The variable Trt_i is a binary variable that indicates the treatment (e.g., drug of interest) prescribed (or randomized) to individual i. When Trt is dummy coded as a 1 or 0, with 1 indicating membership in the treatment group, the regression coefficient β_0 is the mean of y when $t = 0$, β_1 is the slope or rate of change for the control group, and β_2 is the difference in slopes between the treatment and control groups.

In linear regression models, the errors ε_{ij} are assumed to be normally and independently distributed in the population with zero mean and common variance σ^2. This independence assumption makes the typical general linear regression model unreasonable for longitudinal data. This is because the outcomes y are observed repeatedly from the same individuals, and so it is much more reasonable to assume that errors within an individual are correlated to some degree. Furthermore, the above model posits that the change across time is the same for all individuals since the model parameters (β_0, the intercept or initial level, and β_1, the linear change across time) do not vary by individuals except in terms of treatment assignment. For both of these reasons, it is useful to add individual-specific effects into the model that will account for the data dependency and describe differential time-trends for different individuals. This is precisely what MRMs do. The essential point is that MRMs therefore can be viewed as augmented linear regression models. Note also that here and elsewhere in this chapter, we do not include a main effect for treatment in the model. That is, we assume that at baseline, there is no difference in the expected outcomes between treatment groups. This is a reasonable assumption in a clinical trial where participants are randomized prior to receiving treatment. Alternatively, in an observational study where treatment (or exposure) is not randomized, it usually makes sense to include a main effect for treatment to account for differences between treatment groups at baseline.

3.4.1.1   Random Intercept Model

A simple extension of the linear regression model described in Equation 3.1 is the random intercept model, which allows each subject to deviate from the overall mean response by a person-specific constant that applies equally over time:

$$y_{ij} = \beta_0 + \beta_1 t_{ij} + \beta_2(t_{ij} \times Trt_i) + v_{0i} + \varepsilon_{ij} \qquad (3.2)$$

where v_{0i} represents the influence of individual i on his/her repeated observations. Notice that if individuals have no influence on their repeated outcomes, then all of the v_{0i} terms would equal 0. However, it is more likely that subjects will have positive or negative influences on their longitudinal data, and so the v_{0i} terms will deviate from 0. Since individuals in a sample are typically thought to be representative of a larger population of individuals, the individual-specific effects v_{0i} are treated as random-effects. That is, the v_{0i} are considered to be representative of a distribution of individual effects in the population. The most common form for this population distribution is the normal distribution with mean 0 and variance σ_v^2. In addition, the model assumes that the errors of measurement (ε_{ij}) are conditionally independent, which implies that the errors of measurement are independent conditional on

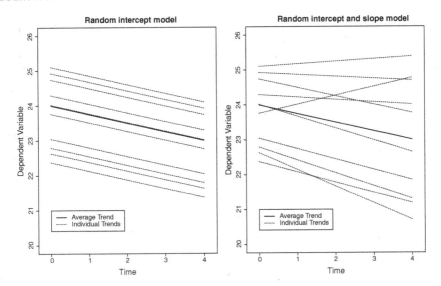

FIGURE 3.1: Simulated longitudinal data based on a random intercept model (left panel) and a random intercept and slope model (right panel). The solid bold line represents the overall population (average) trend. The dashed lines represent individual trends.

the random individual-specific effects v_{0i}. Since the errors now have the influence due to individuals removed from them, this conditional independence assumption is much more reasonable than the ordinary independence assumption associated with the linear regression model in Equation 3.1. The random intercept model is depicted graphically in the left panel of Figure 3.1.

As can be seen, individuals deviate from the regression of y on t in a parallel manner in this model (since there is only one subject effect v_{0i}) (for simplicity, here we assume the treatment effect $\beta_2 = 0$). In this figure the solid line represents the population average trend, which is based on β_0 and β_1. Also depicted are ten individual trends, both below and above the population (average) trend. For a given sample there are N such lines, one for each individual. The variance term σ_v^2 represents the spread of these lines. If σ_v^2 is near-zero, then the individual lines would not deviate much from the population trend and individuals do not exhibit much heterogeneity in their change across time. Alternatively, as individuals differ from the population trend, the lines move away from the population trend line and σ_v^2 increases. In this case, there is more individual heterogeneity in time-trends.

3.4.1.2   Random Intercept and Trend Model

For longitudinal data, the random intercept model is often too simplistic for a number of reasons. First, it is unlikely that the rate of change across time is the same for all individuals. It is more likely that individuals differ in their time-trends; not everyone changes at the same rate. Furthermore, the compound symmetry assumption of the random intercept model is usually untenable for most longitudinal data. In general, measurements at points close in time tend to be more highly correlated than measurements further separated in time. Also, in many studies subjects are more similar at baseline due to entry criteria, and change at different rates across time. Thus, it is natural to expect that variability will increase over time.

For these reasons, a more realistic MRM allows both the intercept and time-trend to vary by individuals:

$$y_{ij} = \beta_0 + \beta_1 t_{ij} + + \beta_2(t_{ij} \times Trt_i) + \upsilon_{0i} + \upsilon_{1i} t_{ij} + \varepsilon_{ij}. \qquad (3.3)$$

In this model, β_0 is the overall population intercept, β_1 is the overall population slope for the group with Trt coded 0, and β_2 indicates how the population slopes vary between treatment groups (by specifically indicating how the slope for Trt coded 1 is different than the slope for Trt coded 0). In terms of the random-effects, υ_{0i} is the intercept deviation for subject i, and υ_{1i} is the slope deviation for subject i (relative to their treatment group). As before, ε_{ij} is an independent error term distributed normally with mean 0 and variance σ^2. As with the random intercept model, the assumption regarding the independence of the errors is one of conditional independence, that is, they are independent conditional on υ_{0i} and υ_{1i}. With two random individual-specific effects, the population distribution of intercept and slope deviations is assumed to be bivariate normal $N(0, \Sigma_\upsilon)$, with the random-effects variance-covariance matrix given by

$$\Sigma_\upsilon = \begin{bmatrix} \sigma_{\upsilon_0}^2 & \sigma_{\upsilon_0 \upsilon_1} \\ \sigma_{\upsilon_0 \upsilon_1} & \sigma_{\upsilon_1}^2 \end{bmatrix}. \qquad (3.4)$$

The model described in Equation 3.3 can be thought of as a personal trend or change model since it represents the measurements of y as a function of time, both at the individual υ_{0i} and υ_{1i} and population β_0 and β_1 (plus β_2) levels. The intercept parameters indicate the starting point, and the slope parameters indicate the degree of change over time. The population intercept and slope parameters represent the overall (population) trend, while the individual parameters express how subjects deviate from the population trends. The right panel of Figure 3.1 represents this model graphically.

As can be seen, individuals deviate from the average trend both in terms of their intercept and in terms of their slope. As with the random intercept model, the spread of the lines around the average intercept is measured by $\sigma_{\upsilon_0}^2$ in Equation 3.4. The variance of the slopes around the average trend is measured by $\sigma_{\upsilon_1}^2$ in Equation 3.4. By allowing the individual slopes to vary, it is now possible for individual trends to be positive even though the overall trend is negative. The term $\sigma_{v_0 v_1}$ in Equation 3.4 measures the association (covariance) between the random intercept and slope. When this quantity is negative, individuals with larger intercepts $(\beta_0 + v_{i0})$ will have steeper slopes $(\beta_1 + v_{i1})$.

3.4.2 Matrix Formulation

A more compact representation of the MRM is afforded using matrices and vectors. This formulation helps to summarize statistical aspects of the model. For this, the MRM for the $n_i \times 1$ response vector $\boldsymbol{y}$ for individual i can be written as:

$$
\underset{n_i \times 1}{\boldsymbol{y}_i} = \underset{n_i \times p}{\boldsymbol{X}_i} \ \underset{p \times 1}{\boldsymbol{\beta}} + \underset{n_i \times r}{\boldsymbol{Z}_i} \ \underset{r \times 1}{\boldsymbol{v}_i} + \underset{n_i \times 1}{\boldsymbol{\varepsilon}_i} \tag{3.5}
$$

with $i = 1 \ldots N$ individuals and $j = 1 \ldots n_i$ observations for individual i. Here, $\boldsymbol{y}_i$ is the $n_i \times 1$ dependent variable vector for individual i, $\boldsymbol{X}_i$ is the $n_i \times p$ covariate matrix for individual i, $\boldsymbol{\beta}$ is the $p \times 1$ vector of fixed regression parameters, $\boldsymbol{Z}_i$ is the $n_i \times r$ design matrix for the random-effects, $\boldsymbol{v}_i$ is the $r \times 1$ vector of random individual effects, and $\boldsymbol{\varepsilon}_i$ is the $n_i \times 1$ residual vector.

For example, in the random intercepts and slopes MRM just considered, for a participant in the treatment group $(Trt_i = 1)$ we would have

$$
\boldsymbol{y}_i = \begin{bmatrix} y_{i1} \\ y_{i2} \\ \ldots \\ \ldots \\ y_{in_i} \end{bmatrix} \text{ and } \boldsymbol{X}_i = \begin{bmatrix} 1 & t_{i1} & t_{i1} \\ 1 & t_{i2} & t_{i2} \\ \ldots & \ldots \\ \ldots & \ldots \\ 1 & t_{in_i} & t_{in_i} \end{bmatrix} \text{ and } \boldsymbol{Z}_i = \begin{bmatrix} 1 & t_{i1} \\ 1 & t_{i2} \\ \ldots & \ldots \\ \ldots & \ldots \\ 1 & t_{in_i} \end{bmatrix}
$$

for the data matrices, and

$$
\boldsymbol{\beta} = \begin{bmatrix} \beta_0 \\ \beta_1 \\ \beta_2 \end{bmatrix} \quad \text{and} \quad \boldsymbol{v}_i = \begin{bmatrix} v_{0i} \\ v_{1i} \end{bmatrix}
$$

for the population and individual trend parameter vectors, respectively. The distributional assumptions about the random-effects and residuals are:

$$
\begin{aligned}
\boldsymbol{v}_i &\sim \mathcal{N}(0, \boldsymbol{\Sigma}_v) \\
\boldsymbol{\varepsilon}_i &\sim \mathcal{N}(0, \sigma^2 \boldsymbol{I}_{n_i}).
\end{aligned}
$$

As a result, it can be shown that the expected value of the repeated measures $\boldsymbol{y}_i$ is

$$
E(\boldsymbol{y}_i) = \boldsymbol{X}_i \boldsymbol{\beta} \tag{3.6}
$$

and the variance-covariance matrix of $\boldsymbol{y}_i$ is of the form:

$$V(\boldsymbol{y}_i) = \boldsymbol{Z}_i \boldsymbol{\Sigma}_v \boldsymbol{Z}_i' + \sigma^2 \boldsymbol{I}_{n_i}. \tag{3.7}$$

For example, with $r = 2$, $n = 3$, and

$$\boldsymbol{X}_i = \begin{bmatrix} 1 & 0 & 0 \\ 1 & 1 & 1 \\ 1 & 2 & 2 \end{bmatrix} \quad \text{and} \quad \boldsymbol{Z}_i = \begin{bmatrix} 1 & 0 \\ 1 & 1 \\ 1 & 2 \end{bmatrix}$$

the expected value of $\boldsymbol{y}$ is

$$\begin{bmatrix} \beta_0 \\ \beta_0 + \beta_1 + \beta_2 \\ \beta_0 + 2\beta_1 + 2\beta_2 \end{bmatrix}$$

and the variance-covariance matrix equals

$$\sigma^2 \boldsymbol{I}_{n_i} + \begin{bmatrix} \sigma_{v_0}^2 & \sigma_{v_0}^2 + \sigma_{v_0 v_1} & \sigma_{v_0}^2 + 2\sigma_{v_0 v_1} \\ \sigma_{v_0}^2 + \sigma_{v_0 v_1} & \sigma_{v_0}^2 + 2\sigma_{v_0 v_1} + \sigma_{v_1}^2 & \sigma_{v_0}^2 + 3\sigma_{v_0 v_1} + 2\sigma_{v_1}^2 \\ \sigma_{v_0}^2 + 2\sigma_{v_0 v_1} & \sigma_{v_0}^2 + 3\sigma_{v_0 v_1} + 2\sigma_{v_1}^2 & \sigma_{v_0}^2 + 4\sigma_{v_0 v_1} + 4\sigma_{v_1}^2 \end{bmatrix}$$

which allows the variances and covariances to change across time. For example, if $\sigma_{v_0 v_1}$ is positive, then clearly the variance increases across time. Diminishing variance across time is also possible if, for example, $-2\sigma_{v_0 v_1} > \sigma_{v_1}^2$. Other patterns are possible depending on the values of these variance and covariance parameters.

Models with additional random-effects are also possible, as are models that allow autocorrelated errors, that is $\varepsilon_i \sim \mathcal{N}(0, \sigma^2 \boldsymbol{\Omega}_i)$, Here, $\boldsymbol{\Omega}$ might, for example, represent an autoregressive (AR) or moving average (MA) process for the residuals. Autocorrelated error regression models are common in econometrics. Their application within an MRM formulation is treated by Chi and Reinsel (1989) and Hedeker (1989), and extensively described in Verbeke and Molenberghs (2000). By including both random-effects and autocorrelated errors, a wide range of variance-covariance structures for the repeated measures is possible. This flexibility is in sharp contrast to the traditional ANOVA models which assume either a compound symmetry structure (univariate ANOVA) or a totally general structure (MANOVA). Typically, compound symmetry is too restrictive and a general structure is not parsimonious. MRMs, alternatively, provide these two and everything in between, and so allow efficient modeling of the variance-covariance structure of the repeated measures.

3.4.3 Generalized Estimating Equation Models

In the 1980s, alongside development of MRMs for analysis of longitudinal and/or clustered data, GEE models were developed (Liang and Zeger 1986, Zeger and Liang 1986). Essentially, GEE models extend generalized linear models (GLMs) to the case of correlated data. Thus, this class of models has become very popular especially for the analysis of categorical and count outcomes, though they can be used for continuous outcomes as well. One difference between GEE models and MRMs is that GEE models are based on quasi-likelihood estimation, and so the full-likelihood of the data is not specified. GEE models are termed marginal models, and they model the regression of y on x and the within-subject dependence (i.e., the association parameters) separately. The term "marginal" in this context indicates that the model for the mean response depends only on the covariates of interest, and not on any random-effects or previous responses. In terms of missing data, GEE assumes that the missing data are Missing Completely at Random (MCAR) as opposed to MAR which is assumed by the models employing full-likelihood estimation.

Conceptually, GEE reproduces the marginal means of the observed data, even if some of those means have limited information because of subject drop-out. Standard errors are adjusted (i.e., inflated) to accommodate the reduced amount of independent information produced by the correlation of the repeated observations over time. By contrast, mixed-effects models use the available data from all subjects to model temporal response patterns that would have been observed had the subjects all been measured to the end of the study. Because of this, estimated mean responses at the end of the study can be quite different for GEE versus MRM, if the future observations are related to the measurements that were made during the course of the study. If the available measurements are not related to the missing measurements (e.g., following dropout), GEE and MRM will produce quite similar estimates. This is the fundamental difference between GEE and MRM, that is, the assumption that the missing data are dependent on the observed responses for a given subject during that subject's participation in the study. It is hard to imagine that a subject's responses that would have been obtained following dropout would be independent of their observed responses during the study. This leads to a preference for full-likelihood approaches over quasi or partial likelihood approaches, and MRM over GEE, at least for longitudinal data. There is certainly less of an argument for a preference for data that are only clustered (e.g., patients nested within clinics), in which case advantages of MAR over MCAR are not as germane.

A basic feature of GEE models is that the joint distribution of a subject's response vector y_i does not need to be specified. Instead, it is only the marginal distribution of y_{ij} at each time point that needs to be specified. To clarify this further, suppose that there are two time-points and suppose that we are dealing with a continuous normal outcome. GEE would only require us to assume that the distribution of y_{i1} and y_{i2} are two univariate normals, rather than assuming that y_{i1} and y_{i2} form a (joint) normal distribution. Thus, GEE avoids the need for multivariate distributions by only assuming a functional form for the marginal distribution at each time point. This leads to a simpler quasi-likelihood approach for estimating the model parameters, rather than the full-likelihood approach of the MRM. The disadvantage, as mentioned above, is that because a multivariate distribution is not specified for the response vector, the assumption for the missing data are more stringent for the GEE than the full-likelihood estimated MRMs.

3.4.4 Models for Categorical Outcomes

Reflecting the usefulness of mixed-effects modeling and the importance of categorical outcomes in many areas of research, generalization of mixed-effects models for categorical outcomes has been an active area of statistical research. For dichotomous response data, several approaches adopting either a logistic or probit regression model and various methods for incorporating and estimating the influence of the random-effects have been developed (Gibbons 1981, Stiratelli et al. 1984, Wong and Mason 1985, Gibbons and Bock 1987, Conaway 1989, Goldstein 2011). Here, we briefly describe a mixed-effects logistic regression model for the analysis of binary data. Extensions of this model for analysis of ordinal, nominal and count data are described in detail by Hedeker and Gibbons (2006).

To set the notation, we again let i denote the sampling units (subjects, clinics, hospitals, counties) and let j denote the clustering of observations within unit i (e.g., repeated measurement occasions within patient i). Assume that there are $i = 1, \ldots, N$ units and $j = 1, \ldots, n_i$ clustered measurements within unit i. Let Y_{ij} be the value of the dichotomous outcome variable, coded 0 or 1. The logistic regression model is written in terms of the log odds (i.e., the logit) of the probability of a response, denoted p_{ij}. Considering first a random-intercept model, augmenting the logistic regression model with a single random-effect yields:

$$\ln\left[\frac{p_{ij}}{1 + p_{ij}}\right] = \boldsymbol{x}'_{ij}\boldsymbol{\beta} + \upsilon_{i0} \qquad (3.8)$$

where x_{ij} is the $(p+1) \times 1$ covariate vector (includes a 1 for the intercept), $\boldsymbol{\beta}$ is the $(p+1) \times 1$ vector of unknown regression parameters, and υ_{i0} is the random unit (e.g., patient or county) effect. These random-effects are assumed to be distributed in the population as $N(0, \sigma_\upsilon^2)$. For convenience and computational simplicity, in models for categorical outcomes the random-effects are typically expressed in standardized form. For this, $\upsilon_{0i} = \sigma_\upsilon \theta_i$ and the model is given as:

$$\ln\left[\frac{p_{ij}}{1 + p_{ij}}\right] = \boldsymbol{x}'_{ij}\boldsymbol{\beta} + \sigma_\upsilon \theta_i. \qquad (3.9)$$

Notice that the random-effects variance term (i.e., the population standard deviation σ_v is now explicitly included in the regression model. Thus, it and the regression coefficients are on the same scale, namely, in terms of the log-odds of a response.

The model can also be expressed in terms of a latent continuous variable y, with the observed dichotomous variable Y being a manifestation of the unobserved continuous y. Here, the model is written as:

$$y_{ij} = \boldsymbol{x}'_{ij}\boldsymbol{\beta} + \sigma_v\theta_i + \varepsilon_{ij} \tag{3.10}$$

in which case the error term ε_{ij} follows a standard logistic distribution under the logistic regression model (or a standard normal distribution under the probit regression model). This representation helps to explain why the regression coefficients from a mixed-effects logistic regression model do not typically agree with those obtained from a fixed-effects logistic regression model, or for that matter from a GEE logistic regression model which has regression coefficients that agree in scale with the fixed-effects model. In the mixed-model, the conditional variance of the latent y given $\boldsymbol{x}$ equals $\sigma_v^2 + \sigma_\varepsilon^2$, whereas in the fixed-effects model this conditional variance equals only the latter term σ_ε^2 (which equals either $\pi^2/3$ or 1 depending on whether it is a logistic or probit regression model, respectively). As a result, equating the variances of the latent y under these two scenarios yields:

$$\boldsymbol{\beta}_M \approx \sqrt{\frac{\sigma_v^2 + \sigma_\varepsilon^2}{\sigma_\varepsilon^2}}\boldsymbol{\beta}_F$$

where $\boldsymbol{\beta}_F$ and $\boldsymbol{\beta}_M$ represent the regression coefficients from the fixed-effects and (random-intercepts) mixed-effects models, respectively. In practice, Zeger et al. (1988) have found that $(15/16)^2\pi^2/3$ works better than $\pi^2/3$ for σ_ε^2 in equating results of logistic regression models.

Several authors have commented on the difference in scale and interpretation of the regression coefficients in mixed-models and marginal models, like the fixed-effects and GEE models (Neuhaus et al. 1991, Zeger et al. 1988). Regression estimates from the mixed-model have been termed "subject-specific" to reinforce the notion that they are conditional estimates, conditional on the random (subject) effect. Thus, they represent the effect of a regressor on the outcome controlling for, or holding constant, the value of the random subject effect. Alternatively, the estimates from the fixed-effects and GEE models are "marginal" or "population-averaged" estimates which indicate the effect of a regressor averaging over the population of subjects. This difference of scale and interpretation only occurs for non-linear regression models like the logistic regression model. For the linear model this difference does not exist.

4

Causal Inference

"Essentially, all models are wrong, but some are useful."
(George Box)

4.1 Introduction

In this chapter, we review methods for drawing causal inference from observational data. Of course, while this is an important goal in epidemiology in general and pharmacoepidemiology in particular, in practice, we rarely achieve it. Rather, we attempt to insulate our findings from bias to the greatest extent possible by conducting analyses with assumptions which when met support causal inferences. It is often difficult if not impossible to know with certainty that such assumptions are ever met. As an example, methods such as propensity score matching and marginal structural models eliminate static and dynamic confounding respectively under the assumption that all relevant confounders have been measured. Of course, this is an untestable assumption. However, we can determine the magnitude of the effect of an unmeasured confounder that would be required to change the conclusion of the analysis and in turn the plausibility of the existence of such an unmeasured confounder. In pharmacoepidemiology, one of the most important unmeasured confounders is severity of illness. We measure concomitant medications, comorbid diagnoses, hospitalizations, and prior experiences of the adverse effect before the drug exposure, but in general, we have no direct measure of the severity of illness of the patient at baseline or following the initial exposure. This limits our ability to draw causal inferences from these observational studies which form the basis for most work in pharmacoepidemiology. In the following sections, we review different design and analytic methods which minimize bias and take us down the path of causal inference.

4.2 Propensity Score Matching

Propensity score matching (Rosenbaum and Rubin 1983) is a remarkable tool for identifying and adjusting for bias in the analysis of observational data. The general idea is to provide a way to balance cases (treated) and controls in terms of multiple potential confounders (e.g., those taking a particular drug versus those not taking the drug for the treatment of a particular condition). Matching on the odds of being treated (i.e., the propensity score), based solely on the confounders, can provide balance between the groups leading to unbiased between group comparisons, conditional on the relevance and completeness of the observed confounders. Equally important, matching on the propensity score can also identify the presence of bias that is inherent in the particular between group comparison of interest that cannot be controlled through simple adjustment. For example, in the now classic example of relationship between smoking and mortality (Cochran 1968), pipe smoking is seen to have the highest risk of mortality not cigarette smoking. However, pipe smokers were on average older than cigarette smokers, so the actual comparison was potentially between a 30 year old cigarette smoker and a 70 year old pipe smoker. Stratification on age produced an unbiased comparison (at least with respect to observed covariates) that showed a clear effect of cigarette smoking on mortality, relative to both cigar and pipe smoking throughout the life cycle. Propensity score matching is therefore a multivariate extension of the single univariate stratification procedure described by Cochran (1968). While propensity score matching assumes that all of the confounders are measured, sensitivity analysis can be used to determine the degree to which conclusions could be altered by unmeasured confounders (i.e., hidden bias).

There are two general methods of correctly implementing propensity score matching (Rubin 2004). First, when the number of subjects in each condition is large ($n > 100$ per group), then stratification on the propensity score into quintiles (see Cochran, 1968 for a description of why quintiles is a good choice) is often the method of choice. Stratification on the propensity score allows one to determine if there is bias due to non-overlap of treatment conditions within quintiles or heterogeneity of the treatment effect across quintiles even if there is complete overlap.

A valid alternative to stratification is matching. There are three general types of matching. The first, direct matching or paired matching or fixed ratio or greedy matching obtains a fixed number (1:1, 2:1, 3:1,...) of nearest available potential control matches for each treated subject (Hansen 2004). A limitation of fixed ratio matching is that as the number matched controls (for each treated subject) increases so does the bias. A variation on direct matching, termed variable matching allows the number of controls to vary from one matched set to another. Ming and Rosenbaum (2000) have shown that variable matching can result in further reduction in bias relative to direct constant ratio approaches. The second approach, optimal matching or full-matching (Rosenbaum 1991, Gu and Rosenbaum 1993), subdivides a sample into a collection of matched sets consisting either of a treated subject and one or more controls or a control subject and one or more treated subjects. A limitation of full-matching is that there can be quite large discrepancies between the number of control and treated subjects within a subsample. Hansen (2004) extended the method of full-matching by introducing restrictions which limit the relative numbers of treated and control subjects in any matched set. The third approach, called fine balance matching (Rosenbaum et al. 2007), combines the ideas of stratification and matching into a single method. The approach begins by constructing a nominal variable with k categories (e.g., age and sex cross classification), for which an exact balance of treated and control subjects is achieved by allocating treated and control subjects into each of the k cells. Next, optimal matching is then performed without regard for the nominal variable (i.e., a matched pair can consist of treated and control subjects from different strata defined by the nominal variable). When there is a large reservoir of controls, direct matching strategies can do nearly as well as optimal matching algorithms (Rosenbaum and Rubin 1985).

Unfortunately, those two classes of statistically valid approaches to propensity score matching (i.e., stratification and matching) represent the minority of cases in which propensity score matching has appeared in the published reports in the medical literature. Rather, propensity scores are used predominantly as a statistical analysis tool by including the propensity score as a covariate in a regression model. There are several problems with this approach. First, it relies upon a strong assumption of linearity between propensity score and the outcome of interest. There is no prior reason to believe that such a simple linear relation exists. Second, unlike matching strategies using the propensity score, the regression approach provides no insight into the degree of balance of potential confounders between cases and controls. There is nothing to alert us to the possibility that we are comparing 40 year old cigarette smokers to 70 year old pipe smokers. Since we cannot rely upon the method to identify bias, we cannot count on the results of the regression based approach to insulate conclusions from bias. Further discussion of this issue and more general overview of the use of propensity score matching in medical research can be found in Rubin (1997), D'Agostino (1998), Rubin (2004), and D'Agostino and D'Agostino (2007).

The issue of missing data in propensity score matching is often overlooked. Propensity score matching assumes that missing observations are missing at random, implying that the mechanism by which data were missing is unrelated to information not contained in the observed data. Following D'Agostino et al. (2001), we can create indicator variables for additional level of missing category for categorical covariates. For continuous missing covariates, a binary variable for whether or not each variable was missing can be added, and in the case of a missing value, a value of zero can be imputed for the missing measurement. An alternative approach to the use of missing value indicators, when the number of potential confounders is relatively small, is to use different regression models based on which set of potential confounders are missing. The propensity scores based on these different regression models can then be combined without bias or introducing extra variability (Rosenbaum and Rubin 1983).

Rosenbaum and Rubin (1984) (Theorem B.1) showed that adjustment for the generalized propensity score in expectation balances the observed covariate information and the pattern of missing covariates, where the generalized propensity score is defined as the probability of treatment assignment given both the observed covariates and the pattern of the missing data. One issue in estimation of a propensity score model is what functional form of the covariates to include in the logistic model. Depending on the application, continuous, discrete, and missing indicators for continuous variables can be included, along with interactions and squared terms. Subsequently it is useful to verify that balancing of the covariate distributions between treated and control patients has been achieved overall and/or within each stratum.

4.2.1 Illustration

Varenicline, a nicotine receptor partial agonist, received FDA approval for use in smoking cessation. Benefits from varenicline in terms of smoking cessation are generally two to three times greater than unassisted attempts at quitting (Cahill et al. 2008, 2009). Post-marketing surveillance evidence that varenicline may be associated with increased risk of neuropsychiatric events, such as depression and suicidal thoughts and behavior, led to an FDA black box warning. Gibbons and Mann (2013) studied efficacy (smoking cessation) of varenicline, and safety (neuropsychiatric events) in both randomized clinical trials (RCTs) and a large observational study conducted by the Department of Defense (DoD) (Meyer et al. 2013). Here we focus on the large-scale observational study, which was designed to compare adverse neuropsychiatric adverse event rates in inpatients and outpatients taking varenicline versus nicotine replacement therapy (NRT) (n=35,800). The DoD study was a retrospective cohort study comparing acute (30 day and 60 day) rates of neuropsychiatric events from the Military Health System. The time-frame (August 1, 2006 to August 31, 2007) was prior to FDA warnings to minimize selection effects and stimulated reporting due to the extensive media coverage of these warnings. There were 19,933 patients treated with varenicline and 15,867 patients treated with NRT. The data were restricted to new users defined by not receiving treatment with either varenicline or NRT for the prior 180 days. The primary endpoints for the observational study were anxiety, depression, drug induced mental disorder, episodic and mood disorder, other psychiatric disorder, post traumatic stress disorder, schizophrenia, suicide attempt, transient mental disorder.

Unadjusted rates of neuropsychiatric disorders were compared between varenicline and NRT using Fisher's exact test. Propensity score matching was used to create a 1:1 matched set of varenicline and NRT treated patients in terms of demographic characteristics, and historical (past year) comorbid physical illness and psychiatric illnesses, and psychiatric and smoking cessation medications (see Table 4.1). Rates were compared using GEE. Table 4.1 reveals that prior to matching, large standardized differences (i.e., greater than 10%) were found for age, Charlson comorbidity score, bupropion, other smoking medications, SSRIs, race, and sex. Following propensity score matching, all standardized differences were less than 3%. This indicates that propensity score matching worked extremely well at balancing the groups in terms of the measured potential confounders.

The unadjusted overall rates of neuropsychiatric events were 2.38% for varenicline and 3.17% for NRT (p<0.0001). Following propensity score matching, the rates were 2.28% for varenicline and 3.16% for NRT (OR=0.72, 95% CI (0.62, 0.83), p<0.0001). Decreases in drug induced mental disorders (OR=0.10, 95% CI (0.04, 0.24), p<0.0001), and other psychiatric disorders (OR=0.20, 95% CI (0.04, 0.91), p<0.04) were also found (see Table 4.2). The only disorder more frequently observed in varenicline treated patients was transient mental disorder; however, there were few such events (9 cases for varenicline 0.05% versus 4 cases for NRT 0.03%), and the results were not statistically significant (0.06% for varenicline versus 0.02% for NRT following propensity score matching). In general, the results with and without propensity score matching were quite similar. When patients with a neuropsychiatric event (i.e., disorder or suicide attempt) in the previous year were excluded, results were also quite similar. The unadjusted overall rates of neuropsychiatric events were 0.53% for varenicline and 1.13% for NRT (p<0.0001). Following propensity score matching, the rates were 0.52% for varenicline and 1.09% for NRT (OR=0.47, 95% CI (0.35, 0.65), p<0.0001).

4.2.2 Discussion

While propensity score matching is an enormously useful and innovative method for exploring and reducing bias in observational studies, it is most often used incorrectly in medical research. A good propensity score analysis examines whether or not balance is achieved, and allows the investigator to make inferences within the balanced sets of cases and controls. We note that direct matching (e.g., 1:1 matching) uses a subset of all available subjects and stratification involves the construction of subclasses that are restricted to only treated and control subjects with substantial overlap in their covariate distributions. However deleting subjects can compromise generalizability, which can also be a source of bias. These are inherent limitations that underlie the analysis of observational data. In contrast, the use of the propensity score as a covariate allows us to use all available subjects in the analysis, which can minimize bias. However, the covariate approach does not alert us to the possibility of hidden bias due to non-overlapping covariate distributions between cases and controls, and the strong assumption of a linear relationship between

TABLE 4.1: Frequency Distributions for Variables Used in Matching

Variables	Before Matching			After Matching		
	Varenicline N=19933 N(%)/Mean(SD)	NRT N=15867 N(%)/Mean(SD)	Standardized Difference	Varenicline N=13215 N(%)/Mean(SD)	NRT N=13215 N(%)/Mean(SD)	Standardized Difference
Age	42.1 (14.3)	35.1 (12.6)	52.31	36.8 (12.4)	36.8 (12.8)	0.41
Charlson comorbidity score	0.37 (0.97)	0.21 (0.77)	18.25	0.23 (0.76)	0.24 (0.83)	1.93
Diagnoses in previous year						
Anxiety	1054 (5.29)	692 (4.36)	4.31	594 (4.49)	619 (4.68)	0.90
Chronic pain	78 (0.39)	36 (0.23)	2.96	29 (0.22)	35 (0.26)	0.92
Delusional disorder	3 (0.02)	5 (0.03)	1.08	3 (0.02)	4 (0.03)	0.47
Depressive disorder	1097 (5.50)	694 (4.37)	5.22	592 (4.48)	630 (4.77)	1.37
Drug-induced mental disorder	45 (0.23)	42 (0.26)	0.79	31 (0.23)	33 (0.25)	0.31
Episodic and mood disorder	879 (4.41)	595 (3.75)	3.34	510 (3.86)	529 (4.00)	0.74
Other non-organic psychosis	34 (0.17)	25 (0.16)	0.32	16 (0.12)	20 (0.15)	0.82
Personality disorder	101 (0.51)	121 (0.76)	3.22	76 (0.58)	83 (0.63)	0.69
PTSD	247 (1.24)	237 (1.49)	2.19	164 (1.24)	173 (1.31)	0.61
Schizophrenia	41 (0.21)	30 (0.19)	0.37	25 (0.19)	25 (0.19)	0.00
Substance abuse	280 (1.40)	382 (2.41)	7.34	225 (1.70)	240 (1.82)	0.86
Suicide attempt	14 (0.07)	21 (0.13)	1.95	13 (0.10)	14 (0.11)	0.24
Transient mental disorder	48 (0.24)	38 (0.24)	0.03	30 (0.23)	32 (0.24)	0.31
Neuropsychiatric (all above)	2595 (13.02)	1762 (11.10)	5.88	1477 (11.18)	1539 (11.65)	1.48
Prescriptions in previous year						
Any antipsychotic medication	560 (2.81)	451 (2.84)	0.20	343 (2.60)	371 (2.81)	1.31
Bupropion	2074 (10.40)	2301 (14.50)	12.43	1419 (10.74)	1507 (11.40)	2.12
Pain medication	14149 (70.98)	10905 (68.73)	4.92	9190 (69.54)	9170 (69.39)	0.33
Any psychiatric medication	7629 (38.27)	5260 (35.42)	5.92	4403 (33.32)	4567 (34.56)	2.62
Sleep medication	2263 (11.35)	1345 (8.48)	9.64	1174 (8.88)	1220 (9.23)	1.21
Other smoking cessation meds	424 (2.13)	1061 (6.69)	22.35	415 (3.14)	434 (3.28)	0.82
SSRIs	2964 (14.87)	1759 (11.09)	11.28	1521 (11.51)	1593 (12.05)	1.69
TCAs	849 (4.26)	502 (3.16)	5.80	419 (3.17)	463 (3.50)	1.85
Marital status						
Married	10746 (53.91)	8831 (55.66)	3.51	7586 (57.40)	7689 (58.18)	1.58
Other	9187 (46.09)	7036 (44.34)		5629 (43.60)	5526 (41.82)	
Race						
White	10071 (50.52)	9388 (59.17)	17.43	7738 (58.55)	7723 (58.44)	0.23
Other	9862 (49.48)	6479 (40.83)		5477 (41.45)	5492 (41.56)	
Sex						
Female	8763 (43.96)	5094 (32.11)	24.61	4814 (36.43)	4737 (35.85)	1.21
Male	11168 (56.04)	10770 (67.89)		8399 (63.57)	8476 (64.15)	

TABLE 4.2: Neuropsychiatric Events Before and After Matching

Diagnosis	Before PS Matching			After PS Matching				
	Varenicline N = 19,933 N (%)	NRT N = 15,867 N (%)	p-value	Varenicline N = 13,215 N (%)	NRT N = 13,215 N (%)	p-value	OR	95% CI
Anxiety Disorder	151 (0.76%)	132 (0.83%)	0.44	92 (0.70%)	110 (0.83%)	0.23	0.84	0.63-1.10
Depressive Disorder	113 (0.57%)	108 (0.68%)	0.18	71 (0.54%)	92 (0.70%)	0.12	0.77	0.57-1.05
Drug Induced Mental Disorder	7 (0.04%)	70 (0.44%)	<0.0001	6 (0.05%)	59 (0.45%)	<0.0001	0.10	0.04-0.24
Episodic and Mood Disorder	190 (0.95%)	152 (0.96%)	0.99	118 (0.89%)	128 (0.97%)	0.56	0.92	0.72-1.18
Other Psychiatric Disorder	3 (0.02%)	10 (0.06%)	0.02	2 (0.02%)	10 (0.08%)	0.04	0.20	0.04-0.91
Post Traumatic Stress Disorder	64 (0.32%)	86 (0.54%)	0.002	45 (0.34%)	65 (0.49%)	0.07	0.69	0.47-1.01
Schizophrenia	10 (0.05%)	15 (0.09%)	0.16	9 (0.07%)	12 (0.09%)	0.66	0.75	0.32-1.78
Suicide Attempt	2 (0.01%)	4 (0.03%)	0.42	2 (0.02%)	3 (0.02%)	0.99	0.67	0.11-3.99
Transient Mental Disorder	9 (0.05%)	4 (0.03%)	0.41	8 (0.06%)	3 (0.02%)	0.23	2.67	0.71-10.06
Neuropsychiatric Disorders (All Above)	475 (2.38%)	503 (3.17%)	<0.0001	301 (2.28%)	417 (3.16%)	<0.0001	0.72	0.62-0.83

the propensity score and the outcome of interest can further bias statistical inferences regarding between group differences in observational studies.

4.3 Marginal Structural Models

In the previous section we used propensity score matching to balance the distributions of measured potential confounders between treated and control conditions in an observational study. The characteristics of interest were static in the sense that they were either measured at baseline or considered to be invariant over time. In many situations of interest in drug safety, this may not be the case. The treatment selection process can be dynamic and the selection of a specific treatment of interest may evolve over time as other characteristics of the patient's experience (e.g., non-response to an alternate treatment or severity of illness change over time). In this case, the simple propensity score may fail to capture the true determinants of treatment and therefore fail to adjust for confounders that vary over time. One solution to this problem is based on the idea of marginal structural models (MSM), Robins et al. (2000). The fundamental idea of MSM is that there are two dynamic models, one for the treatment selection process and the other for the dynamic effect of treatment on the outcome of interest. The first model is used to derive weights which when applied to the second stage model create a pseudo-population which is similar to what would be observed if the treatment assignment were sequentially randomized, thereby eliminating the confounding between characteristics of the individuals which change over time and can affect both the likelihood of future treatment and the outcome of treatment (e.g., changes in severity of depression). This approach is relatively new to the area of drug safety.

The statistical analysis is comprised of two stages. In the first stage, a logistic regression model is used to predict usage of the drug exposure of interest at each of the t time-points conditional on fixed covariates (e.g., demographics and prior history of the adverse event of interest), and time-varying covariates (comorbid conditions, concomitant medications, hospitalizations, and non-pharmacologic treatments such as psychotherapy). The predicted probability of treatment at time-point t is computed as the continued product of probabilities from baseline to time-point t. The inverses of these estimated probabilities are then used as weights $W(t)$ in the second stage analysis that relate actual treatment (dynamically determined on a month by month basis) to the adverse event using either a longitudinal statistical model such as GEE or a mixed-effects logistic regression model for adverse events which are repeatedly experienced (Hedeker and Gibbons 2006) or some form of time-to-event model (e.g., discrete-time survival model (Efron 1988)) for those cases in which we are interested in the time to the first occurrence of the adverse event.

In practice, $W(t)$ is highly variable and sometimes takes extremely small values causing problems in inverse weighting. To overcome this problem, Robins et al. (2000) suggested use of the stabilized weight:

$$SW(t) = \prod_{k=0}^{t} \frac{f\left[A(k) \mid \bar{A}(k-1), V\right]}{f\left[A(k) \mid \bar{A}(k-1), \bar{L}(k)\right]} \tag{4.1}$$

where L is the set of all baseline and time-varying covariates, V is a subset of L consisting of only the baseline covariates (i.e., time invariant effects), $A(k)$ is the actual treatment assignment at time k, $A(k-1)$ is the treatment history, and $f[x]$ is the probability of actual assignment of a treatment at time point k conditioning on both treatment assignment history up to time $(k-1)$ and baseline covariates. The standardized weights should have mean close to 1.0. The net result is that using MSM we are able to control for the effects of time-dependent confounders that are affected by prior treatment. At each time-point the weight is the inverse of the probability of receiving treatment given all factors that affect the likelihood of receiving treatment. Robins et al. (2000) showed that this method creates a pseudo-population that resembles data from a sequentially randomized experiment, under the assumption that all of the factors that determine treatment are observed. Conceptually, MSM is similar to a propensity score which takes on time-specific values and is used as a weight in a second stage analysis rather than used to match treated and control subjects.

A limitation of standard MSM is that it requires all confounders to be observed, measured, and explicitly included in the stage 1 model. In many cases, this assumption may be invalid. For example, depressive severity is not measured, and it is a key determinant of the treatment selection process. One possible solution to this problem is to generalize the MSM approach further, by using a mixed-effects logistic regression to model the treatment selection process in stage 1. Leon and Hedeker (2007) have studied a similar specification using dynamic propensity score stratification and have found evidence that the inclusion of a random-effect in the propensity score dramatically reduces bias associated with unmeasured confounders. This was based on a very simple model specification (random intercept model), which could easily be expanded further to include random-effects over time and clustering within ecological strata such as clinics, hospitals, or geographic units such as counties.

MSM has been used previously in drug safety studies to examine the effectiveness of beta blockers (Delaney et al. 2009), angiotensin receptor blockers on mortality in patients with chronic heart failure (Yang and Joffe 2012), paracalcitral and survival in hemodialysis patients (Miller et al. 2012), the effect of aspirin on cardiovascular mortality (Cook et al. 2002), estrogen and progesterone on coronary heart disease (Toh and Manson 2013), and comparing the effects of different antidepressants on completed suicide in adult veterans (Valenstein et al. 2012).

4.3.1   Illustration

Gibbons et al. (2014) used MSM to adjust for dynamic confounding in the treatment selection process for children and adolescents being treated with antidepressants and its possible association with suicidal behavior (attempts and intentional self harm). They studied this question in parallel in two large medical claims databases (MarketScan and LifeLink) covering over 100 million lives. These datasets contain complete longitudinal information on clinical utilization in inpatient and outpatient settings and all filled prescriptions for insured employees and their dependents. Identical specifications were used for both datasets. They selected all data during the period of 2004 through 2009 for patients with a new diagnosis of depression (ICD-9: 296.2*, 296.3*, 300.4, or 311) in patients ages 5-17. The index date was the date of the depression diagnostic claim. Patients who, during the 6 months prior to study entry, had insurance coverage, no diagnosis of depression, bipolar disorder or schizophrenia, and any antidepressant or antipsychotic medication claims were included. Subjects were followed for up to 180 days. The medical claims data were used to create a monthly person-time dataset, with 6 monthly observation periods from the index depression episode date. A patient who was available during all 6 months of follow-up and did not make a suicide attempt would have 6 monthly observations with an event code of 0 for all 6 records. A patient who had his/her coverage revoked after 3 months and did not make a suicide attempt would have 3 monthly observations with an event code of 0 for all 3 records. A patient who made a suicide attempt in month 4 would have a total of 4 records with event codes of 0 for the first 3 months and a code of 1 on the 4th month. A drug was considered present during a given month if a prescription was filled in that month or a carryover from a prior month was filled (i.e., days supply extended into the next month). If a prescription was filled in the month of a suicide attempt, the drug was considered present if the prescription was filled prior to the attempt. Prior suicide attempts were included as an important covariate in the model and were assessed during the six month period prior to the index date. A suicide attempt on the same day as the index date was treated as a prior suicide attempt.

Table 4.3 presents the distributions of the potential confounders in the two databases. A curious result is that the rate of suicide attempts was almost double for both treated and untreated occasions in the LifeLink database than in the MarketScan database. An even larger discrepancy was seen for suicide attempts in the 6 months prior to the new index episode. While the authors identify regional differences between the two databases that might account for some of this difference, the observation raises questions about the ways and perhaps even the integrity with which such data are collected. On a more positive note; however, it should be noted that although the overall rate of suicide attempts differed between the two datasets, the difference between treated and untreated time-intervals was remarkably similar between the two datasets as were the results of the MSM analysis. Further study of regional differences in suicide rates and factors that may influence differential rates of suicide related claims in different medical claims databases should be a high priority in pharmacoepidemiology.

TABLE 4.3: Distribution of Covariates Used in MSM

Covariates	MarketScan Mean or %	LifeLink Mean or %
Demographics		
Age	14.3	14.1
Female	58.0	56.4
Comorbid Conditions		
Prior Suicide Attempts	0.2	1.3
ADHD	7.7	13.3
Anxiety Spectrum Disorder	7.2	10
Bipolar Disorder	3.9	5.6
Psychotic Disorder	5.6	4.3
Seizure Disorder	0.6	0.9
Conduct Disorder	1.8	3.9
Medication Use		
Antihistamines	1.5	2.4
Antipsychotics	2.7	2.0
Antiepileptics	2.0	2.3
Anxiolytics	1.0	0.8
Lithium	0.2	0.2
Narcotic Analgesics	1.3	1.3
Sedative/Hypnotics	0.4	0.4
Health Service Use		
Psych Hospitalization	3.6	1.9
Psychotherapy Visit	41.9	37.4

Table 4.4 presents the results of the 1st stage treatment selection model. In general, the predictors of treatment were quite similar between the two datasets. The major predictors of increased likelihood of receiving antidepressant treatment were age, and receiving other CNS medications (antiepileptics, antipsychotics, anxiolytics, and sedative/hypnotics). Patients with comorbid anxiety disorder were also at increased likelihood of receiving antidepressant treatment. By contrast, patients diagnosed with bipolar disorder were less likely to receive antidepressant treatment. Given the large sample sizes, the majority of associations were statistically significant. A notable exception was prior suicide attempts, which interestingly neither increased nor decreased the likelihood of receiving treatment.

For the MarketScan Data, there were a total of 55,284 subjects who met criteria for the study. The average age was 14.3 years. 58.0% were female. The overall annualized suicide attempt rate was 12*(173/338922)*100 = 0.61% (0.53% off treatment versus 1.03% on treatment). The average standardized weight was 1.05 (standard deviation (SD) = 0.66). The overall unweighted and

TABLE 4.4: Dynamic Predictors of Antidepressant Treatment

Variable	OR	MarketScan 95% CI	p-value	OR	LifeLink 95% CI	p-value
Month 0	0.71	0.69-0.74	<.0001	0.88	0.86-0.89	<.0001
Month 1	1.50	1.46-1.54	<.0001	1.32	1.30-1.33	<.0001
Month 2	1.30	1.27-1.34	<.0001	1.23	1.22-1.24	<.0001
Month 3	1.20	1.17-1.24	<.0001	1.15	1.13-1.16	<.0001
Month 4	1.12	1.09-1.15	<.0001	1.07	1.06-1.0	<.0001
Sex (Male)	1.06	1.02-1.09	0.002	1.21	1.18-1.23	<.0001
Age	1.63	1.51-1.75	<.0001	1.31	1.26-1.36	<.0001
Age2	0.99	0.98-0.99	<.0001	0.99	0.99-1.00	<.0001
Prior Attempt	1.07	0.77-1.50	0.681	1.02	0.93-1.11	0.707
ADHD	1.07	1.01-1.13	0.014	1.25	1.22-1.29	<.0001
Anxiety	1.58	1.50-1.66	<.0001	1.83	1.78-1.89	<.0001
Bipolar	0.86	0.80-0.93	0.000	0.33	0.31-0.35	<.0001
Conduct Disorder	1.09	0.98-1.21	0.116	1.10	1.05-1.15	<.0001
Psychotic Disorder	1.21	1.14-1.29	<.0001	1.19	1.14-1.24	<.0001
Seizure	1.17	0.99-1.38	0.062	0.91	0.84-0.98	0.015
Narcotic Analgesics	1.07	0.99-1.16	0.081	1.05	1.02-1.08	0.002
Antiepileptics	2.28	2.10-2.47	<.0001	1.80	1.71-1.90	<.0001
Antihistamine	1.41	1.30-1.52	<.0001	1.31	1.27-1.35	<.0001
Lithium	1.19	0.87-1.63	0.269	1.42	1.20-1.67	<.0001
Antipsychotics	4.17	3.90-4.46	<.0001	2.42	2.30-2.56	<.0001
Anxiolytics	2.28	2.07-2.50	<.0001	1.52	1.44-1.60	<.0001
Sedative/Hypnotics	2.86	2.48-3.29	<.0001	1.66	1.53-1.80	<.0001
Psych Hospitalization	0.70	0.65-0.75	<.0001	1.15	1.12-1.18	<.0001
Psychotherapy Visit	1.30	1.27-1.33	<.0001	1.12	1.11-1.13	<.0001

Note: Month 5 is the reference

unadjusted analysis revealed increased risk of suicide attempt with treatment (OR = 1.99, 95% CI = 1.39, 2.85). The unweighted covariate adjusted analysis decreased the risk estimate slightly, but remained significant (OR=1.84, 95% CI = 1.29, 2.64). The weighted MSM analysis revealed a non-significant relationship between antidepressant treatment and suicide attempts (OR=1.21, 95% CI = 0.79, 1.88). For the LifeLink Data, a total of 165,744 subjects met criteria for the study. The average age was 14.1 years. 56.0% were female. The overall annualized suicide attempt rate was 12*(1172/910271)*100 = 1.55% (1.30% off treatment versus 2.54% on treatment). The average standardized weight was 1.05 (SD = 0.55). The overall unweighted and unadjusted analysis revealed increased risk of suicide attempt with treatment (OR=1.94, 95% CI = 1.72, 2.20). The unweighted covariate adjusted analysis decreased the risk estimate but remained significant at (OR=1.66 95% CI = 1.47, 1.87). The weighted MSM analysis revealed a non-significant relationship between antidepressant treatment and suicide attempts (OR=1.05, 95% CI = 0.92, 1.19). Quite similar results were found when the analysis was restricted to SSRIs.

These findings reveal that dynamic confounding in the treatment selection process is responsible for most, if not all of the association between antidepressant treatment and suicide attempts in children and adolescents.

4.3.2 Discussion

The use of between-subject comparisons in pharmacoepidemiology is limited by our ability to access data on all important confounders which may lead one patient down the path of receiving one treatment or another. The ability to perform within-subject comparisons in which periods for which the patient received the treatment are compared to periods in which the patient did not receive the treatment, can eliminate many sources of between-subject bias by using each subject as their own control. Nevertheless, there are dynamic confounders that may influence the likelihood of receiving treatment at a given point in the patient's illness and those variables may in turn be related to the adverse event of interest, producing non-causal association between the drug exposure and the adverse event, even when analyzed within-subjects and adjusting for measured confounders. Marginal structural models provide one approach to insulating such analyses from bias, under the assumption that all dynamic confounders are measured. Future statistical research using random-effects models may help relax this strong assumption, by including unmeasured person-specific effects into the adjustment weighting.

4.4 Instrumental Variables

Instrumental variable (IV) methods are used to estimate causal treatment effects from observational data. In many practical applications, especially with observational studies of adverse drug reactions, there are no data available on all the factors that determine treatment assignment or self-selection into treatment. Thus, it is not always possible to use regression analysis to adjust for covariates or match treatment groups statically (e.g., propensity score matching) or dynamically (e.g., marginal structural models) because key covariates are not observed. IV methods exploit an exogenous source of variation that affects an outcome y only by way of a treatment assignment x. The exogenous source of variation is called the instrument, denoted by z. In economics, instrumental variables are typically framed as structural equation models, which are stochastic models that describe a set of equations representing causal relationship among variables.

Following Angrist et al. (1996), consider the following simple linear system: $y_i = \beta_0 + \beta_1 x_i + u_i$ and $x_i^* = \alpha_0 + \alpha_1 z_i + v_i$. In this model, x is an indicator variable that equals 1 if the latent variable $x^* > c$, where c is a threshold. The latent formulation emphasizes the fact that participating in the treatment is a choice that is affected by the variable z. In the example given in Angrist et al. (1996), x represents veteran status, y is a health outcome (e.g., suicidality in an interval of time), and the instrument z is the observed draft status. The parameter of interest is β_1, which represents the causal effect of veteran status on this health outcome while α_1 measures the strength of the draft status to the probability of being a veteran. The equations above describe a model of choice: whether a person decides to enroll in the army depends on many factors for example, mental health status/suicidality, and some of these factors confound the relationship between treatment and outcome. In economic terminology, the receipt of treatment x is said to be an "endogenous regressor," and as a consequence, x is correlated with the error term ε because the error term contains unobservable confounders. In statistical terminology, the receipt of treatment x is said to be "non-ignorable" (Angrist et al. 1996, Rubin 1978).

The instrument z must satisfy two conditions to be a valid instrument. First, the instrument z must be a good predictor of treatment receipt, or $cov(x_i, z_i) \neq 0$. The second requirement, often called the "exclusion restriction," is that the instrument must be uncorrelated with the error term u, or $cov(u_i, z_i) = 0$. The exclusion restriction implies that the effect of the instrument on the outcome y must be only through an effect on the treatment and not because the instrument is correlated with an unobservable factor that affects the outcome. This automatically holds for the example, as a lottery determines the draft status. Therefore draft status cannot be correlated with any of the factors that confound the relationship between x and y. If draft status were conditionally randomized on some observable characteristic, like age, then the exclusion restriction can still be satisfied by including age as a covariate in both equations. Only the first assumption can be empirically tested, although a sensitivity analysis can be used to determine the extent to which violations of these assumptions could account for the observed results. The validity of the exclusion restriction depends on substantive knowledge about the factors that determine treatment selection and the relationship between the instrument and treatment receipt.

For the system of equations above, the parameter of interest can be estimated by

$$\beta_i^{IV} = \widehat{cov}(y_i, z_i)/\widehat{cov}(x_i, z_i). \tag{4.2}$$

Angrist et al. (1996) reframed IV methods using the Rubin Causal Model (RCM) and principal stratification. In particular, they spelled out the assumptions behind the method and clarified the interpretation of the IV estimand. Rather than measuring the causal treatment effect of x on y in the population, β_i^{IV} estimates a Local Average Treatment Effect (LATE) that applies to those individuals who were treated because of the variation induced by the instrument the "compliers" in the principal stratification framework. In the context of a randomized trial with partial compliance, in which the instrument is treatment assignment, the IV method estimates the treatment effect of those who were induced to comply because they were assigned to the treatment group. In contrast, a comparison of average outcomes between treated and not treated groups provides an intent-to-treat estimate of the treatment effect.

There are several methods for IV estimation, but two-stage least squares appears to be the most popular. Consider the simple ordinary least squares (OLS) regression of of outcome y on treatment x as

$$y = \beta x + u , \tag{4.3}$$

where u is an error term. The regression of y on x yields the OLS estimate $\hat{\beta}$ of β, under the assumption that x is uncorrelated with u as in Figure 4.1.

FIGURE 4.1: Treatment and error are uncorrelated.

However, in some cases, there may be an association between the treatment and the outcome as in Figure 4.2.

$$x \longrightarrow y$$
$$\uparrow \quad \nearrow$$
$$u$$

FIGURE 4.2: Treatment and error are correlated.

For example, in the case of antidepressants and suicidal behavior, depressive severity increases the likelihood of treatment with an antidepressant and depressive severity increases the likelihood of suicidal behavior. Statistically, there is now both a direct effect via βx and an indirect effect via u on x which in turn influences y, both of which can be adjusted for additional covariates. The regression model is now

$$y = \beta x + u(x) \tag{4.4}$$

for which the OLS estimator of β is biased and inconsistent. In economic terms, the inconsistency of the OLS estimator is due to the endogeneity of x because changes in x are associated with both y and the error u. The IV method attempts to generate only exogenous variation in x as in Figure 4.3 which shows the relationships of z, x, y, and u within strata of the observed confounders.

The IV method introduces a variable z which is associated with changes in x but has no direct effect on y. z is associated with x but not with u. z and y

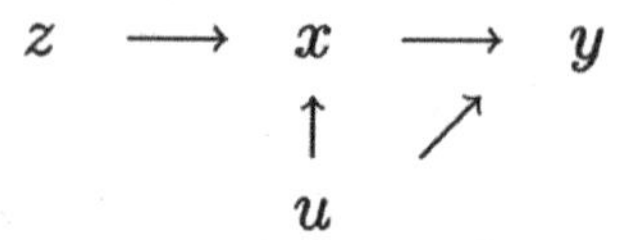

$$z \longrightarrow x \longrightarrow y$$
$$\uparrow \quad \nearrow$$
$$u$$

FIGURE 4.3: The IV method.

are related, but the only through the indirect path of z being correlated with x which in turn determines y. Note that by the previously stated assumptions, z is excluded from being a predictor of y. Mathematically this leads to

$$\beta_{IV} = \frac{dy/dz}{dx/dz}. \tag{4.5}$$

Consistent estimation of dy/dz can be obtained by the OLS regression of y on z with slope estimate $(z'z)^{-1}z'y$, and dx/dz by the OLS regression of x on z with slope estimate $(z'z)^{-1}z'x$, which leads to

$$\beta_{IV} = \frac{(z'z)^{-1}z'y}{(z'z)^{-1}z'x} = (z'x)^{-1}z'y. \tag{4.6}$$

A valid instrument must be a strong predictor of treatment in order to obtain consistent/valid inference. An instrument that is not a strong predictor of treatment is referred to as a "weak instrument." A weak instrument implies an unstable estimate of the LATE treatment effects with poor properties (Bound et al. 1995). A common empirical strategy in the presence of a weak instrument is to augment it with more instruments. Chamberlain and Imbens (2004) proposed random-effects IV estimators for models with one endogenous regressor and many instrumental variables. They add a random-effects structure to the model describing the relationship between the treatment and the instruments, considering the variance of the random coefficients as an unknown parameter. They show that their estimators have better finite sample properties but asymptotically their estimators have the same properties as other alternatives in the literature (Bound et al. 1995).

In pharmacoepidemiology, a natural instrument is the local area (hospital, county, state) rates of prescriptions of the drug(s) of interest as instruments for the treatment selection process for an individual patient in that local area. Other local area characteristics (such as access to health care, income, urban, rural, $\cdots$) can be included as instruments as as well. In addition to the typical econometric modeling described above, mixed-effects regression models can be used to predict person-level drug utilization as a mixture of local area level observed characteristics (i.e., drug prescription rates) and unobserved characteristics that are absorbed into the empirical Bayes estimate of the ecological unit-specific effect. Note that to our knowledge, this has not previously been considered.

4.4.1 Illustration

Davies et al. (2013) examined the use of physician prescribing preferences for instruments for antidepressant prescriptions that they issued their patients. They examined whether physician's previous prescriptions of tricyclic antidepressants (TCAs) versus SSRIs were valid instruments for the patient-level antidepressant treatment selections. As outcomes, they examined hospital admission for self harm or death by suicide. The data were collected from 600 general practices in the United Kingdom representing 11 million patients.

The assumptions of this IV analysis are that (1) the instrumental variable is associated with the actual prescription, i.e., physician's preferences for a particular antidepressant in previous patients are associated with the actual prescription that they issue for the current patient, (2) the instrumental variable does not directly affect the outcome i.e., physician's preferences for a particular antidepressant are unlikely to affect their patient's outcomes, and (3) the instrumental variable is not associated with unmeasured confounding conditional on measured confounding, i.e., physician's preferences for a particular antidepressant may not be associated with potential confounding factors (e.g., an individual with a history of suicidal behavior) because patients' choices of physicians are "quasi-random," and the preference based on previous prescriptions is not associated with the next patient's characteristics.

A total of 897,983 patients prescribed either an SSRI or TCA were identified during the period of January 1995 through June 2010. There were a total of 6,555 physicians drawn from 612 practices. A total of 484,858 patients were given a TCA and 401,877 were given a SSRI. Within 3 months of the first prescription, there were 608 cases of death by suicide or hospital admission for self harm (600 per 100,000). Evidence for confounding with baseline characteristics was strong. Those prescribed TCAs were 21.3 percentage points more likely to be over 40 and 22.5 percentage points more likely to have had more than five prescriptions of any type in the year before the antidepressant prescription was issued. Overall medical comorbidities were also 8.8 percentage points higher based on the Charlson index. By contrast, these differences were far more muted when based on physician preferences, with differences of 2.5%, 2.1%, and 1.2% for the difference between TCA and SSRI prescriptions for patients older than 40, more than five prescriptions and Charlson index (see Table 4.5). The difference in covariate imbalance between actual and prior prescriptions as measured by the Mahalanobis difference was 83% lower for prior relative to actual prescriptions. This indicates that not only is physician preference a good instrument in that it is strongly related to actual prescriptions, it is also unrelated to the observed confounding factors adding support to the validity of the exclusion restriction which also includes unobserved confounders and cannot be empirically proven.

Prior prescriptions were found to be strongly associated with actual prescriptions. Physicians who previously prescribed a TCA were 14.9 percentage points more likely to prescribe TCAs. Physicians who previously prescribed

TABLE 4.5: Potential Confounders in Prior Year - TCAs vs. SSRIs

Variable	Actual Prescription		Prior Prescription		Risk Difference per 100	
	TCAs (%)	SSRIs (%)	TCAs (%)	SSRIs (%)	Actual Prescription	Physician's Prior Prescription
N	484,858	401,877	484,692	402,043		
BMI $> 25 \ kg/m^2$	57.7	50.7	55.0	54.1	7.08	0.92
Hospitalized	0.4	0.3	0.4	0.4	0.10	-0.02
> 13 consultations	76.8	58.6	69.2	67.7	18.42	1.50
Older than 40	71.9	50.8	63.5	61.0	21.28	2.50
> 5 prescriptions	71.1	48.9	62.0	59.9	22.45	2.13
Male	37.7	39.6	38.8	38.3	-1.83	0.46
Ever smoked	40.9	56.8	47.2	49.3	-16.11	-2.15
Depression diagnosis	43.2	62.0	50.6	53.1	-19.01	-2.56
Prior self-harm	5.8	5.8	5.9	5.7	-0.04	0.16
Prior hypnotic	16.5	12.8	14.6	15.1	3.78	-0.59
Prior antipsychotic	2.4	2.0	2.3	2.2	0.42	0.05
Charlson index > 0	42.1	33.4	38.7	37.5	8.83	1.18
% Treated before 2004	50.8	45.9	50.8	45.8	4.95	5.04
Mahalanobis distance(MD)	18.5	16.8	17.9	17.6	1.75	0.29
% Reduction in MD						-83%

paroxetine were 27.7 percentage points more likely to prescribe paroxetine to their next patient. In terms of the outcome, fewer patients prescribed TCAs had a hospital admission for self-harm or died by suicide than those prescribed SSRIs (risk difference per 100 patients prescribed [RD], -0.11; 95% confidence interval -0.14, -0.08. In contrast, the risk difference calculated using one prior prescription as the instrumental variable was attenuated by approximately 50% toward the null (RD = -0.04; 95% CI, -0.21, 0.13), although the CI was wider (less precise) and the null hypothesis of no difference between the conventional and instrumental variable analyses could not be rejected (Hausman test: p=0.45).

These findings reveal that at least to some extent, the observed difference between patients treated with TCAs and SSRIs is moderated by patient characteristics which form the basis for differential treatment decisions. The results of this study also suggest that treatment preference data can be used as a valid instrument in drug safety studies and that further application in this area is warranted. Expanding the current analysis by including preferences by hospital and physician or even looking at state and county level preferences may lead to the construction of even stronger instruments. Using random-effects models which can incorporate both fixed and random-effects at multiple levels (e.g., doctor, hospital, state) may also be useful in that we can capture both observed and unobserved determinants of treatment selection that may be independent of patient-level characteristics and even more highly related to actual treatment received.

4.5 Differential Effects

In the previous sections, we have described several approaches to minimizing bias in analysis of observational data. Propensity score matching and marginal structural models can remove bias associated with observed (i.e., measured) confounders, but not unobserved confounders. By contrast, instrumental variables can remove bias due to observed and unobserved confounders; however, a good instrument is not always available. While matching removes differences in observed confounders by comparing people who are similar, differential comparisons compare people who are inherently different in an attempt to match them on unmeasured confounders. Here we describe a general methodology termed "differential effects" by Rosenbaum (2006), which are immune to certain unobserved biases, called "generic unobserved bias" when they affect different treatments in similar ways. Studying each treatment individually might lead to biased conclusions, but when both treatments are examined simultaneously in people who took only one or the other, unobserved bias can in many cases be controlled. As such, differential comparisons focus on those subjects who received only one of the two treatments, either *a* or *b*, ignoring those subjects who received neither or both. If the unobserved confounders affect both treatments equally, then they are termed generic biases and the differential effect is unbiased. Again, study of either treatment in isolation (relative to no treatment) would exhibit bias and potentially misleading conclusions. The basic idea is to stratify the sample on the basis of observed confounders and then compare people who took one of two possible treatments within these strata in the hopes that the unmeasured confounders equally affect both treatments and are therefore also controlled. The trick is to construct a comparison in which the unobserved confounder does not differentially affect one treatment alternative over the other. Note that if both treatments are known or even suspected to affect the outcome in the same way, they might both have substantial effects yet zero differential effects. As such, it is important to choose the comparators wisely. For example, in looking at the relationship between SSRIs and suicidal behavior, we might select psychotherapy as a comparator, since they are both used in the treatment of depression, but one has a potential pharmacologic adverse effect and the other cannot. The caveat; however, is that if antidepressants are used to treat more severely ill patients than psychotherapy and depressive severity is unmeasured, then this can lead to differential bias (a bias that affects the two treatments differently), a bias for which differential effects are not immune. Here the best we can do is to conduct a sensitivity analysis to determine the magnitude of the unmeasured confounder that would be required to produce the observed data.

Rosenbaum motivates his discussion with the problem of studying injuries resulting from car accidents. He points out that a problem in studying accidents is that car crashes vary in severity and that adequate data on speed, road traction, traffic patterns are rarely available. Seat belts may reduce injury, but individuals who use seat belts may be more cautious drivers which may in turn reduce the force of the crash and resulting injury. To study this problem and fix ideas, Rosenbaum considers an example originally described by Evans (1986), in which the fatality of two people traveling in the front seat of a car during a crash that produced at least one fatality is considered. Table 4.6 presents results of crashes where only one person died and only one person was wearing a seat belt, stratified into nine categories by age.

In Table 4.6 there were a total of 189+111=300 crashes in which the driver was unbelted, with odds of 189/111 of 1.7:1 that the unbelted driver died, whereas in the 153+363=516 crashes in which the driver was belted and the passenger was unbelted, the odds were 363/153 or 2.4:1 that the unbelted passenger died. In all of these cases, the unmeasured characteristics were the same for the driver and passenger because they were in the same car. This is called a double pairs design. Risk may be different in the passenger and driver seats, but both are studied and can be adjusted for. Unbelted drivers with belted passengers may be different than belted drivers with unbelted passengers, so there may be differential biases in addition to the generic biases that are removed in this design.

TABLE 4.6: Car Accident Mortality Data from Evans (1986)

	Age Stratum s Driver, Passenger	Driver Not belted Passenger Belted	Belted Not belted
Driver died, passenger survived	$s=1$	75	36
Driver survived, passenger died	16 to 24, 16 to 24	22	92
Driver died, passenger survived	$s=2$	6	6
Driver survived, passenger died	(16 to 24, 25 to 34)	4	20
Driver died, passenger survived	$s=3$	2	4
Driver survived, passenger died	(16 to 24, $\geq$35)	2	17
Driver died, passenger survived	$s=4$	12	8
Driver survived, passenger died	(25 to 34, 16 to 24)	6	15
Driver died, passenger survived	$s=5$	22	24
Driver survived, passenger died	(25 to 34, 25 to 34)	17	30
Driver died, passenger survived	$s=6$	3	6
Driver survived, passenger died	(25 to 34, $\geq$35)	6	21
Driver died, passenger survived	$s=7$	4	8
Driver survived, passenger died	($\geq$35, 16 to 24)	0	8
Driver died, passenger survived	$s=8$	5	9
Driver survived, passenger died	($\geq$35, 25 to 34)	2	16
Driver died, passenger survived	$s=9$	60	52
Driver survived, passenger died	($\geq$35, $\geq$35)	52	144
Driver died, passenger survived	All strata	189	153
Driver survived, passenger died	combined	111	363

Rosenbaum (2006) formalizes the distinctions between no bias, generic bias, and differential bias in the following way. Assume a finite population of N units divided into S strata $s = 1, \ldots, S$ that are defined by one or more pre-treatment covariates x. The strata are assumed to be homogeneous in the observed covariates such that $x_{si} = x_{sj}$ for all s. There are two factors, each at treatment or control levels, where $Z_{sik} = 1$ if the ith unit in stratum s receives treatment k, for $k = 1, 2$ and $Z_{sik} = 0$ otherwise. For example in our example, $Z_{si1} = 1$ and $Z_{si2} = 0$ indicates that the driver was belted and the passenger was unbelted. Let $\pi_{absi} = pr(Z_{si1} = a, Z_{si2} = b)$. In a completely randomized experiment $\pi_{11si} = \pi_{10si} = \pi_{01si} = \pi_{11si}$, for all s and i. The π_{absi} describe a units chance of exposure to treatment in the population. For each unit i in stratum s, there are four potential responses $(r_{11si}, r_{10si}, r_{01si}, r_{00si})$ only one of which is observed r_{absi}. For example, r_{absi} is a pair of binary variables indicating whether the driver and passenger would survive under seat belt pattern a, b. The effect of the ith unit in stratum s of treatment combination a, b as opposed to treatment combination $a'b'$ is a comparison of potential response r_{absi} to potential response $r_{a'b'si}$. For example, in crash (s, i), $r_{11si} = (1, 1)$ and $r_{10si} = (1, 0)$ then both the driver and the passenger would have lived if both had worn a seat belt, whereas only the driver would have survived if only the driver had worn a seat belt.

The differential effect is the comparison of r_{10si} with r_{01si}. Note that there may be no differential effect, but a substantial overall effect where, for example, a single unbelted person might be lethal to both occupants such that $r_{00si} = r_{10si} = r_{01si} = (0, 0)$, but if both wore a seat belt both would have survived $r_{11si} = (1, 1)$. Each unit receives only one treatment combination

$Z_{si1} = a$ and $Z_{si2} = b$ and we observed the response r_{absi}. Letting R_{si} be the one observed response of the ith unit in stratum s, then

$$
\begin{aligned}
R_{si} &= Z_{si1}Z_{si2}r_{11si} + Z_{si1}(1 - Z_{si2})r_{10si} \\
&\quad + (1 - Z_{si1})Z_{si2}r_{01si} + (1 - Z_{si1})(1 - Z_{si2})r_{00si}. \qquad (4.7)
\end{aligned}
$$

In Rosenbaum's framework, treatment assignment is said to be free of unobserved bias (i.e., it is ignorable) if π_{absi} does not depend on i. This is of course true under randomization, but may not be for an observational study. In an observational study that is free of unobserved bias, the π_{absi} may vary across strata based on observed covariates, but not for characteristics that were not measured. In this case, it is reasonable to combine the results across the strata, adjusting for the strata as is done for example using the Mantel-Haenszel method. In essence, this is identical to a stratified randomized experiment, where subjects within strata are randomized to the four treatment patterns. Of course, in our example, the propensity to wear seat belts depends on other factors beyond age, such as safe-driving practices, and, therefore, the condition is not satisfied in an observational study.

Unobserved generic bias occurs when there is a relevant unobserved covariate u_{si}, which we would have liked to have controlled for through stratification, but were unable to do so because it was not measured. u_{si} might reflect the safe driving practices of the driver of the car. Let $\rho_{si} = \pi_{10si}/\pi_{01si}$ which is the odds of treatment pattern $(Z_{si1} = 1, Z_{si2} = 0)$ relative to pattern $(Z_{si1} = 0, Z_{si2} = 1)$. In our example, ρ_{si} is the odds of a belted driver and unbelted passenger relative to an unbelted driver and belted passenger. Rosenbaum (2006) defines the case of generic unobserved bias if ρ_{si} varies with s, but not with i

$$
\rho_{si} = \frac{\pi_{10si}}{\pi_{01si}} = \lambda_s \qquad (4.8)
$$

for all s and i. The key here is to identify those cases in which there may be bias from unobserved u_{si} but it is only generic unobserved bias, because it only depends on s. When the condition above is not true, Rosenbaum calls this "differential unobserved bias." Here, two units i and i' within the same stratum s may have different values of ρ_{si} and $\rho_{si'}$.

Rosenbaum (2006) provides some general methods to test the assumption of a generic bias and perform sensitivity analyses to determine the magnitude of an unobserved confounder that would be required to produce the observed difference. The general idea may in fact be quite useful in pharmacoepidemiologic studies. For example, the rate of suicide attempts can be contrasted for patients who received either an SSRIs or a TCAs, but not both. In parallel, the rate of suicide attempts can be contrasted for patients who received SSRIs+psychotherapy or TCAs+psychotherapy but not both, and similarly for other concomitant treatments. If SSRIs are stimulating suicide attempts, we expect to see an excess of suicide attempts in many if not most comparisons of SSRIs with other treatments for depression. In contrast, if there is an excess of suicide attempts among people treated with SSRIs vs. no treatment, but not an excess compared to other treatments for depression, then this pattern is compatible with confounding by indication. While use of multiple treatments is a reasonable measure of depressive severity and/or treatment resistance, there may be additional unobserved biases that remain between the two treatments (e.g., SSRI vs. TCA). These would arise if the clinical indications for an SSRI differed from those for a TCA, and no doubt that is true to some extent. For example, suicidal patients are often treated with SSRIs rather than TCAs because overdose of SSRIs is non-fatal. We can explore the effects of additional hidden bias through sensitivity analysis (Rosenbaum 2006). Suppose we find when comparing TCA versus SSRI, suicide rates seem similar. A sensitivity analysis asks how large the differential biases have to be to alter this conclusion. Similarly if suicide is more common with SSRIs, we can determine how large the differential bias would have to be if, in fact, there is no difference. Thus we can determine the robustness of our findings to remaining unobserved differential bias. As previously noted, comparison between SSRIs and psychotherapy are of particular interest because it controls for pharmacologic effects. If suicide and/or suicide attempt rates are similar, it rules out the possibility of a pharmacologic adverse effect.

Additional covariates can be added to this approach using the method of differential propensity scores (Rosenbaum 2006). The differential propensity score is the usual propensity score (Rosenbaum 2002) confined to the individuals who took one of the treatments but not both. In this case, the differential propensity score equals the propensity score that would have been calculated if the unobserved covariate had been measured. Available covariates include, age, sex, race, marital status, diagnosis, comorbidity, previous attempts, previous history of depression, antidepressant treatment history. Thus we can (1) remove bias due to measured characteristics, (2) remove generic bias due to common effects of depressed people seeking treatment, and (3) assess magnitude of differential bias (e.g., due to differences in people who seek antidepressant treatment versus those who seek psychotherapy) necessary to change conclusions.

Returning to the example on car accidents, Rosenbaum (2006) notes the increased relative risk of 1.4 of an unbelted passenger death relative to an unbelted driver, when only one was unbelted and the accident resulted in a single death. Under the assumption of generic unobserved bias, the null hypothesis is the distribution of $S = 9$ independent hypergeometric distributions, which he tests using the Mantel Haenszel test (Mantel and Haenszel 1959). Under the null hypothesis and if there were only generic unobserved biases, we would expect 128.7 unbelted driver fatalities rather than the 189 that were observed (p<0.0001). Rosenbaum concludes that "Wearing seat belts may be associated with unmeasured safe-driving practices, but if these biases are generic, affecting passenger and driver the same way, then there is no doubt that seat belts save lives." He then conducts a sensitivity analysis to determine the magnitude of the unobserved differential bias that would be required to change this conclusion. Specifically, we need to determine if there was a covariate u_{si} that was not measured, how large of an imbalance would be required between a belted driver and unbelted passenger $(\bar{Z}_{sj1}, \bar{Z}_{sj2} = (1,0))$ versus an unbelted driver and belted passenger $(\bar{Z}_{sj1}, \bar{Z}_{sj2} = (0,1))$ in order to produce the overall observed difference which leads to the conclusion of a protective effect of seat-belts. The answer can be found by convolution of S extended hypergeometric distributions as described by Rosenbaum (1995). Let Λ be the multiplier of the increased likelihood of $(\bar{Z}_{sj1}, \bar{Z}_{sj2} = (1,0))$ versus $(\bar{Z}_{sj1}, \bar{Z}_{sj2} = (0,1))$. If $\Lambda = 1$ then there is no differential bias. For $\Lambda = 2$, p=0.0000071; $\Lambda = 3$, p=0.043; and $\Lambda = 4$, p=0.55. As such, it would require a differential bias of $\Lambda = 4$ or an unmeasured confounder which made a belted driver and unbelted passenger 4 times more likely than an unbelted driver and belted passenger to have produced the appearance of a protective effect of wearing seat-belts.

We can extract some additional information from this example, using the methods to be described in Chapter 6 on full-likelihood random-effects meta-analysis. In meta-analysis, the strata represent studies; however, we can use those same methods to examine differential effects, where the strata represent common observed covariate values. The advantage is that we cannot only estimate the overall protective effect of seat-belts and the differential effect between passengers and drivers as fixed-effects, but we can also estimate the corresponding random-effects which describe variability across the strata in the overall likelihood of death and variability in the differential effect across the covariate strata which represents a measure of the magnitude of the effect of unmeasured covariates which contribute to both the overall and the differential effects (see section 6.3). To do this, we rearrange the data in terms of the number of fatalities when the driver was belted and the number of fatalities when the passenger was belted, and the corresponding total sample sizes (see Table 4.7). Given the design, N minus the number of belted driver fatalities is the number of driver fatalities when the driver was unbelted. So for example in age stratum 1, there were 22 driver fatalities when the driver was belted and 97-22=75 driver fatalities when the driver was unbelted (see Table 4.6).

Applying these methods to the current problem reveals that based on Bayesian Information Criterion (BIC, Schwarz (1978)), the best fitting model was a random intercept model. This finding suggests that the strata differ in the overall incidence of fatalities, but the difference between passenger and driver fatality was not significant. Overall, there is a 51% reduction in fatalities when a seat-belt was worn (OR=0.49, 95% CI 0.40, 0.60, p<0.0001). The estimated fatality rate among passengers was reduced by 39% (OR=0.61, 95% CI=0.45, 0.81) when belted and among drivers by 57% (OR=0.43, 95% CI=0.24, 0.78). The difference between fatality rates between belted drivers and passengers was 29% (OR=0.71, 95% CI=0.52, 0.95, p=.03). There does appear to be a differential effect in terms of the rate of fatalities between belted drivers and passengers. However, the variability in this difference across the strata due to unmeasured variables was not significant. The estimated random

TABLE 4.7: Reformatted Car Accident Mortality Data

Age Stratum s	Passenger Belted		Driver Belted	
	# Died	N	# Died	N
16 to 24, 16 to 24	22	97	36	128
16 to 24, 25 to 34	4	10	6	26
16 to 24, ≥35	2	4	4	21
25 to 34, 16 to 24	6	18	8	23
25 to 34, 25 to 34	17	39	24	54
25 to 34, ≥35	6	9	6	27
≥35, 16 to 24	0	4	8	16
≥35, 25 to 34	2	7	9	25
≥35, ≥35	52	112	52	196

intercept variance was 0.032, so even at two standard deviation units above the mean effect for wearing a seat-belt, there is still a reduction in fatality of $100(1 - e^{-.72 - 2\sqrt{0.032}}) = 30\%$. A forest plot of the odds ratios of deaths for belted drivers to passengers is displayed in Figure 4.4. The overall odds ratio for the difference between drivers and passengers in Figure 4.4 is based on the Dersimonian and Laird estimator which is close to but not identical to the full-likelihood estimate.

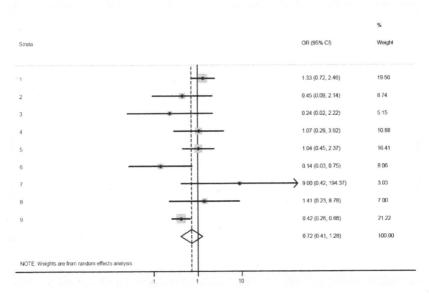

FIGURE 4.4: Forest plot: Odds ratio of death (belted driver/passenger).

5

Analysis of Spontaneous Reports

"The person who takes medicine must recover twice, once from the disease and once from the medicine."
(William Osler, M.D.)

5.1 Introduction

An important source of signals in drug safety has been, and will continue to be, the observations of clinicians who report adverse drug reactions (ADRs). Automated methods are routinely used to mine databases of spontaneous reports to detect drug safety signals. Data mining is the discovery of interesting, unexpected, or valuable structures in large datasets. Modern data mining combines statistics with ideas, tools, and methods from computer science, machine learning, database technology, and other classical data analytical technologies (Hand 1998). In the context of signal detection in the pharmaceutical sector the interest is to detect local structures or patterns and to determine if they are real or chance occurrences. Patterns are usually embedded in a mass of irrelevant data. Interesting patterns can arise due to artifacts of the data recording process or genuine discoveries about underlying mechanism. Therefore, deciding whether a pattern is 'interesting' should be done using knowledge from experts to understand exactly what is being described. Increasing number of large databases maintained by various regulatory agencies and pharmaceutical companies around the world provide opportunity for some novel exploration in post marketing drug safety.

The World Health Organization (WHO) database is the largest international database of case reports of spontaneous reporting of suspected ADRs. To improve the detection of previously unknown serious ADRs and knowledge about regulatory action taken in response to ADR reports, FDA introduced the MedWatch program in June 1993. Each of the databases, held by Uppsala Monitoring Center (UMC) and FDA AERS database, now contains over two million reports of ADRs. Similar databases exist in various European and other countries including India, China, Taiwan, and Iran. These spontaneous reporting system (SRS) databases are overwhelming and complex for safety reviewers using only traditional statistical methods. The data-mining algorithms (DMAs) have been developed to screen large SRS databases for statistical dependencies between drugs and AEs. Each of the signal detection methods has its distinguishing features and no single method is suitable for all circumstances.

Several statistical methods are available for post marketing safety surveillance. Hauben and Zhou (2003) grouped them into two categories: denominator-dependent methods and numerator-based methods. Spontaneous reporting centers and drug safety research units routinely use various numerator based methods such as empirical Bayes screening (EBS) (a variant of which is used by the FDA), Bayesian Confidence Propagation Neural Network (BCPNN used by the WHO), reporting odds ratios (RORs), incidence rate ratio (IRR), and proportional reporting ratio (PRR). Denominator based methods include cumulative sum techniques, time scan method and Poisson methods.

5.2   Proportional Reporting Ratio

The Proportional Reporting Ratio (PRR) is the simplest method available for signal detection. Its computational form is similar to the well-known relative risk calculation for 2×2 tables in epidemiology. However, studies have shown that it can be as powerful as other sophisticated methods available when applied to events that are not rare. Let us assume that there are a total of N reports in the database of which n reports involve a particular drug (or drug group) of interest, E reports involve interesting events, and x reports involve both the drugs and events of interest. These counts are summarized in the following 2×2 contingency table.

TABLE 5.1: Contingency Table of a Drug-Adverse Event Pair.

	Does the event involve a drug(s) of interest?		
	yes	no	total
Events	x	$E - x$	E
Non-events	$n - x$	$N-n-E+x$	$N - E$
Total	n	$N - n$	N

The PRR of events E is defined as follow (Evans et al. 2001, Bate and Evans 2009).

$$PRR = \frac{\frac{x}{n}}{\frac{E-x}{N-n}} \tag{5.1}$$

The standard error of the $ln(PRR)$ is

$$SE[ln(PRR)] = \sqrt{\frac{1}{x} + \frac{1}{n-x} - \frac{1}{E} - \frac{1}{N-E}}. \qquad (5.2)$$

The 95% confidence interval for $ln(PRR)$ is then estimated as $ln(PRR) \pm 1.96 \times SE[ln(PRR)]$ and, taking the exponential, the following result is obtained for the 95% confidence interval for PRR.

$$\text{95\% CI for PRR} = \left(\frac{PRR}{e^{(1.96 \times SE[ln(PRR)])}}, PRR \times e^{(1.96 \times SE[ln(PRR)])} \right) \qquad (5.3)$$

A lower 95% CI of a PRR higher than 1.0 indicate a disproportionate reporting of events involving a particular drug. One of the limitations of PRR is that the large number of reports of particular kind effectively inflate the denominator for that drug reducing the magnitude of PRR for other signals with that drug. The PRR method generates a large volume of potential signals when applied to large databases. To counter this problem remedial measures such as triage criteria can be applied to reduce the volume of signals that are evaluated.

Example

Roxicodone is indicated for the management of moderate to severe pain where the use of an opioid analgesic is appropriate. As with other opioids in clinical use, serious adverse reactions such as cardiac arrest may be associated with roxicodone therapy. In the first quarter of 2010, the FDA received 213488 reports of serious drug-ADRs combinations. Among those 6360 reported cardiac arrest, 100 involved roxicodone and 31 reported both roxicodone and cardiac arrest. The relevant frequency counts are presented in Table 5.2. The calculation of the PRR is as follows.

TABLE 5.2: Example of PRR Calculation - Roxicodone and Cardiac Arrest

	Does the event involve Roxicodone?		
	yes	no	total
Cardiac arrest	31	2988	3019
All other events	69	210398	210469
Total	100	213388	213488

$$PRR = \frac{31}{100} \bigg/ \frac{2988}{213388} = 22.13$$

and

Lower 95% CI limit of ln[PRR] = 2.80.

There is no gold standard on the thresholds that should be adopted for signal detection. The lower limit of 95% CI of $ln[PRR] > 0$ is one reasonable choice of threshold. Using this threshold, the lower limit of 95% CI for the logarithm is positive, the signal is generated on the basis of PRR. This does not imply any kind of causal relationship between roxicodone and the occurrence of the adverse event of cardiac arrest. Further analysis by pharmacovigilance experts must now determine the validity of this signal. The initial decision on whether a drug-event pair should be further investigated depends on thresholds applied to the estimates of the PRR and other statistics.

5.2.1   Discussion

PRR is a statistical aid to signal generation from spontaneous reporting system databases. PRR indicates differential reporting of possible reactions for a given drug compared to all other drugs in the database. It is crucial to remember that a signal identified based on the PRR is indicative of the disproportionate reporting of events and not their occurrence (Moore et al. 2003, 2005). The validity of the PRR rests on equal reporting rates for the different drugs. However, all adverse drug reactions are not reported in spontaneous report databases and the reporting rate for a particular drug is highly dependent on the public perception of the safety of the drug (notoriety bias) and the time since its approval (Weber effect) (Weber 1984). Consequently, PRR may vary significantly over different time frame of evaluations. Furthermore, PRR can be highly unreliable due to extreme sampling variability when observed frequencies of drug-ADR combination are small, resulting in high false-positive rates. Remedial measures such as considering only drug-ADR combinations with 3 or more cases and raising the PRR threshold to 2 have been suggested to reduce the false-positive signals (Evans et al. 2001). Alternative Bayesian methods (covered in the next sections) have shown to be less sensitive to the sampling variation.

5.3   Bayesian Confidence Propagation Neural Network (BCPNN)

Bayesian Confidence Propagation Neural Network (Bate et al. 1998) can handle large data sets, is robust in handling missing data, and may be used with complex variables. It allows finding and quantifying relationships between drugs and AEs that differ significantly from the background of interrelationships in the database. For an individual report in the database, a prior probability that a specific ADR is listed in it is denoted by $P(A)$, a prior probability that a specific drug is listed is denoted by $P(D)$ and a prior probability that the drug - AE pair are present together in it is denoted by $P(A,D)$. The strength of the association between an AE and a drug is measured by the information component (IC) defined as (Bate et al. 1998):

$$IC = log_2 \frac{P(A, D)}{P(A)P(D)}. \tag{5.4}$$

As new quarterly data become available, the corresponding posterior probabilities are calculated and the updated IC is used to generate new signals. A convenient choice of the form of prior is the beta distribution for all three densities. In the absence of prior information an *a priori* assumption is made of equal probability distributions for $P(A)$ and $P(D)$. Let α_1 and α_0 be the parameters governing the beta distributions of $P(A)$ and $P(D)$; γ_{11} and γ be the parameters of the beta distribution of $p(A,D)$; c_i, c_j, and c_{ij} be the report counts of *ith* AE, *jth* drug and combination of *ith* drug with the *jth* AE respectively; and C be the total number of reports in the database. The corresponding expected value of each distribution is the estimator of $P(A)$, $P(D)$, and $P(A,D)$. The normal approximation of variance of IC [$V(IC)$] is (Bate et al. 1998, Orre et al. 2000):

$$V(IC) \approx \left(\frac{1}{log2}\right)^2 \left[\frac{C - c_{ij} + \gamma - \gamma_{11}}{(c_{ij} + \gamma_{11})(1 + C + \gamma)} + \frac{C - c_i + \alpha - \alpha_1}{(c_i + \alpha_1)(1 + C + \alpha)} + \frac{C - c_j + \alpha - \alpha_1}{(c_j + \alpha_1)(1 + C + \alpha)}\right], \tag{5.5}$$

where $\alpha = \alpha_1 + \alpha_0$. As more data become available, the estimate of IC becomes more accurate and the confidence interval of IC becomes narrower. An IC with lower 95% CI> 0 that increases with sequential time scans may be used as a criterion for signal detection.

Example

Rosiglitazone is used to treat type 2 diabetes by making patients more sensitive to their own insulin. Since its approval by regulators in the United States and Europe, the use of rosiglitazone has been suspected of increasing the risk of heart attack. Recently, its use has been restricted only to people who are already taking rosiglitazone and people whose blood sugar cannot be controlled by other medications. The FDA AERS database contains thousands of reports of rosiglitazone along with variety of adverse events. Table 5.3 gives the result of the FDA AERS database search for each quarter from 1999 to 2010.

Rosiglitazone was approved by regulators in the United States and Europe in May, 1999. Figure 5.1 shows the time scan obtained when a run was done of rosiglitazone (regardless of its specific role) and cardiac arrest from the third

TABLE 5.3: Reports of Cardiac Arrest for Rosiglitazone in the FDA AERS.

year	qtr	cij	drug	ae	C	P(A)	P(B)	P(A,B)	IC
1999	3	1	14	184	9594	0.00156	0.01928	0.00021	2.789494
1999	4	5	44	195	8216	0.00266	0.02058	0.00029	2.41267
2000	1	15	93	264	9295	0.00411	0.02214	0.00053	2.547596
2000	2	19	115	312	9301	0.00539	0.02378	0.00076	2.565951
2000	3	19	95	323	10037	0.0062	0.02504	0.00093	2.586363
2000	4	19	116	266	9480	0.00687	0.02579	0.00107	2.588706
2001	1	20	149	243	10285	0.00753	0.02609	0.00117	2.575868
2001	2	20	137	244	10016	0.00809	0.02622	0.00126	2.566549
2001	3	24	182	233	10489	0.00867	0.0262	0.00134	2.555625
2001	4	48	218	275	10979	0.00928	0.02616	0.00145	2.578735
2002	1	21	123	325	10567	0.00973	0.02621	0.00154	2.590996
2002	2	36	148	323	13961	0.01005	0.02619	0.00161	2.616864
2002	3	14	124	277	14290	0.01026	0.02606	0.00166	2.634309
2002	4	14	126	295	14405	0.01039	0.02589	0.00168	2.645696
2003	1	15	106	228	13343	0.01046	0.02567	0.0017	2.658048
2003	2	48	292	324	14454	0.01061	0.02547	0.00172	2.669748
2003	3	34	190	383	18769	0.01073	0.02526	0.00174	2.683832
2003	4	11	131	357	18337	0.01078	0.02504	0.00174	2.693402
2004	1	22	147	400	15049	0.01081	0.02487	0.00175	2.699553
2004	2	22	136	367	15421	0.01082	0.02474	0.00174	2.704895
2004	3	39	160	370	18484	0.01081	0.0246	0.00175	2.715509
2004	4	20	146	495	19729	0.01078	0.02448	0.00174	2.722839
2005	1	22	155	429	18188	0.01074	0.02439	0.00174	2.728313
2005	2	15	166	438	18659	0.0107	0.0243	0.00173	2.730239
2005	3	41	185	624	21938	0.01066	0.02426	0.00172	2.732863
2005	4	17	206	565	20912	0.01061	0.02424	0.00171	2.730921
2006	1	35	219	812	21412	0.01058	0.02428	0.0017	2.725387
2006	2	39	221	1065	21327	0.01054	0.02443	0.00169	2.71478
2006	3	12	127	249	12133	0.01052	0.02455	0.00168	2.705021
2006	4	12	111	293	12918	0.01049	0.02464	0.00167	2.69609
2007	1	12	105	255	14761	0.01046	0.02471	0.00167	2.688767
2007	2	18	192	242	12489	0.01044	0.02475	0.00166	2.681364
2007	3	26	204	327	15051	0.01043	0.02479	0.00165	2.674496
2007	4	17	127	295	13266	0.01042	0.02481	0.00164	2.668373
2008	1	5	62	239	16506	0.0104	0.02481	0.00163	2.663666
2008	2	8	81	340	15931	0.01037	0.02481	0.00162	2.659368
2008	3	141	406	461	17770	0.01037	0.02481	0.00163	2.66286
2008	4	102	264	403	16430	0.01037	0.0248	0.00164	2.671438
2009	1	241	665	514	18487	0.01043	0.02481	0.00167	2.69008
2009	2	197	719	581	18246	0.01052	0.02482	0.00171	2.711943
2009	3	352	1210	811	19815	0.01069	0.02486	0.00178	2.740084
2009	4	322	1144	795	21649	0.01092	0.02492	0.00186	2.771054
2010	1	240	815	780	23376	0.01117	0.02498	0.00195	2.801932
2010	2	540	1736	1073	21988	0.01151	0.02508	0.00206	2.837633
2010	3	1462	4370	2174	30847	0.0121	0.02527	0.00227	2.89117

quarter of 1999 to the third quarter of 2010. The lower 95% confidence limit is higher than 0 from the beginning of the scan indicating a possible signal soon after the marketing of the drug. The signal continued to strengthen until 2005 as more data became available and the estimate of IC became more precise. There is a slight decline in IC from the end of 2005 to 2007. Interestingly, in September 2005, GSK concluded its own meta-analysis of data concerning rosiglitazone's effect on diabetics and informed the FDA that the data "may" signal an increased (32%) risk for heart attacks in diabetics. One possible explanation of the decline in IC in that time period could be the cautious use of the drug by the community of endocrinologists due to a mounting evidence regarding the increased cardiovascular risks associated with rosiglitazone. The signal gains strength once again from 2008. A meta-analysis in May 2007 reported that the use of rosiglitazone was associated with

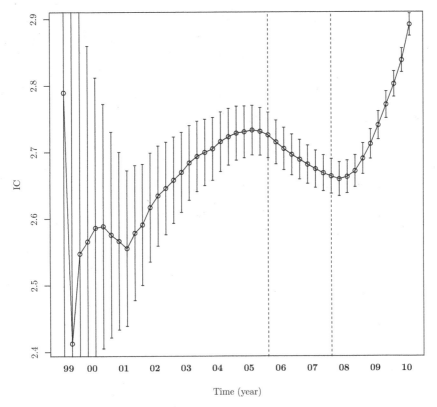

FIGURE 5.1: IC and 95% CI for Rosiglitazone and cardiac arrest.

a significantly increased risk of heart attack. In 2007, four independent, peer-reviewed medical research studies were published showing that rosiglitazone increased diabetics' pre-existing cardiovascular risks. These data, coupled with the FDA's own study led to a black box warning (FDA's most serious drug safety warning) on rosiglitazone's product label to inform consumers of such risks beginning on November 14, 2007. Consequently, the sales of avandia declined and the reporting of cardiac events has increased in FDA's AERS further strengthening of signal from 2008.

Example

Digoxin is commonly indicated for atrial fibrillation and atrial flutter with rapid ventricular response. Due to the narrow margin between effectiveness and toxicity, it is suspected of several severe adverse effects including severe allergic reaction. The retrospective time scan of Digoxin and rash is shown in Figure 5.2 and the details of IC computation is given in Table 5.4 for each quarter from 1998 to 2010.

TABLE 5.4: Reports of Rash for Digoxin in the FDA AERS.

year	qtr	cij	drug	ae	C	IC	P(A)	P(B)	P(A,B)
1998	1	7	270	223	8703	0.1976	0.03113	0.02573	0.00092
1998	2	6	242	214	7729	0.0283	0.03115	0.02630	0.00084
1998	3	4	197	180	7628	-0.0286	0.03033	0.02598	0.00077
1998	4	4	201	212	8433	-0.0705	0.02940	0.02579	0.00072
1999	1	7	288	248	9666	-0.0893	0.02907	0.02571	0.00070
1999	2	7	316	278	9495	-0.1165	0.02914	0.02586	0.00070
1999	3	7	281	245	9594	-0.1275	0.02918	0.02593	0.00069
1999	4	5	269	209	8216	-0.1425	0.02930	0.02596	0.00069
2000	1	3	237	230	9295	-0.1643	0.02929	0.02594	0.00068
2000	2	1	246	227	9301	-0.1984	0.02922	0.02590	0.00066
2000	3	3	239	190	10037	-0.2248	0.02908	0.02575	0.00064
2000	4	5	250	172	9480	-0.2396	0.02894	0.02554	0.00063
2001	1	2	234	146	10285	-0.2513	0.02876	0.02525	0.00061
2001	2	2	258	168	10016	-0.2643	0.02860	0.02494	0.00059
2001	3	5	245	154	10489	-0.2688	0.02843	0.02460	0.00058
2001	4	3	234	245	10979	-0.2751	0.02823	0.02433	0.00057
2002	1	6	241	343	10567	-0.2819	0.02804	0.02418	0.00056
2002	2	6	285	387	13961	-0.2889	0.02782	0.02409	0.00055
2002	3	3	293	340	14290	-0.2988	0.02758	0.02402	0.00054
2002	4	6	258	362	14405	-0.3061	0.02732	0.02397	0.00053
2003	1	8	252	346	13343	-0.3089	0.02706	0.02395	0.00052
2003	2	3	355	449	14454	-0.3184	0.02683	0.02397	0.00052
2003	3	6	312	490	18769	-0.3273	0.02657	0.02400	0.00051
2003	4	12	311	442	18337	-0.3287	0.02630	0.02403	0.00050
2004	1	10	276	549	15049	-0.3292	0.02604	0.02411	0.00050
2004	2	5	246	457	15421	-0.3307	0.02577	0.02420	0.00050
2004	3	5	272	531	18484	-0.3334	0.02549	0.02430	0.00049
2004	4	5	292	559	19729	-0.3371	0.02521	0.02441	0.00049
2005	1	9	272	674	18188	-0.3408	0.02493	0.02454	0.00048
2005	2	14	322	656	18659	-0.3414	0.02466	0.02470	0.00048
2005	3	5	246	665	21938	-0.3429	0.02438	0.02486	0.00048
2005	4	6	296	639	20912	-0.3452	0.02409	0.02502	0.00047
2006	1	5	309	802	21412	-0.3500	0.02382	0.02520	0.00047
2006	2	5	239	695	21327	-0.3553	0.02354	0.02538	0.00047
2006	3	9	163	412	12133	-0.3580	0.02328	0.02555	0.00046
2006	4	6	170	365	12918	-0.3594	0.02303	0.02570	0.00046
2007	1	2	159	423	14761	-0.3613	0.02279	0.02584	0.00046
2007	2	6	147	402	12489	-0.3622	0.02257	0.02597	0.00046
2007	3	1	153	370	15051	-0.3634	0.02235	0.02609	0.00045
2007	4	3	118	317	13266	-0.3641	0.02213	0.02618	0.00045
2008	1	5	128	387	16506	-0.3636	0.02192	0.02627	0.00045
2008	2	4	1203	463	15931	-0.3695	0.02181	0.02635	0.00044
2008	3	6	855	472	17770	-0.3782	0.02175	0.02642	0.00044
2008	4	6	271	391	16430	-0.3856	0.02169	0.02648	0.00044
2009	1	5	223	419	18487	-0.3919	0.02162	0.02653	0.00044
2009	2	8	479	434	18246	-0.3979	0.02156	0.02657	0.00043
2009	3	6	539	388	19815	-0.4039	0.02152	0.02660	0.00043
2009	4	6	352	471	21649	-0.4093	0.02147	0.02661	0.00043
2010	1	4	394	468	23376	-0.4145	0.02142	0.02662	0.00043
2010	2	6	423	458	21988	-0.4194	0.02138	0.02662	0.00043
2010	3	9	399	587	30847	-0.4229	0.02132	0.02660	0.00042

The time scan starts with positive IC with lower 95% confidence well below 0. The IC decreases throughout the time scan towards a distinct negative value. As the number of reports of the drug and AE increase, the associated 95% confidence intervals diminish. The figure demonstrates the diminishing possibility of a causal relationship between Digoxin and rash. This definite

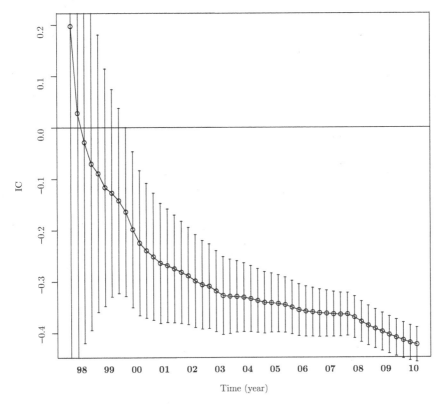

FIGURE 5.2: IC and 95% confidence for digoxin and rash over a period of time.

negative IC represents a situation where joint reporting of Digoxin and rash are not frequent relative to the expected frequency under independence. Therefore association between Digoxin and rash would not be signaled based on IC criteria.

5.4 Empirical Bayes Screening

Empirical Bayes screening was originally developed by William DuMouchel (DuMouchel 1999) and applied to FDA databases of spontaneous reports as a tool to detect signals of AEs that were gender specific. This method computes the baseline (expected) frequency under row and column independence assumption for multiple two-way tables. As Hauben and Zhou (2003) noted, under such assumption the proportional representation of an AE for a particular drug, and the proportional representation of that AE in the entire database should be the same. Therefore, the higher is the magnitude of discrepancy between the two, stronger is the signal for the drug-event combination.

Following DuMouchel (1999), let each observed count N_{ij} of drug-event combinations in the database be a draw from a Poisson distribution with varying unknown means μ_{ij}. However, as a measure of disproportionality, the interest is not on μ directly but on the ratio $\lambda_{ij} = \frac{\mu_{(ij)}}{E_{ij}}$. Furthermore, instead of estimating each individual λ_{ij}, they are assumed to follow a common prior distribution. DuMouchel (1999) suggested the following mixture of two gamma distributions as a candidate for such prior distribution.

$$\pi(\lambda; \alpha_1, \beta_1, \alpha_2, \beta_2, P) = P\, g(\lambda; \alpha_1, \beta_1) + (1 - P)g(\lambda; \alpha_2, \beta_2), \quad (5.6)$$

where

$$g(\lambda; \alpha, \beta) = \beta^\alpha \lambda^{\alpha-1} e^{-\beta\lambda}/\Gamma(\alpha).$$

The gamma distribution is an easy choice because it is the conjugate distribution of the Poisson. Thus the posterior distribution of each λ is again the gamma distribution of (5.6) but with updated parameters as follows:

$$\lambda|N = n \sim \pi(\lambda; \alpha_1 + n, \beta_1 + E, \alpha_2 + n, \beta_2 + E, Q_n) \quad (5.7)$$

where $E = \frac{N_{i.}N_{.j}}{N}$ is the expectation of N_{ij} under row and column independence for row total $N_{i.}$ and column total $N_{.j}$. The Q_n is a posterior probability that λ came from first component of the mixture, given $N = n$. It has the following expression.

$$Q_n = \frac{P\, f(n, \alpha_1, \beta_1, E)}{Pr(N = n)} \quad (5.8)$$

In expression (5.8), $Pr(N = n)$ is the marginal distribution of each N_{ij} for the known $\boldsymbol{\theta} = (\alpha_1, \beta_1, \alpha_2, \beta_2, P)$ and E. It is a mixture of two negative-binomial distributions, $f(\alpha, \beta, E)$. The $f(\alpha, \beta, E)$ and $P(N = n)$ have the following expressions

$$f(\alpha, \beta, E) = (1 + \beta/E)^{-n}(1 + E/\beta)^{-\alpha} \times \frac{\Gamma(\alpha + n)}{\Gamma(\alpha)n!} \quad (5.9)$$

$$P(N = n) = P\, f(n; \alpha_1, \beta_1, E) + (1 - P)f(n; \alpha_2, \beta_2, E). \quad (5.10)$$

The following empirical Bayes measure (*EBlog2*) is used to rank the "interestingness" of cell counts.

$$EBlog2_{ij} = E[log_2\lambda_{ij}|N_{ij}] = \frac{E[log(\lambda_{ij})|N_{ij}]}{log(2)}, \quad (5.11)$$

where

$$E[log(\lambda_{ij})|N_{ij} = n] = Q_n[\Psi(\alpha_1 + n) - log(\beta_1 + E_{ij})]$$
$$+ (1 - Q_n)[\Psi(\alpha_2 + n) - log(\beta_2 + E_{ij})],$$

and $\Psi(x)$ is the derivative of $log[\Gamma(x)]$, also known as the digamma function. Alternatively, $EBGM_{ij} = e^{E[log(\lambda_{ij})|N_{ij}=n]}$ has been suggested which has a direct interpretation as the geometric mean of a "true" reporting rate (DuMouchel 1999). Additionally, the lower $5th$ percentile of the posterior distribution of λ ($EB05$) can be used for ranking the cell counts and $EB05 > 2$ has been recommended as a cut-off for signal detection (Szarfman et al. 2002).

The estimate of $\boldsymbol{\theta}$ is required to evaluate (5.8) and (5.11). The estimate is obtained by considering the marginal distribution of each N_{ij} which is given in (5.10). The likelihood function is the product of density functions of each N_{ij} expressed as the function of $\boldsymbol{\theta}$:

$$L(\boldsymbol{\theta}) = \prod_{ij} \{P\, f(N_{ij}, \alpha_1, \beta_1, E_{ij}) + (1 - P)f(N_{ij}; \alpha_2, \beta_2, E_{ij})\}. \quad (5.12)$$

The estimate of $\boldsymbol{\theta}$ is the maximum likelihood estimator obtained from maximization of $L(\boldsymbol{\theta})$. The maximization involves an iterative search in five-dimensional space; therefore, it must be handled carefully and the starting values of the parameters must be chosen appropriately so that the algorithm converges in a reasonable number of iterations. The authors of the method have recommended $\theta = (\alpha_1 = 0.2, \beta_1 = 0.1, \alpha_2 = 2, \beta_2 = 4, P = 1/3)$ for the starting values.

Example

The AERS database for the first quarter of year 2010 contains adverse event reports of 114681 cases received by the FDA from 01-OCT-2009 to 31-DEC-2009. Each case involves multiple drugs and adverse events, which means that a number of reported drug-ADR combinations is much larger than 114681. After applying a set of pre-defined exclusion criteria, the number of drug-AE combinations reports reduced to 213488. We chose this time period arbitrarily and performed an unstratified analysis for the purpose of illustration. For the proper analysis, one must choose all data available for the time interval of interest and perform an appropriate stratified analysis. To initiate computation, the initial values of the hyperparameters are set at $\alpha_1 = 0.2, \beta_1 = 0.06, \alpha_2 = 1.4, \beta_2 = 1.8$, and $P = 0.1$, and the resulting estimates of the hyperparameters are: $\alpha_1 = 0.009, \beta_1 = 0.011, \alpha_2 = 2.000, \beta_2 = 1.235$, and $P = 0.733$. We calculate $EBlog2$ to rank each drug-ADR in the database. The top 20 and bottom 20 drug-ADR combinations and their corresponding $EBlog2$ values are listed in Table 5.5. The table shows that the ranking based on EBlog2 and $RR = n_{11}/E$ are not exactly the same. Although RR is easily interpretable, it suffers from the extreme sampling variation when baseline and observed frequencies are small. The EBGM estimates are interpreted as the shrinkage estimator of "true" RR and are not as susceptible to sampling variability as RR.

5.5   Multi-item Gamma Poisson Shrinker

The Gamma Poisson Shrinker presented in the Section 5.4 ranks the drug-AE pair by the EBGM. However, it is not capable of finding higher order associations which is usually the case when two or more drugs in combination produce severe adverse events. The most recent example of such interaction is the case of percocet, a drug that is used for controlling breakthrough pain. Another drug, acetaminophen, in general is a very safe medication, but unfortunately, high doses of acetaminophen lead to liver damage. It is also a common ingredient in many commonly used over-the-counter drugs including cough medication. Percocet combines acetaminophen with a short acting narcotic. The FDA advisory panel has recently recommended a ban on percocet because patients who take percocet for long periods of time often need higher doses to achieve the same pain reduction effect. As a consequence, they are getting more acetaminophen, raising the possibility of serious damage to their livers, specially if they are also using one of the OTC drugs containing acetaminophen.

Multi-item Gamma Poisson shrinker (MGPS) (DuMouchel and Pregibon 2001) is a natural extension of GPS for detecting such multi-drug-AE associations. It uses the same estimation technique with some additional steps. The term item in MGPS includes both the drugs and the AEs. Let N_j be the number of reports that include only one item (e.g., drug j); let N_{jk} be the number of reports that include both item j and item k and so forth, where $1 < j < k < J$, and J is the total number of items under consideration. Using DuMouchel and Pregibon (2001) notation, we define the following quantities:

$$
\begin{aligned}
P_j &= \frac{N_j}{N}, & \text{proportion of reports involving item } j \\
P_{jk} &= \frac{N_{jk}}{N}, & \text{proportion of reports involving item } j \text{ and item } k \\
P_{1\cdots J} &= \frac{N_{1\cdots K}}{N}, & \text{proportion of reports involving items } 1, \cdots, J \\
E_j &= N P_j, & \text{baseline frequency of reports involving item } j \\
E_{jk} &= N P_j P_k, & \text{baseline of reports involving item } j \text{ and item } k \\
E_{1\cdots J} &= N P_1 \cdot P_K, & \text{baseline of reports involving items } 1, \cdots, J.
\end{aligned}
$$

The equations (5.6) to (5.12) with corresponding values of $N_{1\cdots k}$ and $E_{1\cdots k}$

TABLE 5.5: The Top 20 and Bottom 20 Drug-ADR.

drug	event	count	expected count	EBlog2	EBGM	n11/E	log2 (n11/E)	drug margin	event margin
DRN 6583	AEN 1035	27	0.0095	10.3616	1315.673	2839.496	11.471	35	58
DRN 1650	AEN 4731	14	0.0012	10.1586	1143.013	11860.444	13.534	18	14
DRN 6856	AEN 1492	22	0.0088	10.1141	1108.257	2508.940	11.293	48	39
DRN 1721	AEN 2223	13	0.0013	10.0358	1049.708	10166.095	13.311	21	13
DRN 3843	AEN 1035	15	0.0041	9.9456	986.115	3680.828	11.846	15	58
DRN 58	AEN 2499	19	0.0137	9.5705	760.320	1386.286	10.437	133	22
DRN 6449	AEN 153	9	0.0034	9.2469	607.550	2668.600	11.382	80	9
DRN 4794	AEN 4881	21	0.0239	9.2138	593.767	878.551	9.779	243	21
DRN 4800	AEN 35	11	0.0077	9.1599	572.008	1421.530	10.473	59	28
DRN 5802	AEN 3237	7	0.0010	9.1305	560.484	7116.267	12.797	15	14
DRN 6449	AEN 402	8	0.0030	9.1058	550.971	2668.600	11.382	80	8
DRN 6449	AEN 570	8	0.0030	9.1058	550.971	2668.600	11.382	80	8
DRN 6449	AEN 576	8	0.0030	9.1058	550.971	2668.600	11.382	80	8
DRN 6931	AEN 4148	19	0.0233	9.0904	545.116	814.840	9.670	262	19
DRN 3774	AEN 2409	8	0.0040	8.9989	511.613	1976.741	10.949	54	16
DRN 170	AEN 5061	10	0.0081	8.9910	508.804	1241.209	10.278	172	10
DRN 6931	AEN 797	15	0.0184	8.9645	499.559	814.840	9.670	262	15
DRN 4794	AEN 1362	17	0.0228	8.9492	494.274	746.769	9.545	243	20
DRN 6449	AEN 3207	7	0.0026	8.9402	491.210	2668.600	11.382	80	7
DRN 4762	AEN 35	7	0.0028	8.9260	486.400	2541.524	11.311	21	28
DRN 302	AEN 3518	6	4.8689	0.2920	1.224	1.232	0.301	1399	743
DRN 338	AEN 413	16	13.0414	0.2918	1.224	1.227	0.295	947	2940
DRN 5546	AEN 983	6	4.8702	0.2917	1.224	1.232	0.301	695	1496
DRN 2742	AEN 5005	9	7.3228	0.2916	1.224	1.229	0.298	416	3758
DRN 5973	AEN 2105	5	4.0525	0.2916	1.224	1.234	0.303	971	891
DRN 5268	AEN 200	6	4.8706	0.2915	1.224	1.232	0.301	438	2374
DRN 3569	AEN 3963	5	4.0527	0.2915	1.224	1.234	0.303	1391	622
DRN 3172	AEN 1056	20	16.3130	0.2915	1.224	1.226	0.294	3198	1089
DRN 6649	AEN 4465	3	2.4139	0.2914	1.224	1.243	0.314	1952	264
DRN 77	AEN 3721	4	3.2346	0.2913	1.224	1.237	0.306	1621	426
DRN 1577	AEN 5028	4	3.2349	0.2912	1.224	1.237	0.306	494	1398
DRN 5107	AEN 1963	7	5.6916	0.2909	1.223	1.230	0.299	1819	668
DRN 8029	AEN 16	5	4.0552	0.2908	1.223	1.233	0.302	1235	701
DRN 5986	AEN 3349	16	13.0512	0.2908	1.223	1.226	0.294	1468	1898
DRN 7819	AEN 4410	4	3.2366	0.2906	1.223	1.236	0.306	1512	457
DRN 77	AEN 2294	6	4.8747	0.2906	1.223	1.231	0.300	1621	642
DRN 5986	AEN 200	20	16.3243	0.2905	1.223	1.225	0.293	1468	2374
DRN 5880	AEN 465	11	8.9681	0.2901	1.223	1.227	0.295	1166	1642
DRN 6167	AEN 1008	5	4.0583	0.2900	1.223	1.232	0.301	380	2280
DRN 5880	AEN 1440	17	13.8781	0.2899	1.223	1.225	0.293	1166	2541

are used to estimate the EBGM for corresponding kth order of multi-item associations. However, interpreting the higher order association is more complicated. As the originator of the method pointed out "when an analyst finds that the frequency of a triple or quadruple is much greater than independence would predict, what exactly has been found? Suppose a triplet ABC is unusually frequent. Is that just because AB and/or AC and/or BC are unusually frequent, or is there something special about the triple that all three occur frequently in transactions [reports]. In general, it would be quite valuable to automatically pick out the multi-item associations that cannot be explained by the pairwise association in the item set."

This problem is addressed by using the log-linear models with all two factor interaction terms. The log-linear models can be used to model 2^J frequency tables, where $J > 2$. Denote the counts in the table by $m_{j_1 j_2 \cdots j_J}$, where each j take a value of 1 if that particular report contains the jth item. A model that allows for two-way association is as follows:

$$\log(\mu_{j_1 j_2 \cdots j_J}) = \alpha + \beta_1 j_1 + \beta_2 j_2 + \cdots + \beta_3 j_J + \gamma_{12} j_1 j_2$$
$$+ \gamma_{13} j_1 j_3 + \gamma_{23} j_2 j_3 + \cdots + \gamma_{J-1,J} j_J j_{J-1} j_J. \tag{5.13}$$

The all-two-factor model implies

$$E(m_{j_1 j_2 \cdots j_J}) = \mu_{j_1 j_2 \cdots j_J} = a b_1^{j_1} b_2^{j_2} \cdots b_3^{j_J} c_{12}^{j_1 j_2} c_{13}^{j_1 j_3} c_{23}^{j_2 j_3} \cdots c_{J-1,J}^{j_J - 1 j_J},$$

where multiplicative terms are the exponential of the parameters of equation (5.13). According to such a model, expected counts of the reports containing none of the item and all of the items are $E(m_{00 \cdots 0}) = a$ and $E(m_{11 \cdots 1}) = ab_1 b_2 \cdots b_3 c_{12} c_{13} c_{23} \cdots c_{J-1,J}$, respectively. In estimating the parameters of all-two-way log-linear models, it is recommended to use the expected shrinkage estimate of two way counts given by $\mu_{jk} = EBGM_{jk} \times E_{jk}$ which are more stable than the raw counts. In doing so the elements of the 2×2 table become $\mu_{jk}, n_j - \mu_{jk}, n_k - \mu_{jk}, N - n_j - n_k + \mu_{jk}$. Finally, the expected count for each item set greater than 2 from the all-two-factor model based on all two-way distributions is defined as

$$E_{all2F} = E(m_{11 \cdots 1}) = ab_1 b_2 \cdots b_3 c_{12} c_{13} c_{23} \cdots c_{J-1,J}.$$

The number of reports involving the item set which are not explained by the pairwise association of items in the item set is estimated as

$$EXCESS2 = EBGM_{1 \cdots J} \times E_{1 \cdots J} - E_{all2F}.$$

The negative value of EXCESS2 is possible but interpreting such a number is not recommended. Rather, the focus is on large values of EXCESS2 which indicate complex relationship involving more than two items. EXCESS2, however, cannot point to the source that caused the large EXCESS2. For example, if we know that the EXCESS2 measure for ABCD is large we cannot know whether it is due to ABC, ABD, or ABCD. It requires more complex analyses that involve higher order log-linear model (Wu et al. 2003).

5.6 Bayesian Lasso Logistic Regression

Confounding by co-medication and masking are two issues that severely limit the use of disproportional reporting analyses. Confounding by co-medication occurs when two or more drugs are involved. For example, drug A and B may appear together more often with the report of a particular ADR, which would elevate disproportional reporting signals for each individual drug A and B. However, in reality, only the drug B is associated with the ADR. Because, drug A is used together with drug B, the association between drug A and the ADR appears stronger than it really is. Whereas, masking occurs when a strong association between a drug and a particular ADR weaken the signal for other related combinations involving that ADR. For example, NSAID drugs and GI bleeding is known to show a strong association, which attenuates the disproportional reporting signals for other reactions involving NSAIDs. A regression based analysis provides a way to correct for these issue to a certain degree. As the outcome of interest is a dichotomous variable (ADR present or absent), logistic regression is a natural choice. An entire spontaneous report database is screened by studying each ADR reported in that database one at a time. In order to accomplish this task, imagine (following the notation in Caster (2007)) that n reports in the database are structured in the following manner:

$$\left\{ ([a_{11}, \ldots a_{1r_1}]^T, [d_{11}, \ldots d_{1s_1}]^T), \ldots, ([a_{n1}, \ldots a_{nr_n}]^T, [d_{n1}, \ldots d_{ns_n}]^T) \right\},$$

where a_{ij} and d_{ik} represent the j-th ADR and k-th drug, respectively, in the i-th report. Such that $a_{ij} \in A = \{\alpha_1, \ldots, \alpha_{|A|}\}$, the set of all ADRs; $d_{ik} \in D = \{\delta_1, \ldots, \delta_{|D|}\}$, the set of all drugs; and $|A|$ and $|D|$ denote the number of ADRs and drugs in the database, respectively. According to the ordinary logistic regression model, a model describing the probability of the j-th ADR conditional on the set of drug indicator variables $\boldsymbol{x}_i$ is

$$P(y_i = 1|\boldsymbol{x}_i) = \frac{exp(\beta_0 + \boldsymbol{\beta}^T \boldsymbol{x}_i)}{1 + exp(\beta_0 + \boldsymbol{\beta}^T \boldsymbol{x}_i)}, \tag{5.14}$$

where

$$y_i = \begin{cases} 1 & \text{if } a_{ij} = \alpha_j \text{ for some } k \in \{1, \ldots, r_i\} \\ 0 & \text{otherwise} \end{cases}$$

and

$$x_{ip} = \begin{cases} 1 & \text{if } d_{il} = \delta_p \text{ for some } l \in \{1, \ldots, s_i\} \\ 0 & \text{otherwise} \end{cases}$$

if x_{ip} is the p-th element of $\boldsymbol{x}_i$. In general, the maximum likelihood method provides the solution of $\boldsymbol{\beta}$. The maximization of likelihood function is achieved by implementing the Newton-Raphson algorithm. The algorithm is convenient and attractive because the Hessian matrix involved in the computation can be used to calculate the standard error of $\hat{\boldsymbol{\beta}}$. However, one of the steps in the optimization involves inversion of the Hessian matrix which poses a major computational burden for high dimensional problems. Screening a SRS database is one such problem that involves a large number of drugs often exceeding the order of 10^4. Therefore, the computational complexity and numerical ill-conditioning hinder the use of ordinary logistic regression for analysis of SRS. To overcome these issues, Genkin et al. (2007) proposed the Bayesian logistic regression that is analogous to the lasso logistic regression (LLR). The LLR imposes the following L_1 constraint on the parameters:

$$\sum_{j=0}^{p} |\beta_j| \le t. \tag{5.15}$$

From the Bayesian prospective, the same constraint on the parameters is achieved by placing the following Laplace prior distribution on the β_j, independently.

$$f(\beta_j | \lambda) = \frac{1}{2} exp(-\lambda |\beta_j|) \tag{5.16}$$

This prior distribution has mean 0, mode 0, and variance $2/\lambda^2$. Furthermore, the hyperparameter λ is a one-to-one transformation of bound t (Hastie et al. 2001) which allows it to be used as a tuning parameter. This prior and the logistic likelihood function yield the following posterior log-likelihood:

$$l(\boldsymbol{\beta}) = K - \sum_{i=1}^{n} log\left(1 + exp(-\boldsymbol{\beta}^T \boldsymbol{x}_i y_i)\right) - \sum_{j=0}^{p}\left(log\frac{2}{\lambda} + \lambda|\beta_j|\right), \tag{5.17}$$

where K is the normalizing constant, and $|D|$ denotes the number of drugs reported in the i-th report. The maximum a posteriori (MAP) estimate of β is obtained by maximizing this posterior log-likelihood. A key advantage of this approach is that the Laplace prior (5.16) favors sparseness in the fitted model, which means that the posterior point estimates for many of the model parameters are not only shrunken toward the zero but are expected to be exactly zero. This feature along with an efficient algorithm allows the effective use of LLR for screening SRS databases. The cyclic coordinate descent algorithm (Luenberger 1984) tuned for Gaussian prior (Zhang and Oles 2001) and modified further for the Laplace prior distribution (Genkin et al. 2007) can be used for efficient calculation of a mode of the posterior log-likelihood equation (5.17). As noted by Genkin et al. (2007) and Caster (2007), the cyclic coordinate descent algorithm breaks down a multidimensional optimization problem into a series of univariate optimization problems. Particularly, it optimizes an objective function with respect to only one parameter at a time, holding all other variables constant. After this one dimensional optimization, it proceed to perform optimization with respect to the next parameter. The first pass of the iteration continues until the optimization with respect to the last parameter. When all variables have been visited, the algorithm returns to the first variable and starts over again. Multiple passes are made until some pre-defined convergence criterion is met.

When fitting LLR, each pass of one-dimensional optimization involves finding β_j^{new}—one at a time—that maximizes the posterior log-likelihood, assuming that all other β_j's are held at their current value. For the posterior log-likelihood equation (5.17), finding β_j^{new} is equivalent to finding the z that optimizes (Caster 2007):

$$g(z) = \sum_{i=1}^{n} log\left(1 + exp((\beta_j - z)x_{ij}y_i - \boldsymbol{\beta}^T \boldsymbol{x}_i y_i)\right) + \lambda|z|. \tag{5.18}$$

A closed form solution for $g(z)$ does not exist. Hence, a numerical optimization procedures such as Newton-Raphson must be implemented to obtain iterative solution. With a careful manipulation of the Zhang and Oles (2001) implementation for Gaussian prior, Genkin et al. (2007) derived the following update equation

$$\Delta\beta_j = \begin{cases} -\Delta_j & \text{if } \Delta v_j < -\Delta_j \\ \Delta v_j & \text{if } -\Delta_j \leq \Delta v_j \leq \Delta_j \\ \Delta_j & \text{if } \Delta_j \leq \Delta v_j \end{cases} \tag{5.19}$$

for

$$\Delta v_j = \frac{\displaystyle\sum_{i=1}^{n} \frac{x_{ij}y_i}{1 + exp(\boldsymbol{\beta}^T \boldsymbol{x}_i y_i)} - \lambda\, sgn(\beta_j)}{\sum_{i=1}^{n} x_{ij}^2 F(\boldsymbol{\beta}^T \boldsymbol{x}_i y_i, \Delta_j x_{ij})},$$

where, for some $\delta > 0$, $F()$ is defined as

$$F(r, \delta) = \begin{cases} 1/4 & \text{if } |r| \leq \delta \\ 1/(2 + exp(|r| - \delta) + exp(\delta - |r|)), & \text{otherwise.} \end{cases} \tag{5.20}$$

Two outstanding issues require further adjustments. First, when $\beta_j = 0$, Δv_j is undefined because $sgn(\beta_j)$ is undefined. In such situation, $sgn(\beta_j)$ is assigned 1 or -1 depending on the value that decreases $g()$ when $\beta_j=0$. Second, $g()$ is not guaranteed to decrease if the update changes the sign of β_j. When such situations arise, β_j^{new} is set to 0. More details on the implementation of the algorithm and selection of the hyperparameter values are provided in Genkin et al. (2007) and Caster (2007).

LLR was originally developed for regression prediction. The use of LLR in SRS analysis is entirely different from the prediction problem. Therefore, the usual techniques for determining optimal values of the hyperparameters, such as cross-validation, are not applicable in this type of analysis. Furthermore, signal generation from SRS requires setting a signaling threshold, which is not included in the development of the LLR method.

Caster (2007) assumed a prior variance of 1 and signaling threshold of $\beta > 0$ when evaluating the LLR for signal generation. The simulation study considered a scenario where a drug A is highly associated with ADR X while another drug B—reported more frequently with drug A—is at the most weakly associated with the X. Results demonstrated that the LLR is capable of correctly flagging the true association between A and X while suppressing a spurious relationship (due to co-medication) between B and X. In contrast, information criterion (IC) measure indiscriminately flagged both A and B as potential suspects for the ADR X. These analyses suggested that the LLR is capable of correcting a potential confounding by co-medication. Additionally, Caster (2007) applied the LLR to the WHO drug safety database focusing on three ADRs: Lactic Acidosis, Hypertriglyceridaemia, and Haemorrhagic Cystitis, that are known to have issues with confounding by co-medication.

The analysis of lactic acidosis revealed similar results as observed in simulation studies. Three classes of anti-diabetes drugs were considered (1) biguanides, (2) slfonylurea, and (3) thaizolidinediones. Among these drug classes, biguanides are known to cause lactic acidosis (two drugs in this class were withdrawn from the market). Sole reports of the drugs in the biguanide class were relatively high and were flagged by both LLR and IC. However, sole reports of the drugs in slfonylurea class were much lower than the reports containing these drugs and one of the biguanides. This suggests high frequency of co-medication of slfonylurea with biguanides (Metformin in particular). Consequently, slfonylurea received low signal scores (below a threshold) by the LLR, whereas they received positive scores (exceeding a threshold) by IC. On the other hand, for the drugs in the thaizolidinediones class, there were very few—sole or co-medicated—reports of lactic acidosis. As a result, the thaizolidinediones received lowered signal scores by both methods, even though there were more sole reports than co-medicated reports.

Anti-HIV drugs were considered for the analysis of hypertriglyceridaemia events. Unlike the lactic acidosis example, there was no obvious confounder in this case, as the drugs were all co-medicated without having a substantial number of sole drug reports. As a result, all Anti-HIV drugs received lower signal scores by the LLR, whereas they received higher scores by IC. Caster (2007) explained this result as "signal sharing" where the LLR allows all drugs to share the same signal. In contrast, the IC measure does not adjust for co-medication and assigns high signal scores for all drugs.

The LLR was also evaluated in the presence of masked effects. As mentioned before, masking is the attenuation of signal for a drug and ADR due to the presence of a strong signal for that drug and some other ADR. Results of the simulation indicate that, in the presence of masking, the LLR is capable of generating a stronger signal compared to the IC measure. However, the difference in the signal score between two methods were not as dramatic as it was in the co-medication situation.

To study the LLR's ability to control masking for the WHO safety database, Caster (2007) selected the drug cerivastatin. The potential ADR of this drug causing rabdomyolysis leading to severe kidney damage was established in 2001. Since then the cerivastatin-rabdomyolysis combination has been seriously over-reported. Such over-reporting is a recipe for the weakening of signals for other drugs involving rabdomyolysis. The LLR (using lower 95% confidence interval as signaling threshold) found 21 new drugs, not found by IC, that are potentially causing this particular ADR. Of which, six were also found to be reported in the literature. However, Caster (2007) cautions that the new associations found may not be entirely due to unmasking, as the results depend on the selected signaling threshold and hyperparameter value. As a result of systematic comparison between the LLR and IC, Caster (2007) recommended prior variance of 0.2 which provides the same precision (fraction of generated signals that are correct) as IC while increases recall (fraction of true associations signaled by the method) by 10%. Caster et al. (2010) study concluded that the LLR based analysis eliminated false positives and false negatives due to other covariates. LLR identified some established drug safety signals earlier than disproportionality-based methods. However, it also failed to identify some other known drug safety issues as early as other established measures. Due to this failure and the lack of empirical basis for estimated regression coefficients, Caster et al. (2010) recommends using LLR in parallel to other methods for ADR surveillance.

5.7 Random-effect Poisson Regression

Random-effect Poisson regression is a straightforward application of statistical theory to post-marketing safety data analysis (see Gibbons et al. 2008). It requires spontaneous reports as well as external data in the form of estimated background incidence of AEs and level of drug utilization. The method can be implemented using either empirical Bayes (EB) or full Bayes estimation of rate multipliers for each drug within a class of drugs, for a particular AE, based on a mixed-effects Poisson regression model. Point estimates and 95% confidence (posterior) intervals are obtained for the rate multiplier for each drug (e.g., antidepressants), which are then used to determine whether a particular drug has an increased risk of association with a particular AE (e.g., suicide). Confidence (posterior) intervals that do not include 1.0 provide evidence for either significant protective or harmful associations of the drug and the AE.

Suppose there are c drugs under study and the adverse effect of each drug is counted at J time points. Let t_j be the jth time point and y_{ij} be the number of AE counts for drug i at time point j. Also, let n_{ij} be the number of subjects who took drug i at time point j and $log(n_{ij})$ is an offset. Denote the mean number of AEs of drug i at time j by λ_{ij}. The mixed-effect Poisson regression model is:

$$f(y_{ij}; \lambda_{ij}) = \frac{e^{-\lambda_{ij}} \lambda_{ij}^{y_{ij}}}{y_{ij}!} \tag{5.21}$$

where the mean parameter λ_{ij} is linked to linear predictors through the log link,

$$
\begin{aligned}
\eta_{ij} &= log(\lambda_{ij}) \\
&= log(n_{ij}) + \boldsymbol{x}_j^T \boldsymbol{b}_i \\
&= log(n_{ij}) + \boldsymbol{x}_j^T \boldsymbol{\beta}_i + \boldsymbol{x}_j^T \boldsymbol{u}_i, \tag{5.22}
\end{aligned}
$$

where $\boldsymbol{x}_j^T$ is a $p \times 1$ vector of the time covariate $[t_j^0, t_j^1, \cdots, t_j^{p-1}]$, $\boldsymbol{b}_i$ is uncentered random coefficient vector with $\boldsymbol{b}_i \sim G(\boldsymbol{\Phi})$, the $\boldsymbol{b}_i$s are independent over drugs, G is the assumed distribution for the $\boldsymbol{b}_i$, with distribution depending on a vector of hyperparameters, $\boldsymbol{\Phi}$, and $\boldsymbol{u}_i$ is a random-effect centered at 0, such that $\boldsymbol{u}_i = \boldsymbol{b}_i - \boldsymbol{\beta}$.

Three approaches may be used to estimate the Poisson regression model: empirical Bayes (EB), parametric full Bayes (FB) approach, and a semiparametric FB approach. The main differences among three approaches reside on how G is specified and estimated. In the EB and FB approaches, G is assumed to be a normal distribution, with $\boldsymbol{\Psi}$ defined by mean vector and covariance-matrix parameters. In the EB approach, $\boldsymbol{\Psi}$ is inferred by point-estimation using maximum marginal likelihood, while in the parametric FB approach, a prior is placed on $\boldsymbol{\Psi}$, and inference focuses on the posterior distribution of $\boldsymbol{\Psi}$. In the semiparametric FB approach, a prior is placed directly on G, with support on the set of all (measurable) distributions G, with this prior defined by hyperparameter $\boldsymbol{\Psi}$.

The main focus in statistical inference is the rate multiplier for each drug. It is an exponential of the centered random intercept, $e^{u_{01}}$, as defined below. Posterior distributions are used in all FB approaches for the inference of the random-effect (rate multiplier). EB assumes that the variance of the random-effect is known in obtaining the posterior distribution of u_{i0} although in fact it is estimated with imprecision, while the FB approaches do not impose such assumption.

5.7.1   Rate Multiplier

A mean of the linear predictor over time for drug i is

$$
\begin{aligned}
\bar{\eta}_i &= \frac{1}{J} \sum_{j=1}^{J} \eta_{ij} \tag{5.23}
\end{aligned}
$$

$$
\begin{aligned}
&= \frac{1}{J} \sum_{j=1}^{J} log(n_{ij}) + \frac{1}{J} \sum_{j=1}^{J} \boldsymbol{x}_j^T \boldsymbol{\beta}_i + \frac{1}{J} \sum_{j=1}^{J} \boldsymbol{x}_j^T \boldsymbol{u}_i \tag{5.24}
\end{aligned}
$$

$$
\begin{aligned}
&= \bar{n}_i + \bar{\beta} + \bar{u}_i \tag{5.25}
\end{aligned}
$$

where $\bar{n}_i = \frac{1}{J}\sum_{j=1}^{J} log(n_{ij})$, $\bar{\beta} = \frac{1}{J}\sum_{j=1}^{J} \boldsymbol{x}_j^T \boldsymbol{\beta}_j$, and $\bar{u}_i = \frac{1}{J}\sum_{j=1}^{J} \boldsymbol{x}_j^T \boldsymbol{u}_i$. Taking exponentials of both sides of (5.25),

$$
\begin{aligned}
\bar{\lambda}_i &= e^{\bar{n}_i} \\
&= e^{\bar{n}_i} e^{\bar{\beta}} e^{\bar{u}_i} \\
&= e^{\bar{n}_i} \bar{\lambda} m_i
\end{aligned}
\tag{5.26}
$$

where $e^{\bar{\lambda}} = e^{\bar{\beta}}$ and $m_i = e^{\bar{u}_i}$. The $\bar{\lambda}_i$, $\bar{\lambda}$, and m_i are called a rate of drug i, a mean rate (over drugs), and a rate multiplier for drug i, respectively. A multiplier of 1 reflects a drug with an adverse event report rate equal to the overall rate for the drugs, a multiplier of 2 reflects a doubling of the rate, and a multiplier of 0.5, half of the rate. Although $\bar{\lambda}$ is called a mean rate, it is not a mean of rates over drugs but an exponential of a mean of log rates.

Unlike other methods that do not require a denominator, this procedure requires either an exact denominator or a proxy denominator. For example, if complete medical records database such as the Veterans Administration (VA) database is used as an alternative to the AERS system, we can determine the number of subjects who were prescribed a particular drug. This is an example of an exact denominator. No such denominator is available for the AERS data; however, a proxy denominator such as the number of prescriptions of a particular drug during a time interval of interest can be obtained from a variety of sources including the National Ambulatory Medical Care Evaluation Survey (NAMCES) and National Hospital Ambulatory Medical Care Evaluation Survey (NHAMCES) and IMS Health databases. In general, large sample sizes are required to justify the use of these methods.

Example

In September 2004, the FDA's Neuro-Psychopharmacologic Advisory Committee and Pediatric Advisory Committee concluded that there was sufficient evidence to support a causal link between antidepressants and pediatric suicidality. One month later in October 2004, the FDA ordered pharmaceutical companies to add to antidepressant advertisements, package inserts, and information sheets developed for patients and clinicians, a "black box" warning (a statement in prominent, bold-faced type and framed by a black border) regarding pediatric use. In 2006 the FDA extended the black box warning to young adults, ages 18-25 (Thomas 2006). Although the black box warning is for all antidepressants, concern has focused primarily on the newer antidepressants SSRIs and SNRIs as compared to TCAs, which predominantly affect the noradranergic system. In this example, we analyzed all available spontaneous reports of suicidality associated with antidepressant use in the U.S., between 1998-2004.

To illustrate the method (Gibbons et al. 2008), analyzed MedWatch data (1998-2004) for antidepressants (generic, brand name(s)) categorized into three classes SSRIs (citalopram, celexa; paroxetine, paxil; fluoxetine, prozac, sarafem; fluvoxamine, luvox; sertraline, zoloft;), SNRIs (nefazodine, serzone; mirtazapine, remeron; bupropion, wellbutrin; venlafaxine, effexor), and TCAs (amitriptyline, elavil, endep; amoxapine, asendin; clomipramine, anafranil; desipramine, norpramine, pertofrane; doxepin, adapin, sinequan; imipramine, janimine, tofranil; nortriptyline, aventyl, pamelor; protriptyline, triptil, vivactil; trimipramine, rhotrimine, surmontil). The AE of interest was suicide, as reported by a hospital, health care provider, pharmaceutical company, or patient. The total dataset consisted of 28,317,382 records which included all reported AE's and drug combinations. To obtain a denominator (i.e., population at risk as measured by estimates of the national number of prescriptions for each drug or drug class by year), estimates of the national prescription rates from the NAMCES and NHAMCES were used. Each year 3,000 physicians are randomly selected to provide data on approximately 30 patient visits over a randomly selected 1-week period (NAMCES). Each year 500 nationally representative hospitals are surveyed for a randomly selected 4-week period (NHAMCES). All prescriptions that are written during these periods are recorded and extrapolated to obtain estimates of national rates. These estimates do not provide information on whether the prescriptions were either filled or taken. Furthermore, the NAMCES data are a survey of office visits and not individual patients; therefore, the estimates may over-represent frequent users of the health care system. Finally, estimates of prescription rates for older drugs that are infrequently prescribed may have increased uncertainty given the small number of physicians sampled (i.e., 3,000).

Figure 5.3, presents a plot of the empirical Bayes estimates and their confidence limits for each drug, for all ages combined. It reveals that as a class, SSRIs and SNRIs have rate multipliers that are significantly less than 1.0, which means lower than the national average suicide adverse event report rate for antidepressants. By contrast, as a class TCAs have rate multipliers that are significantly above the national average suicide rate for antidepressants. Most notable are the TCAs amoxapine (asendin), desipramine (norpramine), and trimipramine (surmontil) that have rates 4 to 5 times higher than the average for antidepressants. The TCAs clomipramine (anafranil) and doxepin (sinequan) also have rate multipliers that are significantly above the average rate for the class of antidepressants (exp(EB)=1.5 or 50% increase). Based on these data, the safest TCA is amitriptyline (elavil). By contrast, all of the SSRIs and SNRIs with the exception of mirtazapine (remeron) and fluvoxamine (luvox) are significantly below the average suicide adverse event report rate for antidepressants. The SNRI nefazedone (serzone) had the lowest spontaneously reported rate for completed suicide. As in the previous analyses, these data do not support the hypothesis that SSRIs and SNRIs are associated with increased risk of suicide. When adjusted for numbers of prescriptions, TCAs appear to have the highest risk of suicide adverse event reports, as compared to SSRIs and SNRIs.

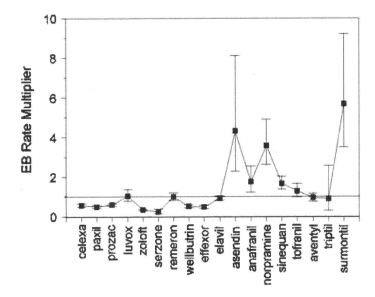

FIGURE 5.3: Bayes estimates and confidence intervals - multiplier of overall rate.

5.8 Discussion

ADR surveillance using statistical methods is still an area of active research. After several years of effort by many researchers, no single method can claim absolute superiority. This is partly because of the complexity of the SRS data and uncontrolled collection of self-reported entries riddled with the problems of under-reporting, over-reporting, and duplicate reporting. Further, as a consequence of modern advances in medicine, patients are more likely to be treated with multiple drugs and not surprisingly multiple drugs are mentioned in almost all the spontaneous reports. These characteristics of SRS data present both challenges and opportunities for methodological developments. More recently, various techniques have emerged that have focused primarily on the minimization of false discovery rate (Ahmed et al. 2009, 2010a,b, 2012) and identification of drug-drug interaction (Eugène et al. 2000, Almenoff et al. 2003, Norén et al. 2008, Villerd et al. 2010, Qian et al. 2010, DuMouchel and Harpaz 2012). Despite use of several different well established methods, automatic signal detection methods cannot and are not designed to replace pharmacovigilance expertise. However, their ability to efficiently explore large spontaneous reporting system databases and detect relevant signals quickly compared with traditional pharmacovigilance makes them powerful tools. As access to higher quality and more complete data streams (medical claims, electronic health records, ...) become available, these methods may prove even more useful for ADR discovery and large scale screening.

6

Meta-analysis

"Our figures show approximately four and one half million hospital admissions annually due to the adverse reactions to drugs. Further, the average hospital patient has as much as thirty percent chance, depending how long he is in, of doubling his stay due to adverse drug reactions."
(Milton Silverman, M.D. Professor of Pharmacology, University of California)

6.1 Introduction

The impact of meta-analysis in drug safety has never been greater than in the recent years. High profile cases against blockbuster drugs such as vioxx and avandia have brought meta-analysis to the forefront of the discussion in the drug safety community. It has become both an indispensable and a highly controversial tool for analyzing rare outcomes in medical and pharmaceutical research. It is indispensable because each individual study or trial is usually not large enough to contain a sufficient number of events for a meaningful analysis. For example the rate of suicidal events (ideation and behavior) is approximately 0.001. In order to estimate and test the efficacy or the safety of drugs in relation to such events with acceptable precision, a large number of subjects must be included in the trial. Meta-analyses combine results from many similar studies and provide a combined estimate with large effective sample size. Meta-analyses are also controversial because of the potential for various biases and for inappropriate methodological choices. There are two primary methodological choices of meta-analyses in the frequentest domain: (1) fixed-effects meta-analyses which assume that the variation in observed effect estimates across the studies are due to sampling variability alone; and (2) random-effect meta-analyses which assume that there is a systematic component in the variation of observed effect estimates across the studies and is quantified by a heterogeneity parameter. Bayesian meta-analysis is also popular for combining results from multiple studies. For each methodology there are a multitude of estimation techniques, each with their respective strengths and weaknesses.

6.2 Fixed-effect Meta-analysis

Let θ_i be a measure of effect size and σ_i^2 be the variance of the corresponding measure in the ith of K studies included in the meta-analysis. Many different metrics can be used to measure effect size, for example, the Pearson product-moment correlation coefficient; standardized mean difference; odds ratios, risk ratios, risk differences, etc. Regardless of a metric used, the true effect size θ is estimated by combining effect sizes from individual studies as follows:

$$\hat{\theta} = \frac{\sum_{i=1}^{K} w_i \theta_i}{\sum_{i=1}^{K} w_i}, \tag{6.1}$$

where,

$$w_i = \frac{1}{\sigma_i^2}. \tag{6.2}$$

Clearly, individual studies are weighted by the inverse of a variance w_i, so that the contribution of each study reflects the precision of individual measures of the effect size. The sampling variance of this combined effect size is the reciprocal of the sum of weights. So, its standard error is:

$$SE(\hat{\theta}) = \sqrt{\frac{1}{\sum_{i=1}^{K} w_i}}. \tag{6.3}$$

The null hypothesis of $H_0 : \theta = \tilde{\theta}$ is tested against the alternate hypothesis $H_1 : \theta \neq \tilde{\theta}$ using the following Wald test:

$$z = \frac{\hat{\theta} - \tilde{\theta}}{SE(\hat{\theta})}. \tag{6.4}$$

The $(1 - \alpha)100\%$ confidence interval for the effect size is constructed as $\hat{\theta} \pm z_{(1-\alpha/2)} \times SE(\hat{\theta})$, where $z_{(1-\alpha/2)}$ is a $(1-\alpha/2)$ percentile point of the standard normal distribution.

6.2.1 Correlation Coefficient

The commonly used metric of effect size to measure linear association between two continuous variables is the correlation coefficient, ρ. The estimated correlation within an individual study of size n_i is denoted by r_i, which asymptotically follows $N\left(\rho, \frac{(1-\rho^2)^2}{n_i}\right)$. Most often, however, r_i is normalized using Fisher's transformation to obtain a random variable z which has variance independent of the unknown parameter ρ. The transformation has the following expression:

$$z_{r_i} = \frac{1}{2} log \frac{1 + r_i}{1 - r_i}. \tag{6.5}$$

The transformed variable z follows $N(\xi, \sigma^2)$, where $\xi = \frac{1}{2} log \frac{1+\rho}{1-\rho}$ and $\sigma^2 = \frac{1}{n-3}$. The combined transformed correlation coefficient across K studies given by the weighted average estimator of equation (6.1) is:

$$z = \frac{\sum_{i=1}^{K} w_i z_{r_i}}{\sum_{i=1}^{K} w_i},$$

(6.6)

where, $w_i = n_i - 3$. The variance of the overall z is $\sum_{i=1}^{K} n_i - 3K$ and the $(1-\alpha)100\%$ CI is $z \pm z_{(1-\alpha/2)} \Big/ \sqrt{\sum_{i=1}^{K} n_i - 3K}$.

6.2.2   Mean Difference

Studies with continuous outcomes often compare the mean outcome from two populations. The two populations may differ with respect to the treatment regimen, program intervention, or exposure. Let $\bar{x}_{1i}$ and $\bar{x}_{2i}$ be the estimated mean outcomes; s_{1i}^2 and s_{2i}^2 be the variances; and n_{1i} and n_{2i} be the sample sizes in the first and the second population, respectively. The impact of the exposure or the intervention is estimated by the difference between outcome means of each group, $\bar{x}_{d_i} = \bar{x}_{1i} - \bar{x}_{2i}$. A pooled variance across two groups is $s_{p_i}^2 = \frac{(n_{1i}-1)s_{1i}^2 + (n_{2i}-1)s_{2i}^2}{n_{1i}+n_{2i}-2}$ and an estimated variance σ_{di}^2 of $\bar{x}_{d_i}$ is as follows:

$$\sigma_{di}^2 = \frac{n_{1i} + n_{2i}}{n_{1i} n_{2i}} s_{p_i}^2.$$

(6.7)

The estimate of common mean difference ($\hat{\theta}$) across K studies is estimated using the general expression in (6.1) as follows:

$$\hat{\theta} = \frac{\sum_{i=1}^{K} w_i \bar{x}_{d_i}}{\sum_{i=1}^{K} w_i},$$

(6.8)

where,

$$w_i = \frac{1}{\sigma_{di}^2}, \quad \text{and} \quad Var(\hat{\theta}) = \frac{1}{\sum_{i=1}^{K} w_i}.$$

(6.9)

There are alternative expressions available for $Var(\hat{\theta})$, which are not covered in this text.

6.2.3   Relative Risk

Prospective studies of a binary outcome, measure effect size as a ratio of risks for the two groups. The measure is called relative risk or the risk ratio (RR). It is a measure with straight forward interpretation and with wide application in epidemiological studies. The outcome of the *ith* trial with binary outcome can be summarized in the following 2×2 contingency table.

TABLE 6.1: Contingency Table of a Drug-Adverse Event Pair in *ith* Trial/Study.

	Event		
	yes	no	total
Treatment	x_{Ti}	$n_{Ti} - x_{Ti}$	n_{Ti}
Control	x_{Ci}	$n_{Ci} - x_{Ci}$	n_{Ci}
Total	m_{Ei}	m_{NEi}	N_i

In Table 6.1 x_{Ti} and x_{Ci} are the number of individuals presented with adverse events in the treatment and the control conditions, respectively. Further, n_{Ti} and n_{Ci} are the number of participants in the treatment and the control groups, respectively. The RR of an adverse event for a study is calculated as follows:

$$RR_i = \frac{x_{Ti}/n_{Ti}}{x_{Ci}/n_{Ci}}. \qquad (6.10)$$

Although, computation of relative risk is easy, its variance estimation is not straight forward, and the domain is not symmetric about its null value. Therefore, the logarithmic transformed relative risk, $ln(RR)$ is commonly used instead of RR which better approximates the large sample distribution and also includes the entire real line in its domain. Since the logarithm is a monotonically increasing function, $ln(RR)$ can be easily transformed back to its original scale. Log transform creates some undesirable complexity in meta-analysis. As $ln(0)$ is not defined, studies without an event in either group cannot be included in the meta-analysis. In order to avoid such complexity, a small constant a called a continuity correction, is added to the cell count of the elements in Table 6.1. The estimate of $ln(RR_i)$ with continuity correction for an individual study is expressed as follows:

$$ln(\widehat{RR_i}) = ln\left[\frac{(x_{Ti} + a)/(n_{Ti} + a)}{(x_{Ci} + a)/(n_{Ci} + a)}\right]. \qquad (6.11)$$

Variance of the estimate in (6.11) following the delta method is as follows:

$$\widehat{Var}[ln(RR_i)] = \frac{1}{x_{Ti} + a} - \frac{1}{n_{Ci} + a} + \frac{1}{x_{Ci} + a} - \frac{1}{n_{Ci} + a}. \qquad (6.12)$$

There are two ways of combining relative risks from multiple studies or trials. One way is to use the general inverse variance method described in equations (6.1) to (6.4). The other way is to use the Mantel-Haenszel method which was originally developed for combining odds/risk ratios across the stratified 2×2 tables. The Mantel-Haenszel method is attractive because it naturally accommodates zero event studies as long as events are observed in one of the two treatment arms. A study is eliminated only when the event is not observed in both treatment arms.

6.2.3.1 Inverse Variance Method

Derivation of an estimate of the combined risk ratio in the inverse variance method follows from the general expression of the fixed-effect estimate of effect size, where $ln(\widehat{RR_i})$ replaces θ_i and $\widehat{Var}[ln(RR_i)]$ replaces σ_i^2 in equation (6.1). Consequently, the combined estimate, $ln(\widehat{RR})$, from K studies is given by

$$ln(\widehat{RR}) = \frac{\sum_{i=1}^{K} \frac{1}{\widehat{Var}[ln(RR_i)]} \left[ln\frac{(x_{Ti}+a)}{(n_{Ti}+a)} - ln\frac{(x_{Ci}+a)}{(n_{Ci}+a)} \right]}{\sum_{i=1}^{K} \frac{1}{\widehat{Var}[ln(RR_i)]}}, \qquad (6.13)$$

and the variance of $ln(\widehat{RR})$ is

$$(6.14)$$

$$Var[ln(\widehat{RR})] = \sum_{i=1}^{K} \frac{1}{\widehat{Var}[ln(RR_i)]}. \qquad (6.15)$$

A null hypothesis of $RR = 1$ is tested using the Wald statistic in equation (6.4) and $(1-\alpha)100\%$ confidence interval of the combined relative risk is calculated as $\left[\widehat{RR} \, exp\left(z_{(1-\alpha/2)}\sqrt{Var[ln(\widehat{RR})]} \right), \frac{\widehat{RR}}{exp\left(z_{(1-\alpha/2)}\sqrt{Var[ln(\widehat{RR})]} \right)} \right].$

6.2.3.2 Mantel-Haenszel Method

The Mantel-Haenszel method is an heuristic estimate of the assumed common risk ratio across the studies. A distinct advantage of this method over the inverse variance method is that it allows studies with zero event in one treatment arm without needing continuity correction. The Mantel-Haenszel method estimate of the common risk ratio is

$$\widehat{RR}_{MH} = \frac{\sum_{i=1}^{K} x_{Ti} n_{Ci}/N_i}{\sum_{i=1}^{K} x_{Ci} n_{Ti}/N_i}, \qquad (6.16)$$

which can be expressed as a weighted average estimate as follows:

$$\widehat{RR}_{MH} = \frac{\sum_{i=1}^{K} w_i \widehat{RR}_i}{\sum_{i=1}^{K} w_i}, \qquad (6.17)$$

where

$$w_i = x_{Ci} n_{Ti}/N_i. \qquad (6.18)$$

Unlike the inverse variance method, the weights in equation (6.18) are not reciprocals of the variances of relative risk estimates from individual studies. Therefore, the variance of the common RR estimate is not as simple. Several approximations of the asymptotic variance have been proposed. The most accurate estimate is the Robins-Breslow-Greenland estimate of variance for $ln(\widehat{RR}_{MH})$. It has the following form:

$$\widehat{Var}[ln(\widehat{RR}_{MH})] = \frac{\sum_{i=1}^{K} \frac{n_{Ti} n_{Ci}}{N_i^2} m_{Ei}}{\left(\sum_{i=1}^{K} \frac{x_{Ti} n_{Ci}}{N_i}\right) \left(\sum_{i=1}^{K} \frac{x_{Ci} n_{Ti}}{N_i}\right)}. \tag{6.19}$$

The null hypothesis of equal risks in treatment and control subjects, i.e., $RR_{MH} = 1$, may be tested by the following 1 degree of freedom χ^2-test, which is obtained based on the assumption of a conditional binomial distribution for the events x_{Ti} in Table 6.1:

$$X_{MH}^2 = \frac{\left[\sum_{i=1}^{K} (x_{Ti} - n_{Ti} m_{Ei})/N_i\right]^2}{\sum_{i=1}^{K} \frac{n_{Ti} n_{Ci} m_{Ei} m_{NEi}}{N_i(N_i - 1)}}. \tag{6.20}$$

6.2.4 Odds Ratio

Large scale drug safety studies are not conducted routinely unless mandated by the FDA. Initial safety concerns often originate from the combined evidences of studies which are conducted to assess efficacy of a treatment. Drug safety studies are, therefore, usually retrospective in nature. The effect size measure commonly used in the retrospective studies of a binary outcome is the odds ratio. Odds ratios share many of the same numerical issues of the relative risk including a non-symmetry about its null value, a need for logarithmic transformation, and a problem with zero studies. Therefore, similar approaches are employed to obtain an estimate of the common odds ratio across multiple studies. When the event is rare (less than 5%) the OR and RR are quite similar.

The observed frequencies of events from the retrospective studies can be summarized in the same way as Table 6.1.

6.2.4.1 Inverse Variance Method

The simplest estimation of combined odds ratio once again follows from the general expression of fixed-effect estimate of effect size, where $ln(\widehat{OR}_i)$ replaces the θ_i and $\widehat{Var}[ln(OR_i)]$ replaces the σ_i^2 in the equations (6.1). Thus, the combined estimate $ln(\widehat{OR})$ from K studies is given by

$$ln(\widehat{OR}) = \frac{\sum_{i=1}^{K} \dfrac{1}{\widehat{Var}[ln(OR_i)]} ln\left[\dfrac{(x_{Ti}+a)(n_{Ci}-x_{Ci}+a)}{(x_{Ci}+a)(n_{Ti}-x_{Ti}+a)}\right]}{\sum_{i=1}^{K} \dfrac{1}{\widehat{Var}[ln(OR_i)]}}, \quad (6.21)$$

and the variance of $ln(\widehat{OR})$ is

$$Var[ln(\widehat{OR})] = \sum_{i=1}^{K} \frac{1}{\widehat{Var}[ln(OR_i)]}, \quad (6.22)$$

where

$$\widehat{Var}[ln(OR_i)] = \frac{1}{x_{Ti}+a} + \frac{1}{x_{Ci}+a} + \frac{1}{n_{Ti}-x_{Ti}+a} + \frac{1}{n_{Ci}-x_{Ci}+a}.$$

The null hypothesis is tested using the Wald statistic in equation (6.4) and the $(1-\alpha)100\%$ confidence interval of the combined odds ratio is calculated

as $\left[\widehat{OR}\, exp\left(z_{(1-\alpha/2)}\sqrt{Var[ln(\widehat{OR})]}\right), \dfrac{\widehat{OR}}{exp\left(z_{(1-\alpha/2)}\sqrt{Var[ln(\widehat{OR})]}\right)}\right].$

6.2.4.2 Mantel-Haenszel Method

The Mantel-Haenszel method estimate of common odds ratio is

$$\widehat{OR}_{MH} = \frac{\sum_{i=1}^{K} x_{Ti}(n_{Ci}-x_{Ci})/N_i}{\sum_{i=1}^{K} x_{Ci}(n_{Ti}-x_{Ti})/N_i}, \quad (6.23)$$

which can be expressed as a weighted average estimate as follows:

$$\widehat{OR}_{MH} = \frac{\sum_{i=1}^{K} w_i \widehat{OR}_i}{\sum_{i=1}^{K} w_i}, \quad (6.24)$$

where

$$w_i = \frac{x_{Ci}(n_{Ti}-x_{Ti})}{N_i}. \quad (6.25)$$

Again the weights in equation (6.25) are not reciprocals of the variances of odds ratio estimates from individual studies. The Robins-Breslow-Greenland estimate of variance for $ln(\widehat{OR}_{MH})$ is of the following form:

$$\widehat{Var}[ln(\widehat{OR}_{MH})] = \frac{S_3}{2S_1^2} + \frac{S_5}{2S_1 S_2} + \frac{S_4}{2S_2^2}, \quad (6.26)$$

where $S_1 = \sum_{i=1}^{K} \dfrac{x_{Ti}(n_{Ci}-x_{Ci})}{N_i}$, $S_2 = \sum_{i=1}^{K} \dfrac{x_{Ci}(n_{Ti}-x_{Ti})}{N_i}$,

$$S_3 = \sum_{i=1}^{K} \frac{x_{Ti}(n_{Ci}-x_{Ci})(x_{Ti}+n_{Ci}-x_{Ci})}{N_i^2},$$

$$S_4 = \sum_{i=1}^{K} \frac{x_{Ci}(n_{Ti} - x_{Ti})(x_{Ci} + n_{Ti} - x_{Ti})}{N_i^2}, \text{ and}$$

$$S_5 = \sum_{i=1}^{K} \frac{x_{Ci}(n_{Ti} - x_{Ti})(x_{Ti} + n_{Ci} - x_{Ci}) + x_{Ti}(n_{Ci} - x_{Ci})(x_{Ci} + n_{Ti} - x_{Ti})}{N_i^2}.$$

A null hypothesis of equal odds in treatment and control subjects, i.e., $OR_{MH} = 1$, may be tested by the following χ^2-test:

$$X_{MH}^2 = \left[\sum_{i=1}^{K} \frac{x_{Ti}(n_{Ci} - x_{Ci}) - x_{Ci}(n_{Ti} - x_{Ti})}{N_i} \right]^2. \tag{6.27}$$

6.2.4.3   Peto Method

Peto method is popular for combining results when the events are moderately rare. For this method studies without events do not present numerical difficulty. Let us define the following quantities for the 2×2 table in 6.1

$$E_i = \frac{(x_{Ti} + x_{Ci})n_{Ti}}{N_i}, \tag{6.28}$$

and

$$V_i = \frac{(x_{Ti} + x_{Ci})(N_i - x_{Ti} - x_{Ci})n_{Ti}n_{Ci}}{N_i^2(N_i - 1)}. \tag{6.29}$$

For the fixed marginal totals, E_i and V_i are the mean and the variance of x_{Ti} which follow hypergeometric distribution under the null hypothesis of odds ratio equal to one. Then for K independent tables, the pooled estimate of $\ln(OR)$ is as follows:

$$\ln(\widehat{OR})_{Peto} = \frac{\sum_{i=1}^{K}(x_{Ti} - E_i)}{\sum_{i-1}^{K} V_i}, \tag{6.30}$$

and

$$Var[\ln(\widehat{OR})_{Peto}] = \frac{1}{\sum_{i-1}^{K} V_i}. \tag{6.31}$$

The combined odds ratio estimated using this method, however, is not a consistent estimator. It performs well only for balanced designs with odds ratio close to 1.

6.3   Random-effect Meta-analysis

Random-effect meta-analysis takes a slightly different approach than its fixed-effect counterpart in that the overall effect size parameter θ is viewed as the mean of a random quantity as opposed to a fixed constant. The random quantity in question is the "true" effect size θ_i in the individual studies included in the meta-analysis. Additionally, the θ_i's are assumed to be a sample of effect sizes from a population of all possible studies with mean effect size θ and variance τ^2. The observed effect size $\hat{\theta}_i$ is regarded as a realized value of the random quantity θ_i. Hence, in random-effect meta-analysis there is not a single "true" population parameter. Each θ_i is a "true" parameter for the ith study. The aim is to estimate a mean effect size of these individual "true" effect sizes. The most commonly used distribution to model the behavior of random effect sizes is a normal distribution. Thus, it is assumed that $\hat{\theta}_i \sim N(\theta_i, \sigma^2)$ and $\theta_i \sim N(\theta, \tau^2)$ which lead to the following estimate of the overall mean effect size, $\hat{\theta}$:

$$\hat{\theta} = \frac{\sum_{i=1}^{N} w_i \hat{\theta}_i}{\sum_{i=1}^{N} w_i}, \tag{6.32}$$

where,

$$w_i = \frac{1}{\sigma_i^2 + \tau^2}. \tag{6.33}$$

The sampling variance of the mean effect size is the reciprocal of the sum of weights and the standard error is:

$$SE(\hat{\theta}) = \sqrt{\left(\frac{1}{\sum_{i=1}^{N} w_i} \right)}. \tag{6.34}$$

Therefore, the sampling variance of the random-effect estimate of the mean effect size is a function of both the sampling error of $\hat{\theta}_i$ about θ_i and the underlying variability of the θ_i. In the context of meta-analysis, the underlying variability of θ_i is called the study heterogeneity and measured by the heterogeneity parameter τ^2. Addition of the heterogeneity parameter in the weights of the expression (6.33) inflates the standard error of the mean effect estimate.

In equation (6.33), τ^2 is assumed to be known. However, in practice it must be estimated from the sample of studies included in the meta-analysis. Several estimates of between-study variance are available. Among those estimates most commonly used estimate, Q, is based on the weighted sum of squared errors. The Q-statistic also known as Cochran's Q-test has the following form:

$$\hat{Q} = \sum_{i=1}^{K} w_{i0}(\theta_i - \hat{\theta})^2, \quad \text{where } w_{i0} = \frac{1}{\sigma_i^2}, \text{ and} \qquad (6.35)$$

$$E(\hat{Q}) = \tau^2 \sum_{i=1}^{K} w_{i0} - \frac{\tau^2 \sum_{i=1}^{K} w_{i0}^2}{\sum_{i=1}^{K} w_{i0}} + \sum_{i=1}^{K} w_{i0}\sigma_i^2 - \frac{\sum_{i=1}^{K} w_{i0}^2 \sigma_i^2}{\sum_{i=1}^{K} w_{i0}} \qquad (6.36)$$

$$= \tau^2 \sum_{i=1}^{K} w_{i0} - \frac{\tau^2 \sum_{i=1}^{K} w_{i0}^2}{\sum_{i=1}^{K} w_{i0}} + (K - 1). \qquad (6.37)$$

Using the expression (6.36), an estimate of τ^2 is obtained by matching first order moment of Q with $\hat{Q}$; i.e., $\hat{Q} = E(Q)$ and rearranging the terms (Der-Simonian and Laird 1986). The process yields the following estimate of τ^2:

$$\hat{\tau}^2 = \frac{\hat{Q} - (K - 1)}{\displaystyle\sum_{i=1}^{K} w_{i0} - \frac{\sum_{i=1}^{K} w_{i0}^2}{\displaystyle\sum_{i=1}^{K} w_{i0}}}. \qquad (6.38)$$

If the estimate yields a negative value, then it is set to zero because the between-study variance cannot be negative. The estimator in (6.38) is a single step non-iterative solution. However, it has downward bias that increases with the decreasing event rates. Other alternative estimators of heterogeneity are discussed in the following section.

The only difference between expressions to calculate the overall effect size in the fixed-effect and the random-effect analysis is the additional τ^2 term in the expression of the weight in equation (6.33). When the between-study variance is absent or small, the fixed-effect and random-effect estimates of the overall mean are the same. A statistical test of significance of heterogeneity relies on the Q-statistic in equation (6.35). For a large number of studies, Q follows a χ^2 distribution with $K - 1$ degrees of freedom. Thus, a critical value of the test of heterogeneity, at α level of significance, is the $(1 - \alpha)100^{th}$ percentile point of the χ_{K-1}^2 distribution. Although, it is a widely used test of heterogeneity, statistical power of this test has been shown to be inadequate, especially for small values of τ^2 and for non-Gaussian outcomes. Alternatively, the I^2 statistic is used to quantify heterogeneity (Higgins and Thompson 2002). It is independent of a number of studies and the treatment effect metric. The I^2 statistic is derived from Q as follows:

$$I^2 = max\left\{0, \frac{Q - (K - 1)}{Q}\right\}. \qquad (6.39)$$

I^2 is interpreted as the percentage of variability due to heterogeneity between studies. I^2 value of 30% indicates the presence of moderate heterogeneity and 50% indicates the presence of strong heterogeniety. The value of the I^2

statistic depends on the precision of the estimate of individual effect sizes of the included studies. The value increases with number of patients included in the studies in a meta-analysis regardless of the underlying study heterogeneity (Rucker et al. 2008). Therefore, I^2 values must be interpreted cautiously.

6.3.1 Sidik-Jonkman Estimator of Heterogeneity

The Sidik-Jonkman (Sidik and Jonkman 2005) estimator is simple, non-iterative and always non-negative. It has less bias when the heterogeneity variance is moderate to large. The estimation method is developed in the framework of a linear regression model with no covariates. The estimate, τ^2_{SH}, is found by using the weighted residual sum of squares as follows:

$$\hat{\tau}^2_{SH} = \frac{1}{K-1} \sum_{i=1}^{K} v_i^{-1} (\hat{\theta}_i - \bar{\theta})^2, \tag{6.40}$$

where $v_i = r_i + 1$ and $r_i = \sigma_i^2 / \tau^2$. The estimator $\hat{\tau}^2_{SH}$ depends on the unknown parameter τ^2 through r_i. A crude estimate of τ^2 for defining r_i for the computation of $\hat{\tau}^2_{SH}$ from equation (6.40) is obtained as:

$$\hat{\tau}^2_0 = \frac{1}{K} \sum_{i=1}^{K} (\hat{\theta}_i - \bar{\theta})^2, \tag{6.41}$$

where $\bar{\theta} = \frac{1}{K} \sum_{i=1}^{K} \hat{\theta}_i$. An interval estimate of $\hat{\tau}^2_{SH}$ is found by assuming that $(K-1)\hat{\tau}^2_{SH}/\tau^2$ has approximately a χ^2-distribution with $K-1$ degrees of freedom. Thus, an approximate $(100-1)\alpha\%$ confidence interval for τ^2 given α is obtained as

$$\frac{(K-1)\hat{\tau}^2_{SH}}{\chi^2_{K-1,1-\alpha/2}} \leq \tau^2 \leq \frac{(K-1)\hat{\tau}^2_{SH}}{\chi^2_{K-1,\alpha/2}}. \tag{6.42}$$

Figure 6.1 shows the SJ estimates of τ^2 for varying baseline risk rates in binary event studies. It reveals the overestimating tendency of the SJ estimator at the null value of heterogeneity for the rare events. On the other hand, for moderate event rates, the SJ estimator shows remarkable accuracy.

6.3.2 DerSimonian-Kacker Estimator of Heterogeneity

The original non-iterative estimate of τ^2 can be improved by a two-step process (DerSimonian and Kacker 2007). First, the intermediate estimate of τ^2 is obtained using equation (6.38). Second, the weights w_{i0} in (6.36) are replaced by w_i in (6.33) where τ^2 is substituted with the estimate $\hat{\tau}^2$ obtained in the

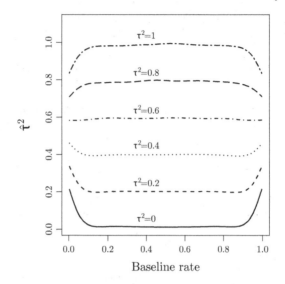

FIGURE 6.1: Sidik-Jonkman estimator of heterogeneity for different baseline risks.

first step. The resulting two-step estimator (τ_{DSK}^2) has following expression.

$$
\hat{\tau}_{DSK}^2 = \frac{\left(\sum_{i=1}^{K} w_i (\theta_i - \hat{\theta})^2 \right) - \left(\sum_{i=1}^{K} w_i \sigma_i^2 - \dfrac{\sum_{i=1}^{K} w_i^2 \sigma_i^2}{\sum_{i=1}^{K} w_i} \right)}{\sum_{i=1}^{K} w_i - \dfrac{\sum_{i=1}^{K} w_i^2}{\sum_{i=1}^{K} w_i}}.
\tag{6.43}
$$

An additional step usually improves the estimate of heterogeneity. The second step of the process depends on having a non-zero estimate of intermediate τ^2. In rare event studies, equation (6.38) often fails to detect even moderate heterogeneity resulting in a zero intermediate estimate and consequently a zero final estimate of heterogeneity. Thus, for rare event studies, the advantage of a two-step estimate is diminished.

6.3.3   REML Estimator of Heterogeneity

Fully iterative solution of heterogeneity is obtained using maximum likelihood theory. According to the standard random-effect model in Section 6.3,

$\hat{\theta}_i$ follows a $N(\theta, \tau^2 + \sigma_i^2)$ distribution. The log-likelihood function is

$$l(\theta, \tau^2 | \hat{\theta}_i) = -\frac{1}{2} \sum_{i=1}^{K} ln[2\pi(\sigma_i^2 + \tau^2)] - \frac{1}{2} \sum_{i=1}^{K} \frac{\theta_i - \theta}{\sigma_i^2 + \tau^2}, \quad \tau^2 \geq 0. \quad (6.44)$$

The maximum likelihood estimator is found by maximizing this likelihood function with respect to θ and τ^2. Unfortunately, closed form solution of the estimating equation does not exist. Hence, the solution is obtained by iterating between the following two equations until convergence (Hardy and Thompson 1996).

$$\theta_{MLE} = \sum_{i=1}^{K} \frac{\hat{\theta}_i}{(\sigma_i^2 + \hat{\tau}_{MLE}^2)} \bigg/ \sum_{i=1}^{K} \frac{1}{(\sigma_i^2 + \hat{\tau}_{MLE}^2)}. \quad (6.45)$$

$$\tau_{MLE}^2 = \sum_{i=1}^{K} \frac{(\hat{\theta}_i - \theta_{MLE})^2 - \sigma_i^2}{(\sigma_i^2 + \hat{\tau}_{MLE}^2)^2} \bigg/ \sum_{i=1}^{K} \frac{1}{(\sigma_i^2 + \hat{\tau}_{MLE}^2)^2}. \quad (6.46)$$

A 95% confidence interval of τ^2 is obtained by a profile likelihood ratio test statistic. It is defined as a set of $\tilde{\tau}^2$ estimates which satisfy the following condition:

$$l(\tilde{\theta}, \tilde{\tau}^2) \geq l(\theta_{MLE}, \tau_{MLE}^2) - 3.84/2. \quad (6.47)$$

Alternatively, the estimate and confidence interval of τ^2 may be obtained using the restricted maximum likelihood (REML) estimate which overcomes a tendency of ML methods to underestimate variances. The following restricted likelihood l_R of τ^2 is given by Viechtbauer (2007):

$$l_R = -\frac{1}{2} \sum_{i=1}^{K} ln(\sigma_i^2 + \tau^2) - \frac{1}{2} ln \sum_{i=1}^{K} \frac{1}{\sigma_i^2 + \tau^2} - \frac{1}{2} \sum_{i=1}^{K} \frac{(\hat{\theta}_i - \hat{\theta})^2}{\sigma_i^2 + \tau^2} \quad (6.48)$$

where $\hat{\theta} = \sum_{i=1}^{K} \frac{\hat{\theta}_i}{(\sigma_i^2 + \hat{\tau}^2)} \big/ \sum_{i=1}^{K} \frac{1}{(\sigma_i^2 + \hat{\tau}^2)}$. Then the REML estimate of τ^2 is obtained by iteratively solving the following estimating equation:

$$\tau_{REML}^2 = \sum_{i=1}^{K} \frac{(\hat{\theta}_i - \hat{\theta}_{REML})^2 - \sigma_i^2}{(\sigma_i^2 + \hat{\tau}_{REML}^2)^2} \bigg/ \sum_{i=1}^{K} \frac{1}{(\sigma_i^2 + \hat{\tau}_{REML}^2)^2} + \frac{1}{\sigma_i^2 + \hat{\tau}_{REML}^2}. \quad (6.49)$$

A 95% confidence interval based on profile likelihood ratio test is given by a set of $\tilde{\tau}^2$ which satisfy following condition

$$l_R(\tilde{\tau}^2) \geq l_R(\tau_{REML}^2) - 3.84/2. \quad (6.50)$$

6.3.4   Improved PM Estimator of Heterogeneity

An alternative fully iterative approach to estimate τ^2 is provided by Paule and Mandel (1982) and is based on the following estimating equation:

$$F(\tau^2) = \sum_i w_i(\hat{\theta}_i - \hat{\theta})^2 - (k-1) = 0. \tag{6.51}$$

A unique solution of (6.51), $\hat{\tau}^2_{PM}$, can be determined by numerical iteration starting with $\tau^2 = 0$. If $F(\tau^2)$ is negative for all positive τ^2, $\hat{\tau}^2_{PM}$ is set to 0. This method is a natural approximation to the restricted maximum likelihood method. When the normality assumption holds and the estimate of within-study variances are regarded as the true within-study variance, Paule and Mandel's approach is statistically optimal. But the assumption of normality is not required to apply this method which makes it more robust when that assumption does not hold (DerSimonian and Kacker (2007)). Note that $\hat{\tau}^2_{PM}$ is based on $\hat{\sigma}_i$ which varies from study to study.

Studies with binary outcome usually report number of success and sample size in each arm. In such cases, the variance estimator may be improved by borrowing strength from all studies when estimating each within-study variance $\hat{\sigma}^2_i$ as follows:

$$\begin{aligned}
\hat{\sigma}^2_i(*) &= \frac{1}{(n_{Ti}+1)}\left[e^{\left(-\bar{\mu}-\bar{\theta}+\frac{\tau^2}{2}\right)} + 2 + e^{\left(\bar{\mu}+\bar{\theta}+\frac{\tau^2}{2}\right)}\right] \\
&+ \frac{1}{(n_{Ci}+1)}\left[e^{-\bar{\mu}} + 2 + e^{\bar{\mu}}\right],
\end{aligned} \tag{6.52}$$

where $\bar{\mu} = \sum_{i=1}^{K}\hat{\mu}_i$ and $\bar{\theta} = \sum_{i=1}^{K}\hat{\theta}_i$. The $\hat{\mu}_i$ and $\hat{\theta}_i$ are the estimated log odds of success and log odds ratio measure of effect size, respectively. A new estimator, denoted by $\hat{\tau}^2_{IPM}$, is the solution to a modified version of (6.51), where the weights w_i are replaced by the shared-strength weights $w_i(*) = \frac{1}{\tau^2+\hat{\sigma}^2_i(*)}$. This is in line with the Bohning et al. (2002) recommendation of using a population averaged version of the study-specific variances as weights.

6.3.5   Example

Rosiglitazone is widely used to treat patients with type 2 diabetes mellitus. For the past few years the scientific community has expressed concerns regarding its adverse effect on cardiovascular morbidity and mortality. In 2007 a group of scientists from the Cleveland clinic lead by Steven E. Nissen conducted a meta-analysis of 42 trials of rosiglitazone. A total of 15,565 patients were randomly assigned to regimens that included rosiglitazone, and 12,282 were assigned to comparator groups with regimens that did not include rosiglitazone. Myocardial infarction (MI) was one of the adverse event considered. Only 38 of 42 trials had at least one MI event. The remaining four trials were eliminated from further analysis because the effect estimates were not possible for these trials. The following forest plot shows number of patients and number of events in each treatment arm, the estimated odds ratios and associated 95% CI for each trial, and the overall odds ratio and 95% CI estimate using Peto method. The estimates of the overall odds ratio using other estimators are listed in the Table 6.2. Peto method yields the largest and statistically significant estimate of the overall odds ratio (OR=1.43, p=0.03), whereas the other three methods: inverse variance (I), Mantel-Haenszel (MH), and DerSimonian-Laird (DL), yield statistically non-significant (p=0.15) estimates. As we noted earlier the Peto method is susceptible to bias when combining highly unbalanced studies such as studies in this example.

The forest plot shows large heterogeneity in the estimated odds ratio from the individual studies. However, the estimates of between study heterogeneity in the Table 6.3 are near 0 for all but Sidik-Jonkman (SJ) method. The discrepancy in observed and the estimated heterogeneity could be due to two reasons. First, the forest plot shows effect estimates in their original scale, where as heterogeneity is estimated for the effect in the logarithmic scale which attenuates the magnitude of the between study differences. Second, average baseline event rates of MI in these studies are about 6/1000. The usual heterogeneity estimates do not perform well in such rare event cases. In contrast, the SJ estimator showed moderate heterogeneity. However, simulation study has shown that for rare events the SJ estimators have a tendency to overestimate when the true heterogeneity is near 0 (Sidik and Jonkman 2005).

TABLE 6.2: Estimate of Overall Odds Ratio.

Method	OR	95 % CI of OR	p
I	1.24	[0.9201; 1.6814]	0.15
MH	1.24	[0.9275; 1.6572]	0.14
Peto	1.43	[1.0309; 1.9788]	0.03
DL	1.24	[0.9201; 1.6814]	0.15

TABLE 6.3: Estimates and Test of Heterogeneity.

Method	τ^2
DL	0
SJ	0.26
REML	0
ML	0
IPM	0
I^2	0
Q-test pvalue	0.99

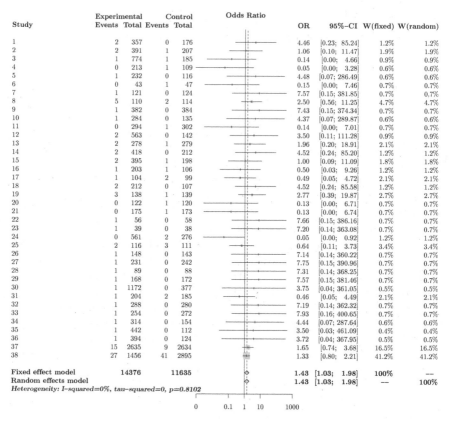

Study	Experimental Events	Experimental Total	Control Events	Control Total	OR	95%-CI	W(fixed)	W(random)
1	2	357	0	176	4.46	[0.23; 85.24]	1.2%	1.2%
2	2	391	1	207	1.06	[0.10; 11.47]	1.9%	1.9%
3	1	774	1	185	0.14	[0.00; 4.66]	0.9%	0.9%
4	0	213	1	109	0.05	[0.00; 3.28]	0.6%	0.6%
5	1	232	0	116	4.48	[0.07; 286.49]	0.6%	0.6%
6	0	43	1	47	0.15	[0.00; 7.46]	0.7%	0.7%
7	1	121	0	124	7.57	[0.15; 381.85]	0.7%	0.7%
8	5	110	2	114	2.50	[0.56; 11.25]	4.7%	4.7%
9	1	382	0	384	7.43	[0.15; 374.34]	0.7%	0.7%
10	1	284	0	135	4.37	[0.07; 289.87]	0.6%	0.6%
11	0	294	1	302	0.14	[0.00; 7.01]	0.7%	0.7%
12	2	563	0	142	3.50	[0.11; 111.28]	0.9%	0.9%
13	2	278	1	279	1.96	[0.20; 18.91]	2.1%	2.1%
14	2	418	0	212	4.52	[0.24; 85.20]	1.2%	1.2%
15	2	395	1	198	1.00	[0.09; 11.09]	1.8%	1.8%
16	1	203	1	106	0.50	[0.03; 9.26]	1.2%	1.2%
17	1	104	1	99	0.49	[0.05; 4.72]	2.1%	2.1%
18	2	212	0	107	4.52	[0.24; 85.58]	1.2%	1.2%
19	3	138	1	139	2.77	[0.39; 19.87]	2.7%	2.7%
20	0	122	1	120	0.13	[0.00; 6.71]	0.7%	0.7%
21	0	175	1	173	0.13	[0.00; 6.74]	0.7%	0.7%
22	1	56	0	58	7.66	[0.15; 386.16]	0.7%	0.7%
23	1	39	0	38	7.20	[0.14; 363.08]	0.7%	0.7%
24	0	561	2	276	0.05	[0.00; 0.92]	1.2%	1.2%
25	2	116	3	111	0.64	[0.11; 3.73]	3.4%	3.4%
26	1	148	0	143	7.14	[0.14; 360.22]	0.7%	0.7%
27	1	231	0	242	7.75	[0.15; 390.96]	0.7%	0.7%
28	1	89	0	88	7.31	[0.14; 368.25]	0.7%	0.7%
29	1	168	0	172	7.57	[0.15; 381.46]	0.7%	0.7%
30	1	1172	0	377	3.75	[0.04; 361.05]	0.5%	0.5%
31	1	204	2	185	0.46	[0.05; 4.49]	2.1%	2.1%
32	1	288	0	280	7.19	[0.14; 362.32]	0.7%	0.7%
33	1	254	0	272	7.93	[0.16; 400.65]	0.7%	0.7%
34	1	314	0	154	4.44	[0.07; 287.64]	0.6%	0.6%
35	1	442	0	112	3.50	[0.03; 461.09]	0.4%	0.4%
36	1	394	0	124	3.72	[0.04; 367.95]	0.5%	0.5%
37	15	2635	9	2634	1.65	[0.74; 3.68]	16.5%	16.5%
38	27	1456	41	2895	1.33	[0.80; 2.21]	41.2%	41.2%
Fixed effect model		14376		11635	1.43	[1.03; 1.98]	100%	—
Random effects model					1.43	[1.03; 1.98]	—	100%

Heterogeneity: I–squared=0%, tau–squared=0, p=0.8102

                0   0.1   1   10   1000

FIGURE 6.2: Meta-analysis of rosiglitazone trials. The fixed-effect estimate is obtained using the Peto method.

6.3.6   Issues with the Weighted Average in Meta-analysis

The weighted average estimator, such as the DL estimator, has been in use for several decades. Classical statistical theory has established that the weighted average is the most efficient estimator of the population mean of a random variable, on the assumption that the weights used in estimation are not related to the random variable in question. In meta-analysis the validity of this assumption is questionable. While it is not as clear in studies with normally distributed continuous outcomes, the correlation between weights and individual effect estimates in studies with a binary outcome is undeniable. The weighted average estimator of overall effect is biased when such correlation exists. Shuster (2010) derived the following expression for the expected value of the overall effect estimator for the random-effect model (6.33)

$$E(\hat{\theta}) = K \times Cov(W_i\hat{\theta}_i) + \theta, \tag{6.53}$$

where $W_i = w_i / \sum w_i$. He also showed that only the unweighted mean is the unbiased estimator of the overall effect in these conditions. A similar conclusion was reached by Bhaumik et al. (2012) and recommended using unweighted mean with 0.5 continuity correction when necessary. Hence, results of the weighted average estimate must be interpreted with caution.

6.4 Maximum Marginal Likelihood/Empirical Bayes Method

An alternative to the method of moments, is the maximum marginal likelihood (MML) method. A distinct advantage of the MML approach is that studies with zero events in both arms can be included without adjustments such as continuity corrections. Furthermore, the overall treatment effect and the heterogeneity parameter(s) can be simultaneously estimated.

Consider an observed 2×2 Table 6.1 for the ith study for a meta-analysis of K studies. Let p_{ti} and p_{ci} be the event probabilities in treatment and control groups, respectively, of the ith study; $\epsilon_1 \sim N(0, \sigma_\mu^2)$ and $\epsilon_2 \sim N(0, \tau^2)$; and T_{ji} be a treatment indicator variable, i.e., $T_j = 0$ for $j = c$ and $T_j = 1$ for $j = t$. The log-odds of adverse events in the jth group can be modeled as follows. The model allows for heterogeneity in both the baseline risk and the treatment effect.

$$ln \left(\frac{p_{ji}}{1 - p_{ji}} \right) = \mu + \epsilon_{1i} + (\theta + \epsilon_{2i}) T_{ji} \tag{6.54}$$

$$\begin{pmatrix} \epsilon_1 \\ \epsilon_2 \end{pmatrix} \sim N \left(\begin{pmatrix} 0 \\ 0 \end{pmatrix}, \begin{pmatrix} \sigma_\mu^2 & \rho \sigma_\mu \tau \\ \rho \sigma_\mu \tau & \tau^2 \end{pmatrix} \right). \tag{6.55}$$

The likelihood function based on the observations from the ith study is written as follows:

$$l(\boldsymbol{x_i}|\epsilon) = p_{ti}^{x_{ti}} q_{ti}^{n_{ti} - x_{ti}} p_{ci}^{x_{ci}} q_{ci}^{n_{ci} - x_{ci}}, \tag{6.56}$$

where $\boldsymbol{x_i} = (x_{ti}, x_{ci})$ is the vector pattern of responses from study i. Then, for the parameter vector $\boldsymbol{\beta} = (\mu, \theta, \Sigma)$, the marginal likelihood for study i is given by

$$h(\boldsymbol{\beta}; \boldsymbol{x_i}) = h(\boldsymbol{x_i}) = \int_\epsilon l(\boldsymbol{x_i}|\epsilon) g(\epsilon) d\epsilon, \tag{6.57}$$

where $g(\epsilon)$ represents the standard multivariate normal density. Now, the full log-likelihood for k studies can be written as

$$\log L = \sum_{i=1}^{k} \log h(\boldsymbol{x_i}), \tag{6.58}$$

and for an arbitrary parameter vector, $\boldsymbol{\eta}$, the first derivatives of the log-likelihood with respect to $\boldsymbol{\eta}$ are

$$\frac{\partial \log L}{\partial \boldsymbol{\eta}} = \sum_{i=1}^{k} \frac{1}{h(\boldsymbol{x}_i)} \frac{\partial h(\boldsymbol{x}_i)}{\partial \boldsymbol{\eta}} , \tag{6.59}$$

where

$$\frac{\partial h(\boldsymbol{x}_i)}{\partial \boldsymbol{\eta}} = \int_{\epsilon} \frac{\partial \log l(\boldsymbol{x}_i | \epsilon)}{\partial \boldsymbol{\eta}} l(\boldsymbol{x}_i | \epsilon) g(\epsilon) d\epsilon . \tag{6.60}$$

The integration on the random effect space (i.e., ϵ) in the marginal likelihood equation in (6.57) can be approximated numerically using Gauss-Hermite quadrature to any practical degree of accuracy. The integration in Gauss-Hermite quadrature is approximated by a summation on a specified number of quadrature nodes and the corresponding quadrature weights. Both adaptive (based on selecting quadrature nodes in accordance with provisional estimates of the posterior mean and variance) and nonadaptive versions of the algorithm are available Hedeker and Gibbons (2006). Optimal points and weights for the standard normal univariate density were given by Stroud and Secrest (1966), and this method is now in widespread use in nonlinear mixed-effects regression models. Solution of the likelihood equations can be obtained iteratively using the Newton-Raphson algorithm. At convergence, the diagonal elements of the inverse of the information matrix provide the variance of the estimated parameters.

The MML models are fitted using commercial software packages such as SAS, STATA, SuperMix, etc. The linearized approximation can be fitted using the GLIMMIX procedure in SAS or the glmer package in R. The following SAS code illustrates the NLMIXED implementation of the MML meta-analysis.

6.4.1 Example: Percutaneous Coronary Intervention Based Strategy versus Medical Treatment Strategy

Percutaneous coronary intervention or PCI (commonly known as angioplasty) is the standard treatment for patients with acute coronary disease; however, the effects of PCI in the treatment of patients with stable coronary artery disease have not received thorough examination. Schömig et al. (2008) conducted a meta-analysis of 17 RCTs that compared PCI to medication management (MED) in patients with stable coronary artery disease aimed at synthesizing evidence of efficacy of PCI versus MED. Briefly, the study included a total of 7513 patients (3675 PCI and 3838 MED) with the average length of follow-up of 51 months. The sample consisted of mostly elderly men (82%) and 54% had experienced an (MI). In the PCI group, 271 patients died and in the MED group 335 died. Among the 13 studies that reported cardiac mortality, the PCI and MED arms had a combined 115/2814 and 151/2805 cardiac deaths, respectively. Finally, MI rates were provided in all 17 studies, reporting 319 in the PCI group and 357 in the MED group. The original authors used Cochran's Q-test to assess heterogeneity and performed Mantel-Haenszel (MH) and DerSimonian and Laird methods to estimate the overall treatment effect. Tests of heterogeneity (Cochran's Q statistic) were not significant for either total mortality (p=.263) or cardiac mortality (p=.161), but was significant for MI (p=.003). The fixed-effect (MH) model showed a significant protective effect of PCI on total mortality (OR = 0.80, CI = 0.68-0.95), and cardiac mortality (OR = 0.74, CI = 0.57-0.96), and approached significance for MI (OR = 0.91, CI = 0.77-1.06). The random-effect (DL) model showed a significant protective effect of PCI on total mortality (OR = 0.80, CI = 0.64-0.99), an effect that approached significance for cardiac mortality (OR = 0.74, CI = 0.51-1.06), and a nonsignificant effect for MI (OR = 0.90, CI = 0.66-1.23) that was in the same protective direction as the other effects. On the basis of these results, the authors concluded that a PCI-based invasive strategy may improve long term survival compared with a medical treatment in patients with stable coronary artery disease. Table 6.4 shows the frequencies of each type of even for these 17 studies.

TABLE 6.4: Example 1: Data from a Meta-analysis of Studies Comparing PCI to MED in the Treatment of Patients with Stable Coronary Artery Disease.

Study	Number of events in PCI group				Number of events in MED group			
	MI	Cardiac death	All cause mortality	# Obs.	MI	Cardiac death	All cause mortality	# Obs.
1	2	0	0	44	0	1	1	44
2	14	-	16	115	8	-	15	112
3	6	-	9	51	6	-	10	50
4	7	-	2	192	18	-	20	366
5	2	1	1	21	0	1	1	23
6	5	1	1	177	4	1	1	164
7	5	4	6	72	3	2	6	72
8	3	1	2	90	0	2	4	91
9	10	4	6	149	12	14	17	151
10	32	20	43	504	23	24	43	514
11	18	32	45	153	18	33	40	148
12	1	0	0	50	0	0	0	51
13	32	-	19	503	59	-	24	505
14	5	2	2	104	7	1	1	101
15	23	24	28	205	31	25	35	203
16	11	3	6	96	40	22	22	105
17	143	23	85	1149	128	25	95	1138

A re-analysis of the cardiac mortality data is presented in Table 6.6 along with the NLMIXED code snippet used for this analysis in Table 6.5. There were 13 studies with an average of 215 subjects per study per arm. The estimated baseline incidence rate is -3.22 based the MML model, which corresponds to a baseline rate of 4%. The analysis reveals that the primary variance component is for the baseline incidence rate. The estimated odds ratio is 0.75 (95% CI 0.42–1.33), and the estimated treatment variance is 0.23. While the point estimate is similar to the moment-based methods, the full-likelihood method reveals considerably more uncertainty in the estimate.

TABLE 6.5: The NLMIXED Code for PCI Example

```
PROC NLMIXED DATA=pci qpoints= 11;
PARMS b0= −4 b1= −0.1 v0= 1.4 c01= −0.5 v1= 0.2;
eta = b0 + b1*Group + u0 + u1*Group;
expeta = exp(eta);
prob = expeta/(1+expeta);
model x ~ binomial(n,prob);
RANDOM u0 u1 ~ NORMAL([0, 0], [v0, c01, v1]) SUBJECT=studyid;
ESTIMATE 're corr' c01/SQRT(v0*v1);
RUN;
```

TABLE 6.6: Analysis of PCI vs MED for Cardiac Mortality Data

Parameters	Estimate	Std. err	p-val
θ	-0.28	0.217	0.303
$\hat{\sigma}_\mu^2$	1.411	0.737	0.076
$\hat{\sigma}_{\mu\tau}$	-0.267	0.345	0.488
$\hat{\tau}^2$	0.235	0.243	0.348
$\hat{\rho}$	-0.464	0.421	

The MML model also allow flexibility of modeling with single variance components either in the baseline rate or in the treatment effect. However, there is a risk of model mis-specification when using a single variance component. In such cases the effect estimates can be severely biased and the type I error can be substantial Amatya et al. (2014).

6.5   Bayesian Meta-analysis

The Bayesian approach to meta-analysis provides a flexible modeling strategy that naturally accounts for uncertainty in all of the parameter estimates. Unlike the frequentest approach, the Bayesian framework can be easily extended to non-normal distribution of random effects. This approach allows additional information from other trials or studies to be incorporated in the form of a prior distribution. Perhaps the most interesting advantage of the approach is its ability to make predictions about the outcomes of future studies. The Bayesian approach requires computing the posterior distributions of the parameter which often are computationally intensive. Fortunately, rapid development in Monte Carlo technique and computing power have made these complex computations feasible.

The generic Bayesian meta-analysis model places a prior distribution on both the effect parameter and the heterogeneity parameter as follows:

$$\hat{\theta}_i \sim f(\hat{\theta}_i|\theta_i, \sigma_i^2) \tag{6.61}$$

$$\theta_i \sim \pi(\theta_i|\theta, \tau^2) \tag{6.62}$$

$$\theta \sim h(\theta) \tag{6.63}$$

$$\tau^2 \sim h(\tau^2) \tag{6.64}$$

$$p(\theta, \tau, \theta_i|\hat{\theta}_i) \propto h(\theta)h(\tau^2)\prod_{i=1}^{K}\pi(\theta_i|\theta, \tau^2)\prod_{i=1}^{K}f(\hat{\theta}_i|\theta_i, \sigma_i^2) \tag{6.65}$$

Inference regarding a parameter is made from the mode of the posterior distribution (6.65). Computation of the posterior mode in closed form can be very complex. Monte Carlo methods such as Gibbs sampling make computation feasible by exploiting computational power of new computers.

An example of Gibbs sampling is presented in meta-analysis of randomized controlled trials comparing sodium monobuorophosphate (SMFP) to sodium Buoride (NaF) dentifrices (toothpastes) in the prevention of caries development by Abrams and Sanso (1998). Nine studies were included in the analysis of change in the decayed missing (due to caries) filled surface (DMFS) dental index from baseline. The following Bayesian model was used to model the difference in mean responses $\hat{\theta}_i$ for the ith study:

$$\hat{\theta}_i \sim N(\theta_i, \sigma_i^2/n_i), \tag{6.66}$$

$$\theta_i \sim N(\mu, \tau^2), \tag{6.67}$$

$$\tau^2 \sim IG(a, b), \tag{6.68}$$

$$\pi(\sigma_i^2) \propto 1/\sigma_i^2, \tag{6.69}$$

where $n_i = n_{Ti}n_{Ci}/(n_{Ti} + n_{Ci})$, σ_i is the within-study variance and IG(a,b) is an inverse gamma distribution. The μ is assumed to follow a locally uniform prior distribution. When the conditional posterior distribution may be obtained in closed form as in this example, Gibbs sampling may be used to obtain the estimate of posterior mode. The conditional posterior distributions for the model in this example are as follows:

$$P(\theta_i|\mu, \sigma^2, \tau^2, \hat{\theta}, \hat{\sigma}^2, n) = N\left(\theta_i\left|\frac{\hat{\theta}_i n_i/\sigma_i^2 + \mu/\tau^2}{n_i/\sigma_i^2 + 1/\tau^2}, \frac{1}{n_i/\sigma_i^2 + 1/\tau^2}\right.\right)$$

$$P(\mu|\boldsymbol{\theta}, \sigma^2, \tau^2, \hat{\theta}, \hat{\sigma}^2, n) = N\left(\mu\left|\sum\theta_i/K, \tau^2/K\right.\right)$$

$$P(\sigma_i^2|\boldsymbol{\theta}, \mu, \tau^2, \hat{\theta}, \hat{\sigma}^2, n) = IG\left(\sigma_i^2|n_i, 2/[n_i\{(\hat{\theta}_i - \theta_i)^2 + \hat{\sigma}_i^2\}]\right)$$

where $i = 1, \cdots, K$, and

$$P(\tau^2 | \boldsymbol{\theta}, \mu, \boldsymbol{\sigma}^2, \hat{\boldsymbol{\theta}}, \hat{\boldsymbol{\sigma}}^2, \boldsymbol{n}) = IG\left(\tau^2 | K/2 + a, 2/\sum(\theta_i - \mu)^2 + b\right).$$

Then the marginal posterior distribution is estimated by sampling from each of the posterior conditional distributions, in turn conditioning on the current draw of the unknown model parameters. For the complete treatment of this example readers are referred to the original paper (Abrams and Sanso 1998).

6.5.1 WinBugs Example

The example 6.3.5 analyzed 42 trials of rosiglitazone using fixed and random-effect methods. The major issue in meta-analyzing these data is the high proportion of trials without a single event in either treatment arm. Such "zero studies" either must be excluded from the analyses or some form of continuity correction must be applied. Both of these remedies have potential for biasing the final result. Bayesian modeling techniques provide an efficient alternative which naturally accommodate sparse data. WinBugs is a powerful computational tool for Bayesian analyses which shifts the computational burden from analyst to computer. With help of the software program an analyst can focus on modeling aspects of the analyses without having to invest significant amount of effort on the computational details.

One of the adverse effects monitored in the rosiglitazone trials was the incidence of MI among the participants. Let r_{Ti} and r_{Ci} be the MI incidences among n_{Ti} and n_{Ci} participants randomized to treatment and to placebo, respectively. Further, assume that p_{Ti} and p_{Ci} are the probabilities of experiencing MI among participants in ith trial under treatment and placebo, respectively. The observed data may be modeled as follows under the Bayesian framework:

$$
\begin{aligned}
r_{Ti} &\sim binomial(p_{Ti}, n_{Ti}) \\
r_{Ci} &\sim binomial(p_{Ci}, n_{Ci}) \\
\mu_i &= logit(p_{Ci}) \\
logit(p_{Ti}) &= \mu_i + \theta_i \\
\theta_i &\sim N(\theta, \tau^2).
\end{aligned}
$$

The model presented above can be easily implemented in the WinBugs program (Warn et al. 2002). There are three components of the program: first, the model segment; second, the observed data; and third, initial values of the stochastic nodes. Together they form a complete program as follows:

```
model
{

    for (i in 1:k){
    r.c[i] ~ dbin(pi.c[i], n.c[i]);
    r.t[i] ~ dbin(pi.t[i], n.t[i]);
```

```
    mu[i] <- logit(pi.c[i]);
    logit(pi.t[i]) <- mu[i] + delta[i];
    delta[i] ~ dnorm(theta, precision.tau);
    pi.c[i] ~ dunif(0,1);
    }
theta ~ dnorm(0, 0.1);
precision.tau <- 1/(tau*tau);
tau ~ dunif(0, 2);
}


# data
list( n.t=c(357, 391, 774, 213, 232, 43, 121, 110, 382, 284,
294, 563, 278, 418, 395, 203, 104, 212, 138, 196, 122, 175, 56,
39, 561, 116, 148, 231, 89, 168, 116, 1172, 706, 204, 288, 254,
314, 162, 442, 394, 2635, 1456),
n.c =c( 176, 207, 185, 109, 116, 47, 124, 114, 384, 135, 302,
142, 279, 212, 198, 106, 99, 107, 139, 96, 120, 173,
58, 38, 276, 111, 143, 242, 88, 172, 61, 377, 325, 185,
280, 272, 154, 160, 112, 124, 2634, 2895),
r.t = c(2, 2, 1, 0, 1, 0, 1, 5, 1, 1, 0, 2, 2, 2, 2, 1, 1, 2, 3,
0, 0, 0, 1, 1, 0, 2, 1, 1, 1, 1, 0, 1, 0, 1, 1, 1, 1, 0,
1, 1, 15, 27),
r.c = c(0, 1, 1, 1, 0, 1, 0, 2, 0, 0, 1, 0, 1, 0, 1, 1, 2, 0, 1,
0, 1, 1, 0, 0, 2, 3, 0, 0, 0, 0, 0, 0, 0, 2, 0, 0, 0, 0,
0, 0, 9, 41), k=42)


# initial values
list( theta = 0.5, tau=0.01, pi.c = c(0.886, 0.483, 0.439,
0.191, 0.845, 0.187, 0.071, 0.025, 0.234, 0.522, 0.167, 0.812,
0.492, 0.196, 0.894, 0.759, 0.041, 0.917, 0.251, 0.139,
0.944, 0.775, 0.932, 0.273, 0.470, 0.813, 0.366, 0.184,
0.830, 0.834, 0.856, 0.941, 0.203, 0.391, 0.853, 0.358,
0.576, 0.781, 0.591, 0.004, 0.432, 0.335),
delta = c(0.004, 0.003, 0.001, 0.000, 0.004, 0.001, 0.000,
0.005, 0.001, 0.000, 0.002, 0.002, 0.001, 0.001, 0.004, 0.000,
0.001, 0.003, 0.001, 0.004, 0.004, 0.002, 0.003, 0.003, 0.001,
0.002, 0.001, 0.001, 0.001, 0.001, 0.003, 0.001, 0.004, 0.005,
0.002, 0.003, 0.003, 0.001, 0.002, 0.003, 0.003, 0.001)
```

The WinBugs program computes posterior distributions of parameters based on MCMC methods. Therefore, it is important to monitor convergence and adequate mixing of simulation using tools available in the program. After convergence, the posterior mode of each parameter can be calculated based on the posterior simulation discarding the burn-in runs. The posterior distributions of θ and τ (not τ^2) are displayed in Figure (6.3).

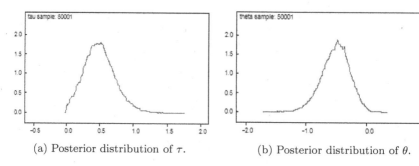

(a) Posterior distribution of τ.   (b) Posterior distribution of θ.

FIGURE 6.3: Posterior distributions of τ and θ.

TABLE 6.7: Bayesian Meta-Analyses of 42 Rosiglitazone Trials.

	Mean	2.5%	25%	50%	75%	97.5%
OR	0.613	0.395	0.536	0.617	0.713	0.905
τ^2	0.228	0.012	0.101	0.226	0.380	0.816

    The posterior estimate of combined odds ratio and heterogeneity from the above modeling is given in Table 6.7. The results in Table 6.7 show a posterior estimate of the odds ratio of 0.613 with 95% credible interval of (0.395, 0.904), which is markedly different from the moment-based estimators in Table 6.2. What could be the reason for such a dramatic discrepancy which essentially alters the conclusion in the opposite direction? An answer can be found in Figure 6.4. The figure displays the effect of changing parameters of the prior distribution of a probability of MI incidence for subjects randomized to placebo. At the population level it is a prevalence of MI in diabetic patents. The figure illustrates that the posterior log odds ratio remains below 0 as the prior becomes increasingly vague as is the case for the results in Table 6.7. However, one might argue that the prevalence of MI cannot possibly be higher than 0.1% and apply an informative prior of uniform(0, 0.01). Use of such prior results in a positive log odds ratio and is in closer agreement with the moment-based results. The figure essentially shows that if one is willing to bet *a priori* that the prevalence of MI is extremely rare, less than 6/1000, in a diabetic population, then the observed data support an elevated risk of MI among rosiglitazone users. In the absence of such prior information, the observed data do not support the conclusion obtained for the moment-based analyses.

    This example clearly demonstrates the effect of the prior distribution on the conclusion of the meta-analysis. One way to minimize such influence is to use a hierarchical Bayesian approach. In this approach a hyper-prior is placed on the prior distribution of p_c. Continuing with the rosiglitazone example, a *beta(a, b)* prior distribution may be used to model p_c and a *gamma(s, r)* hyper-prior may be placed on the parameters of the beta distribution. The fully Bayesian model now becomes:

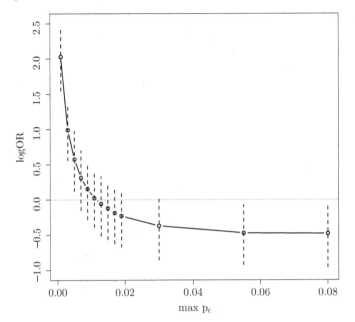

FIGURE 6.4: Posterior mean and 95% credible interval of θ
for varying upper limits of prior distribution of $p_c \sim unif(0, max\ p_c)$.

$$
\begin{aligned}
r_{Ti} &\sim binomial(p_{Ti}, n_{Ti}) \\
r_{Ci} &\sim binomial(p_{Ci}, n_{Ci}) \\
\mu_i &= logit(p_{Ci}) \\
logit(p_{Ti}) &= \mu_i + \theta_i \\
p_{Ci} &\sim beta(a, b) \\
\theta_i &\sim N(\theta, \tau^2) \\
a &\sim gamma(s, r) \\
b &\sim gamma(s, r)
\end{aligned}
$$

where, $gamma(s, r) = \frac{r^s}{\Gamma(s)} x^{s-1} e^{-rs}$ for $x > 0, r > 0$ and $s > 0$. The corresponding WinBugs model segment is written as follows:

```
model {
for (i in 1:k) {
r.c[i] ~ dbin(pi.c[i], n.c[i]);
r.t[i] ~ dbin(pi.t[i], n.t[i]);
```

```
mu[i] <- log(pi.c[i]);
log(pi.t[i]) <- mu[i] + delta[i];
delta[i] ~ dnorm(theta, precision.tau);
pi.c[i] ~ dbeta(alpha,beta);
}
theta ~ dnorm(0, 0.1);
alpha ~ dgamma(0.001,0.25);
beta ~ dgamma(1, 0.25);
precision.tau <- 1/(tau*tau);
tau ~ dunif(0, 2);
}.
```

Estimates obtained from the model are presented in Table 6.8 for different combinations of parameters of the gamma hyper-prior distribution. The posterior means of the log odds ratio are clearly more consistent between 0.11 (OR=1.12) and 0.16 (OR=1.17) over different specifications of hyper-prior distribution. These estimates of log odds ratio are closer to the estimates obtained from the moment-based methods. With regards to τ^2, it is interesting that the value decreases from 0.228 when p_{ic} were treated as independent to 0.06 when p_{ic} were treated as a sample from a common gamma distribution.

TABLE 6.8: Hierarchical Bayesian Analysis of 42 Rosiglitazone Trials Using Different Gamma Hyper-prior Distributions.

s	r	α mean	β mean	log odds ratio (θ) mean	2.5%	97.5%	τ^2 mean	2.5%	97.5%
0.01	6.787	0.411	32.95	0.145	-0.243	0.511	0.063	0.0002	0.523
0.002	15.283	0.484	49.39	0.150	-0.246	0.513	0.062	0.0001	0.587
0.006	10.386	0.445	39.84	0.129	-0.28	0.488	0.070	0.0001	0.546
0.003	5.412	0.391	29.647	0.146	-0.262	0.52	0.069	0.0001	0.618
0.001	1.215	0.353	22.137	0.126	-0.261	0.483	0.070	0.0003	0.621
0.007	5.667	0.398	30.499	0.154	-0.235	0.535	0.065	0.0001	0.627
0.006	1.718	0.35	22.657	0.146	-0.22	0.486	0.064	0.0001	0.635
0.006	6.167	0.404	31.747	0.128	-0.272	0.512	0.068	0.0001	0.702
0.003	16.076	0.488	50.308	0.145	-0.238	0.51	0.066	0.0002	0.578
0.004	6.577	0.409	32.398	0.142	-0.234	0.537	0.060	0.0001	0.624
0.466	7.875	0.423	35.107	0.130	-0.262	0.526	0.064	0.0001	0.615
3.812	1.437	0.406	25.133	0.113	-0.303	0.529	0.064	0.0000	0.517
3.411	5.974	0.453	34.192	0.110	-0.313	0.47	0.072	0.0002	0.616
3.316	11.691	0.511	44.916	0.103	-0.271	0.492	0.064	0.0000	0.496
2.699	19.686	0.57	59.036	0.118	-0.283	0.492	0.066	0.0001	0.477
2.08	2.013	0.385	24.722	0.126	-0.291	0.514	0.069	0.0001	0.530
2.362	9.968	0.483	41.096	0.105	-0.32	0.559	0.068	0.0001	0.581
0.862	4.548	0.4	29.092	0.123	-0.293	0.486	0.068	0.0003	0.593
4.067	14.267	0.544	50.355	0.104	-0.32	0.462	0.066	0.0001	0.584
2.667	0.321	0.373	21.696	0.134	-0.251	0.493	0.062	0.0000	0.656

6.6 Confidence Distribution Framework for Meta-analysis

Confidence distribution (CD) has its roots in Fisher's fiducial distribution theory. Although the history of CD is not new, its utility in modern statistical problems has not been fully explored. Recent interest in CD and its application is facilitated by the formal definition of CD by Schweder and Hjort (2002) and Singh et al. (2005). They defined a confidence distribution for a parameter θ as a function $H_n(\cdot) = H_n(\boldsymbol{X}_n, \cdot)$ on $\aleph \to [0, 1]$ such that (i) for each sample set $\boldsymbol{X}_n$ in the sample set space $\aleph$, $H_n(\cdot)$ is a continuous cumulative distribution function in the parameter space Θ; and (ii) at the true parameter value $\theta = \theta_0$, $H_n(\theta_0) = H_n(\boldsymbol{X}_n, \theta_0)$, as a function of sample set $\boldsymbol{X}_n$, has a uniform distribution $U(0, 1)$. The function $H_n(\cdot)$ is an asymptotic confidence distribution, if (ii) is met only asymptotically. Thus, a confidence distribution is a sample dependent distribution function on the parameter space that has desired frequentest properties. Although, the CD is not a distribution on θ, it contains a wealth of information on θ. In that sense CD is a frequentest's analog of the Bayesian posterior distribution. In the context of hypothesis testing of the form $H_0 : \theta \leq \theta_0$, $H_n(\theta_0)$ provides a p-value regardless of the value of θ_0. Conversely, any pair of confidence quantiles forms the confidence interval $(H_n^{-1}(\alpha_1)), H_n^{-1}(\alpha_2))$ with $\alpha_2 - \alpha_1$ degree of confidence.

The simplest and most direct way to construct a CD is through pivotal statistics. A pivot is a function of a sample $\boldsymbol{X}_n$, the parameter of interest, and some other known parameters, and does not involve any other unknown parameters. It's true CDF is generally analytically tractable and does not involve any unknown parameter. Suppose $Q(\boldsymbol{X}_n, \theta)$ is a such function and G_n is its continuous CDF. Then, the exact CD for θ is given by (Singh et al. 2005, see):

$$H_n(x) = \begin{cases} G_n(Q(\boldsymbol{X}_n, \theta)), & \text{if } Q \text{ is increasing in } \theta \\ 1 - G_n(Q(\boldsymbol{X}_n, \theta)), & \text{if } Q \text{ is decreasing in } \theta \ . \end{cases} \quad (6.70)$$

Example 1: Normal mean and known variance.

Consider estimation of the population mean for the normal distribution with mean μ and known variance σ^2. The standard pivot is $Q(\boldsymbol{X}_n, \mu) = \frac{\bar{X}_n - \mu}{\sigma/\sqrt{n}}$, which has the standard normal CDF, Φ. Using the substitution scheme given in (6.70), the CD for μ is

$$H_n(x) = 1 - \Phi\left(\frac{\bar{\boldsymbol{X}}_n - x}{\sigma/\sqrt{n}}\right) = \Phi\left(\frac{x - \bar{\boldsymbol{X}}_n}{\sigma/\sqrt{n}}\right). \quad (6.71)$$

Example 2: Normal mean and unknown variance.

When the population variance is unknown, a standard pivot is $Q(\boldsymbol{X}_n, \mu) = \frac{\bar{\boldsymbol{X}}_n - \mu}{s_n/\sqrt{n}}$, where s_n is a sample standard deviation. The pivot has Students t-distribution with $n - 1$ degrees of freedom. Following the method in (6.70), the CD for μ can be expressed as:

$$H_n(x) = 1 - P\left(T_{n-1} \leq \frac{\bar{\boldsymbol{X}}_n - x}{s_n/\sqrt{n}}\right) = P\left(T_{n-1} \leq \frac{x - \bar{\boldsymbol{X}}_n}{s_n/\sqrt{n}}\right); \qquad (6.72)$$

where $T_{n-1} \sim t_{df} = n - 1$.

For σ^2, the usual pivot is $Q(\boldsymbol{X}_n, \sigma^2) = (n-1)s_n^2/\sigma^2$ that has χ_{n-1}^2 distribution. Using the above substitution method, the CD for σ^2 is

$$H_n(x) = P\left(\chi_{n-1}^2 \geq (n-1)s_n^2/x^2\right), \quad x \geq 0 \qquad (6.73)$$

where χ_{n-1}^2 is a random variable that has the χ_{n-1}^2 distribution.

6.6.1   The Framework

A unifying framework for meta-analysis through combining CDs from individual studies was proposed by Xie et al. (2011). In contrast to the traditional meta-analysis where a combined estimate is obtained from weighted individual point estimates, the combined confidence distribution function is obtained by appropriately weighting the individual distribution estimators. In doing so, the combined CD achieves various optimality conditions depending on the characteristics of the weights used for combining individual CDs.

A general framework for meta-analysis involves the following recipe for CD combination. Suppose $H_i(\theta) = H_i(\boldsymbol{X}_i, \theta)$, $i = 1, \ldots, k$ are CD functions for the parameter θ from k independent samples $\boldsymbol{X}_i$ with sample size n_i. A combined confidence distribution function (H_c) is constructed as

$$H_c = G_c\{g_c(H_1(\theta), \ldots, H_k(\theta))\}, \qquad (6.74)$$

where $g_c(u_1, \ldots, u_k) = w_1 F_0^{-1}(u_1) + \ldots + w_k F_0^{-1}(u_k)$ is a monotonic function that has cumulative distribution function $G_c(t) = P(g_c(U_1, \ldots, U_k) \leq t)$ for $U_i \sim U[0, 1]$. The cumulative distribution functions $F_0(\cdot)$ are weighted by fixed positive weights $w_i \geq 0$. The recipe (6.74) encompasses most commonly used meta-analysis approaches in this chapter.

6.6.1.1   Fixed-effects Model

A fixed-effects model assumes that individuals in a study are an independent sample from the population sharing the same parameter. Thus, a parameter estimate from each study is a realization from a population of study estimates. The parameter estimates from k studies are assumed to follow an asymptotic normal distribution. Let θ be the central parameter of interest and $\hat{\theta}_i$ is the estimate from the *ith* independent study. Thus,

$$\hat{\theta}_i \sim N(\theta, \sigma_i^2). \tag{6.75}$$

Under the fixed-effects model assumption, the pivot for the *ith* study is

$$Q(\boldsymbol{X}_n, \theta) = \frac{\hat{\theta}_i - \theta}{\sigma_i}.$$

As σ_i is assumed known, $Q(\boldsymbol{X}_n, \theta) \sim N(0, 1)$. Thus, following the equation (6.70), the CD function from the *ith* study is

$$H_i(\theta) = 1 - \Phi\left(\frac{\hat{\theta}_i - \theta}{\sigma_i}\right) = \Phi\left(\frac{\theta - \hat{\theta}_i}{\sigma_i}\right).$$

Then, a combined CD function can be constructed by taking $F_0(t) = \Phi(t)$ and $w_i = 1/\sigma_i$ in (6.74). Such that,

$$g(H_1(\theta) + \ldots + H_k(\theta)) = \frac{1}{\sigma_1}\Phi^{-1}(H_1(\theta)) + \ldots + \frac{1}{\sigma_k}\Phi^{-1}(H_k(\theta)).$$

As $\sum_{i=1}^{k} \frac{1}{\sigma_i}\Phi^{-1}(H_i(\theta)) \sim N\left(0, \sum_{i=1}^{k}\frac{1}{\sigma_k^2}\right)$ implies $G_c(t) = \Phi\left(\frac{t}{\sqrt{\sum_{i=1}^{k}\frac{1}{\sigma_i^2}}}\right)$,

$$H_c(\theta) = \Phi\left\{\frac{\frac{1}{\sigma_1}\Phi^{-1}\left(\Phi\left(\frac{\theta-\hat{\theta}_1}{\sigma_1}\right)\right) + \ldots + \frac{1}{\sigma_k}\Phi^{-1}\left(\Phi\left(\frac{\theta-\hat{\theta}_k}{\sigma_k}\right)\right)}{\left(\sum_{i=1}^{k}\frac{1}{\sigma_i^2}\right)^{1/2}}\right\} \tag{6.76}$$

$$= \Phi\left(\frac{\sum_{i=1}^{k}\frac{\theta-\hat{\theta}_i}{\sigma_i^2}}{\left(\sum_{i=1}^{k}\frac{1}{\sigma_i^2}\right)^{1/2}}\right) = \Phi\left\{\left(\sum_{i=1}^{k}\frac{1}{\sigma_i^2}\right)^{1/2}\left(\theta - \frac{\sum_{i=1}^{k}\hat{\theta}_i/\sigma_i^2}{\sum_{i=1}^{k}1/\sigma_i^2}\right)\right\} \tag{6.77}$$

Equation (6.77) allows the estimation of θ by a normal CD function that has mean $\frac{\sum_{i=1}^{k}\hat{\theta}_i/\sigma_i^2}{\sum_{i=1}^{k}1/\sigma_i^2}$ and variance $\left(\sum_{i=1}^{k}1/\sigma_i^2\right)^{-1}$. Note that these expressions match exactly with the ones in the equation (6.1).

6.6.1.2 Random-effects Model

As described in the Section 6.3, the random-effects model assumes that $\hat{\theta}_i|(\theta_i, \sigma_i^2) \sim N(\theta_i, \sigma_i^2)$ and $\theta_i|(\theta, \tau^2) \sim N(\theta, \tau^2)$, which together leads to $\hat{\theta}_i \sim N(\theta_i, \sigma_i^2 + \tau^2)$ and the following CD for the *ith* study

$$H_i(\theta) = 1 - \Phi\left(\frac{\hat{\theta}_i - \theta}{(\sigma_i^2 + \tau^2)^{1/2}}\right) = \Phi\left(\frac{\theta - \hat{\theta}_i}{(\sigma_i^2 + \tau^2)^{1/2}}\right).$$

Following the derivation in the Section 6.6.1.1 and substituting $w_i = 1/(\sigma_i^2 + \tau^2)^{1/2}$, the combined CD function for random-effects model is given by

$$H_c(\theta) = \Phi \left\{ \left(\sum_{i=1}^{k} \frac{1}{\sigma_i^2 + \tau^2} \right)^{1/2} \left(\theta - \frac{\sum_{i=1}^{k} \hat{\theta}_i/(\sigma_i^2 + \tau^2)}{\sum_{i=1}^{k} 1/(\sigma_i^2 + \tau^2)} \right) \right\},$$

where the mean of combined CD function is $\hat{\theta}_c = \frac{\sum_{i=1}^{k} w_i \hat{\theta}_i}{\sum_{i=1}^{k} w_i}$ and the variance is $\left(\sum_{i=1}^{k} \frac{1}{\sigma_i^2 + \tau^2} \right)^{-1}$. These expressions match equations (6.33) and (6.34) given in the Section 6.3.

Example

The withdrawal of rofecoxib (vioxx) has raised the safety concerns about a potential class effect of cyclooxygenase-2 (COX-2) inhibitors (coxib) and all non-steroidal anti-inflammatory drugs (NSAIDs). Chen and Ashcroft (2007) assessed the risk of MI for all coxibs in the meta-analysis of 38 trials (82,489 patients). As a part of the assessment, they compared all coxibs against non-selective NSAIDs. Table 6.9 contains the cases of MI reported in those trials. The Trials were identified by searching MEDLINE, EMBASE, the Cochrane Database of Systematic Reviews, and the Cochrane Central Register of Controlled Trials. They included trials of coxibs that had been licensed in the UK or US (celecoxib, rofecoxib, valdecoxib, parecoxib, etoricoxib, and lumiracoxib).

The forest plot in Figure 6.5 shows the number of MI events and sample size in each study included in the analysis. A continuity correction of 0.5 was added to treatment arms with a 0 event. The odds ratio estimate of MI comparing Coxibs against NSAIDs is also shown in the figure. Both fixed-effect (OR=1.49, 95% CI: $1.14 - 1.95$) and random-effect (OR=1.44, 95% CI: $1.08 - 1.93$) estimates indicate elevated risk of MI associated with Coxibs compared to NASAIDs. The near identical estimates between fixed- and random-effects estimate is expected as there was no evidence of heterogeneity among the trials ($I^2 = 0.00\%$, p-value for heterogeneity=0.87).

The figure 6.6 shows confidence densities of log odds ratio estimates from eight randomly chosen trials along with the combined confidence density. Table 6.9 lists mean and median log odds ratios, standard deviations, and 95% confidence intervals estimated from the confidence distribution of individual trials. It also shows the corresponding quantities estimated from the combined confidence distribution of the estimates from the 38 trials. The combined odds ratio estimate obtained from CD approach is 1.44 with 95% CI: $1.08 - 1.93$. These estimates are identical to the random-effect estimates obtained from the traditional method because CD approach also utilizes an inverse variance weighted estimate (see (6.77)).

TABLE 6.9: Fixed-Effects CD Estimates of θ and the Corresponding 95% CIs.

Study	mean	median	stddev	LCL	UCL
1	-0.420	-0.420	1.734	-3.818	2.978
2	0.000	0.000	1.733	-3.397	3.397
3	2.367	2.367	1.501	-0.575	5.309
4	0.704	0.704	1.734	-2.694	4.102
5	-0.433	-0.433	1.734	-3.831	2.966
6	-0.011	-0.011	1.417	-2.788	2.766
7	0.265	0.265	1.583	-2.838	3.367
8	1.610	1.610	1.049	-0.446	3.666
9	0.690	0.690	1.736	-2.713	4.092
10	0.551	0.551	0.325	-0.086	1.188
11	-0.687	-0.687	1.734	-4.086	2.712
12	-0.704	-0.704	1.733	-4.101	2.694
13	-0.167	-0.167	0.674	-1.488	1.154
14	0.051	0.051	1.735	-3.348	3.451
15	0.473	0.473	0.383	-0.278	1.225
16	0.004	0.004	1.736	-3.398	3.406
17	0.038	0.038	1.743	-3.378	3.454
18	0.587	0.587	0.395	-0.187	1.361
19	-0.332	-0.332	0.586	-1.481	0.816
20	-0.005	-0.005	1.734	-3.403	3.392
21	-0.703	-0.703	1.416	-3.479	2.073
22	-0.050	-0.050	1.734	-3.448	3.349
23	-0.004	-0.004	1.734	-3.403	3.394
24	-0.330	-0.330	1.003	-2.296	1.637
25	-1.417	-1.417	1.734	-4.816	1.981
26	-0.659	-0.659	1.003	-2.624	1.307
27	-0.007	-0.007	1.227	-2.412	2.399
28	1.109	1.109	1.157	-1.159	3.376
29	-1.113	-1.113	1.736	-4.516	2.290
30	1.705	1.705	0.544	0.638	2.771
31	1.606	1.606	1.096	-0.541	3.754
32	0.661	0.661	1.733	-2.737	4.058
33	-2.999	-2.999	1.485	-5.910	-0.088
34	1.026	1.026	1.462	-1.840	3.892
35	0.293	0.293	1.583	-2.810	3.396
36	-1.047	-1.047	1.416	-3.823	1.729
37	-1.399	-1.399	1.583	-4.501	1.703
38	-0.706	-0.706	1.416	-3.482	2.070
combined CD	0.368	0.368	0.147	0.079	0.656

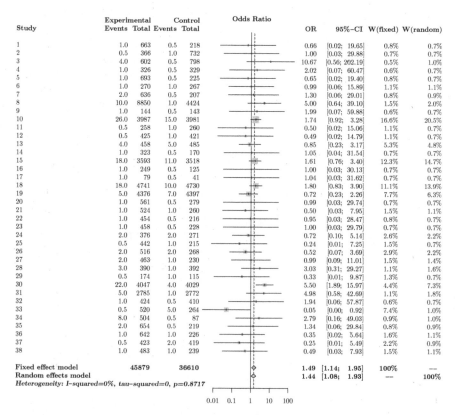

FIGURE 6.5: Assessment of MI risk of Coxib vs. NSAID using traditional moment-based meta-analysis methods.

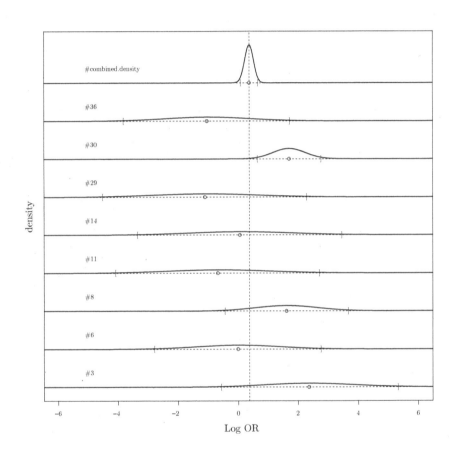

FIGURE 6.6: Fixed-effects CD estimates of θ. Only eight randomly selected studies are shown.

6.6.2 Meta-analysis of Rare Events under the CD Framework

Rare event studies present some unique challenges for traditional meta-analysis methods. A zero event in either or the both treatment arms of a study either necessitates continuity correction or renders the study noninformative. A few different approaches for determining an appropriate continuity correction have been suggested in the literature. However, there is little consensus regarding this issue. The CD framework provides a way to combine all of the rare event studies, including studies with zero event on both treatment arms. The method was developed by Tian et al. (2009) and Liu et al. (2014) for risk difference and odds ratio measures, respectively.

Liu et al. (2014) use exact p-value functions as the CD functions for individual studies and combine them by applying the general CD combination method. Suppose Ψ is the parameter of central interest and a hypothesis of interest is

$$H_0 : \Psi = \Psi^* vs. H_1 > \Psi^*.$$

The p-value function $p(\Psi)$ is a function derived from varying the value of Ψ^* in the parameter space of Ψ. The formal definition of the p-value for the given observations is:

$$p(\Psi; \boldsymbol{X}_n) = \mathbb{P}(T \geq t | \Psi^*), \qquad (6.78)$$

where T is a pivot statistic that has a distribution function $F(T)$, and t is a realized value computed from sample $\boldsymbol{X}_n$. If Ψ^0 is the true value of Ψ, then

$$p(\Psi^0; \boldsymbol{X}_n) = \mathbb{P}(T \geq t | \Psi^0) = 1 - \mathbb{P}(T \leq t | \Psi^0) = 1 - F_0(t), \qquad (6.79)$$

where F_0 is the distribution of T under the null hypothesis. As distribution function implies F_0 to be at least left-continuous, it follows that $\mathbb{P}(T \geq t | \Psi^0) = \mathbb{P}(F_0(T) \geq F_0(t))$. Thus, equation (6.79) can be written as follows:

$$\begin{aligned} \mathbb{P}(T \geq t | \Psi^0) = \mathbb{P}(F_0(T) \geq F_0(t) | \Psi^0) &= 1 - F_0(t) \\ \mathbb{P}(F_0(T) \leq F_0(t) | \Psi^0) &= F_0(t). \end{aligned} \qquad (6.80)$$

Equation (6.80) implies that $F_0(T)$ follows a uniform distribution. This also implies that $1 - F_0(T)$ is uniformly distributed. Thus, $p(\Psi; \boldsymbol{X}_n)$ is uniformly distributed under the null hypothesis. Therefore, the p-value function is a valid confidence distribution.

The p-value function proposed for combining rare event studies is based on mid-p adaptation of Fisher's exact test for the odds ratio. Using this exact test, the p-value function for the odds ratio Ψ is obtained as follows (see Liu et al. 2014) :

$$p_i(\Psi) \equiv p_i(\Psi; x_{Ti}, x_{Ti}) = Pr_\Psi(X_{Ti} > x_{Ti} | T_i = t_i) + \frac{1}{2} Pr_\Psi(X_{Ti} = x_{Ti} | T_i = t_i), \qquad (6.81)$$

where X_{Ti} is assumed to follow a hypergeometric distribution conditional on $T_i = X_{Ti} + X_{Ci}$. Then for $L_i = max(0, t_i - n_{Ci})$ and $U_i = min(n_{Ti}, t_i)$, it follows that

$$Pr_{\Psi}(X_{Ti} = x_{Ti} | T_i = t_i) = \frac{\binom{n_{Ti}}{x_{Ti}} \binom{n_{Ci}}{t_i - x_{Ti}} \Psi^{x_{Ti}}}{\sum_{s=L_i}^{U_i} \binom{n_{Ti}}{s} \binom{n_{Ci}}{t_i - s} \Psi^s}, \quad L_i \leq x_{Ti} \leq U_i.$$

(6.82)

The statistic $p_i(\Psi^0)$ asymptotically follows $U(0, 1)$. However, asymptotically, the probability of having zero events in any study is zero. Additionally, for rare events the deviation of $p_i(\Psi^0)$ from $U(0, 1)$ can be substantial. Nonetheless, Liu et al. (2014) justified using the general idea of a CD combining algorithm in the finite sample setting by providing a way to adjust type I error rate and guidelines for selecting weights that increase the combination efficiency. They also showed that not only can zero events studies be included in this approach, but also they contribute meaningfully by increasing uncertainty in the overall inference outcome.

The impact of zero studies is appropriately adjusted for the sample size of the corresponding studies by using the weights

$$w_i \propto \left[\{n_{Ti}\pi_{Ti}(1 - \pi_{Ti})\}^{-1} + \{n_{Ci}\pi_{Ci}(1 - \pi_{Ci})\}^{-1} \right]^{-1/2}.$$

(6.83)

The w_is require the estimates of π_{Ci} and π_{Ti}. The simple estimate of these probabilities using sample proportions are not stable for the rare events. Liu et al. (2014) proposed to model π_{Ci} using the beta distribution $Beta(\beta_1, \beta_2)$. The parameters of this beta distribution are estimated as follows:

$$(\hat{\beta}_1, \hat{\beta}_2, \hat{\Psi}) = \arg\max_{\beta_1, \beta_2, \Psi} \sum_{i=1}^{k} Log \int_0^1 f_{\psi}(x_{Ci}, x_{Ti} | \pi_{Ci}) f_{\beta_1, \beta_2}(\pi_{Ci}) d\pi_{Ci}, \quad (6.84)$$

where $f_{\beta_1,\beta_2}(\pi_{Ci}) = \pi_{Ci}^{\beta_1 - 1}(1 - \pi_{Ci})^{\beta_2 - 1} / \int_1^0 \pi_{Ci}^{\beta_1 - 1}(1 - \pi_{Ci})^{\beta_2 - 1} d(x_{Ci})$, $f_{\psi}(x_{Ci}, x_{Ti}|\pi_{Ci}) = c(x_{Ci}, x_{Ti})\pi_{Ci}^{x_{Ci}}(1 - \pi_{Ci})^{n_{Ci} - x_{Ci}}\pi_{Ti}^{x_{Ti}}(1 - \pi_{Ti})^{n_{Ti} - x_{Ti}}$, and $\pi_{Ti} = (\Psi\pi_{Ci})/(1 - \pi_{Ci} + \Psi\pi_{Ci})$. The empirical conditional density of π_{Ci} is obtained by substituting the estimates $(\hat{\beta}_1, \hat{\beta}_2, \hat{\Psi})$ for the corresponding parameters in $f_{\beta_1,\beta_2,\Psi}(\pi_{Ci}|x_{Ci}, x_{Ti}) \propto f_{\hat{\psi}}(x_{Ci}, x_{Ti}|\pi_{Ci})f_{\hat{\beta}_1,\hat{\beta}_2}(\pi_{Ci})$ whose mean is taken as the estimate $\hat{\pi}_{Ci}$ of π_{Ci}. Consequently, $\hat{\pi}_{Ti} = (\Psi\pi_{Ci})/(1 - \hat{\pi}_{Ci} + \hat{\Psi}\hat{\pi}_{Ti})$. This estimation approach produces non-zero estimates of π_{Ti} and π_{Ci} even when $x_{Ti} = x_{Ci} = 0$ for the *ith* study. This particular characteristic of the estimation procedure allows inclusion of zero-event studies without continuity correction. In the situation of $x_{Ti} = 0 \ \forall i$, limiting weights are used. These weights are calculated for $\lim_{\hat{\Psi} \to 0}$ as follows:

$$\lim_{\hat{\Psi} \to 0} \left(w_i / \sum_{i=1}^{k} w_i \right)^2 = \frac{n_{Ci}x_{Ci}/(1 - x_{Ci})}{\sum_{i=1}^{k} n_{Ci}x_{Ci}/(1 - x_{Ci})}.$$

The case where $x_{Ci} = 0 \; \forall i$ is handled similarly.

Example

The Coxibs vs. NSAIDs example data contain 15 trials that have zero events on the NSAID arm and 7 trials that have zero event on the Coxib arm. The 15 trials do not yield any information on the magnitude of event rates in the NSAIDs group. Similarly, the 7 trials do not yield any information on the magnitude of event rates in the Coxib group. Thus, the first set of trials lacks any information on how large the odds ratio is and the second set of trials lacks any information on how small the odds ratio is. The lack of such information is reflected in the corresponding confidence curves in the Figure 6.7. For example, trial 16 has zero events in the NSAID arm and provides no information on how large the odds ratio is. Therefore, the upper confidence interval for the log odds ratio goes to ∞. Whereas trial 25 has zero events in the Coxibs arm and provides no information on how small the odds ratio is. Therefore, the lower confidence interval for the log odds ratio goes to $-\infty$. The mean and median log odds ratios, standard deviations, and 95% confidence interval estimates based on exact CD are listed in the Table 6.10. The combined CD estimate of $\theta = 0.527$ (95% CI=0.23 0.83) is also shown in the table (OR=1.694).

6.7 Discussion

The methods covered in this chapter all have their respective strengths and weaknesses. However, most display undesirable characteristics when applied to studies with extremely low event rates as is commonly the case in drug safety. In such cases, the moment-based methods are biased, the MML methods are under powered and the Bayesian methods are highly dependent on choice of prior distribution. A possible alternative, for combining homogeneous effect sizes, is an exact method. It is computationally intensive, but provides inference based on the exact distribution of observations without having to make asymptotic assumptions. Several commercial computer programs, e.g., StatXact, SAS, STATA, etc., are available for exact meta-analysis. Recently, there has been new developments based on the concept of confidence distribution. It has unified different meta-analytic approaches under the idea of fiducial inference (Xie et al. 2011). For rare event studies, it has an attractive feature of not requiring arbitrary continuity correction. In addition, it is capable of dealing with highly outlying studies by incorporating a set of data dependent adaptive weights. However, rigorous evaluation of the CD based method is lacking for rare events in the presence of treatment effect heterogeneity (τ^2). The R-package *gmeta* is freely available from http://stat.rutgers.edu/home/gyang/researches/gmetaRpackage/ which implements this unifying framework for meta-analysis. It is incumbent on analysts to be mindful of available methods and their properties when conducting meta-analysis of drug safety data.

TABLE 6.10: Summary of Individual and Combined Confidence Curves Based on Exact CD Method

	mean	median	stddev	95% LCL	95% UCL
study-01	∞	∞	∞	-4.060	∞
study-02	$-\infty$	$-\infty$	∞	$-\infty$	3.6376
study-03	∞	∞	∞	0.176	∞
study-04	∞	∞	∞	-2.935	∞
study-05	∞	∞	∞	-4.074	∞
study-06	-0.010	-0.011	1.632	-3.669	3.6559
study-07	∞	∞	∞	-2.368	∞
study-08	1.605	1.489	1.109	-0.176	4.6965
study-09	∞	∞	∞	-2.951	∞
study-10	0.551	0.547	0.327	-0.081	1.2117
study-11	$-\infty$	$-\infty$	∞	$-\infty$	2.9522
study-12	$-\infty$	$-\infty$	∞	$-\infty$	2.9350
study-13	-0.169	-0.160	0.696	-1.604	1.2121
study-14	∞	∞	∞	-3.585	∞
study-15	0.474	0.468	0.387	-0.276	1.2585
study-16	∞	∞	∞	-3.632	∞
study-17	∞	∞	∞	-3.599	∞
study-18	0.588	0.580	0.399	-0.182	1.4011
study-19	-0.334	-0.323	0.600	-1.571	0.8424
study-20	∞	∞	∞	-3.642	∞
study-21	-0.652	-0.702	1.631	-4.366	2.9645
study-22	∞	∞	∞	-3.686	∞
study-23	∞	∞	∞	-3.641	∞
study-24	-0.328	-0.329	1.078	-2.595	1.9384
study-25	$-\infty$	$-\infty$	∞	$-\infty$	2.2237
study-26	-0.656	-0.658	1.077	-2.921	1.6090
study-27	0.022	-0.068	1.360	-2.590	3.3819
study-28	1.110	1.022	1.261	-1.136	4.3819
study-29	$-\infty$	$-\infty$	∞	$-\infty$	2.5303
study-30	1.710	1.673	0.553	0.704	2.9270
study-31	1.592	1.501	1.175	-0.372	4.7760
study-32	∞	∞	∞	-2.978	∞
study-33	$-\infty$	$-\infty$	∞	$-\infty$	-0.8859
study-34	∞	∞	∞	-0.968	∞
study-35	∞	∞	∞	-2.342	∞
study-36	-0.967	-1.045	1.631	-4.713	2.6209
study-37	$-\infty$	$-\infty$	∞	$-\infty$	1.2347
study-38	-0.655	-0.705	1.631	-4.369	2.9619
Combined CD	0.527	0.527	0.154	0.230	0.835

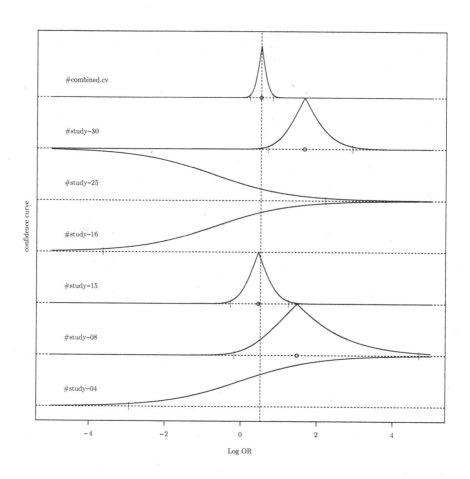

FIGURE 6.7: Plot of confidence curves of six randomly selected trials and combined confidence curves based on exact CD method. The confidence curve is calculated as $cv = 1 - 2|H(\Psi) - 0.5|$.

7

Ecological Methods

"Literature is my legal wife and medicine my mistress. When I get tired of one, I spend the night with the other."
(Anton Pavlovich Chekhov (1860-1904), Russian author, playwright)

7.1 Introduction

Ecological methods investigate group level aggregate data. These methods are motivated mainly due to the relative low cost and convenience of the data, limited availability of individual-level data, design limitations of individual studies, interest in ecologic effect, and simplicity of analysis and presentation (Morgenstern 1995). For very rare events (e.g., death by suicide) that occur at rates on the order of 1 in 10,000, there may be few options for routine drug surveillance. One approach is to use ecological data that attempt to relate changes in prescription rates of particular drugs or classes of drugs to the AE rate of interest. These more global associations clearly do not support causal inferences, but can be hypothesis generating and help support inferences drawn from other studies, in some cases based on surrogate endpoints (e.g., suicide attempts and/or ideation). In some cases, natural experiments such as a black box warning provide an opportunity to evaluate the positive or negative consequences of decreased access to the drug on the event of interest. Here we may compare national rates of the AE before and after the public health warning, to determine if the warning has had the anticipated effect. If the warning is specific to a strata of the population, comparison of changes in that strata versus those for which the warning did not apply provides stronger inferences.

The traditional approach to ecological analysis typically involves either log-linear or Poisson regression analysis of rates over time, using exposure based on prescription rates during the same time-period. Serial correlation can be accommodated using Huber-White robust standard errors that allow for arbitrary autocorrelation pattern (Huber 1967, White 1980, 1982). Where data from multiple countries are combined, both fixed-effects (Ludwig and Marcotte 2005) and random-effects models (Hedeker and Gibbons 2006) can be used to allow each country to have its own linear time trend. For the fixed-effects log-linear model, weighted least squares can be used to adjust for heterogeneity in the residual errors, using each country's population as a weight. A similar approach can be taken using a mixed-effects Poisson regression model where each country's population is used as an offset (see Hedeker and Gibbons 2006).

A more informative approach was suggested by Goldsmith et al. (2002) in which AE rates are stratified by demographic characteristics such as age, race, and sex within counties, and a mixed-effects Poisson regression model is used to analyze the data, treating the county as the unit of analysis. County population is used as an offset in the Poisson regression model. To evaluate drug-AE interactions, county-level prescription rates of the drug or drugs can be added to the model to determine if changes in prescription rates are associated with changes in the AE rate. When longitudinal data are available, we can tease apart between-county effects from within-county effects by expressing prescription rates as two variables, one of the mean over time and the other for the yearly deviations from the mean (also see Chapter 10). The former provides an estimate of the between-county effect whereas the latter provides an estimate of the within-county effect. Both within-county drug effect can be treated as a random-effect in the model, so that the relationship between prescription rates and AE rates can vary from county to county (i.e., treatment heterogeneity). The methodology has been described in detail by Gibbons et al. (2005, 2006).

7.2 Time Series Methods

Post marketing surveillance of therapeutic drugs involves continuous monitoring of safety data over a period of time. A sequence of data points, typically rate of adverse events per unit utilization of drugs at the population level, are aggregated at successive fixed time intervals (e.g., each quarter). These aggregate data represent the average incidence of adverse events during a particular time period. Time series data are naturally generated when drugs are monitored for safety outside the controlled environment of clinical trials.

Let y_t be the number of ADR cases observed over t^{th} time interval. Assume, that the drug utilization during the tth time period is n_t. The drug utilization can be measured directly as the number of individuals exposed to the drug, or using other proxy measures such as number of pills dispensed, number of prescriptions written, number of patients with a relevant condition, etc. Obviously, the validity of estimates and inference of safety depends on the accuracy and relevance of such proxy measures.

The visual display of rates over the monitoring period provides valuable insight into the trends of ADRs. Since 1990, numerous jurisdictions in the United States (US) have reported increases in drug poisoning mortality. Dur-

ing the same time period, the use of opioid analgesics has increased markedly
as part of more aggressive pain management. The study by Paulozzi et al.
(2006) documented a dramatic increase in poisoning mortality rates. Figure
7.1 is the time series plot of unintentional opioid drug poisoning mortality
rates from 1979 to 1998. The figure shows increasing trend in mortality rate
related to opioid poisoning. In this example, the trend is clearly visible without any further statistical aids. Smoothing techniques are used when trends
are not apparent. A common method for obtaining the trend is to use linear filters on a given time series. A simple class of linear filters are moving
averages with equal weights:

$$T_t = \frac{1}{2a+1} \sum_{i=-a}^{a} y_{t+i}.$$

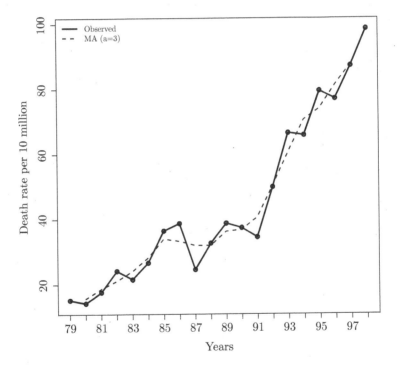

FIGURE 7.1: Unintentional opiate drug poisoning mortality rate.

The filtered value of a time series at a given period t is represented by
the average of the values $\{y_{t-a}, \ldots, y_t, \ldots, y_{t+a}\}$. The smoothed line obtained
by the moving average is more helpful in visualizing trends when high resolu-
tion data are available. Regression models can also be used to fit parametric

models to time series data. A natural candidate model for the time series of counts taking non-negative integer values is the Poisson regression. The Poisson regression model for the event count on the tth time period is

$$ln(\lambda_t) = ln(exposure_t) + \beta_1 t + \boldsymbol{\beta}' \boldsymbol{x}_t, \qquad (7.1)$$

where $\boldsymbol{\beta}$ is a vector of regression coefficients, and $\boldsymbol{x}_t$ is a vector of covariates. The parameters of the model (7.1) are easily estimated by likelihood methods. The model can be used to estimate deterministic trend in the observed data as in Figure 7.2. However, the model is not appropriate for inference because the model requires observations to be i.i.d Poisson random variable. Time series data most certainly violate the i.i.d assumption. The successive observations are more likely to be correlated in time series data that induces over- or under-dispersion in count data. Methods have been developed to allow for both over- or under-dispersion in the Poisson model.

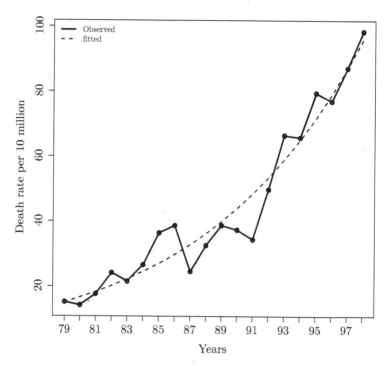

FIGURE 7.2: Unintentional opiate drug poisoning mortality rate.

7.2.1 Generalized Event Count Model

The time series count data in ecological investigation of drug safety are seldom serially correlated. However, the count data are either under- or over-dispersed. Over-dispersion arises due to unobserved heterogeneity and contagion effects. In such situations, pure time series methods may not be necessary to model the count data. When the nature of dispersion is known, a specific distribution can be used to allow such dispersion. For example, a negative-binomial model is used to allow for over-dispersion. Under-dispersion, on the other hand, can occur due to a negative contagion. Truncated event count models with a reparameterized binomial distribution is a possible alternative to deal with under-dispersion. In order to choose an appropriate model, one needs to conduct a test to determine the type of dispersion. Furthermore, the incorrect choice among the different alternatives can lead to inconsistency as well as inefficiency. The generalized event count distribution overcomes the model selection issue. The generalized event count distribution is a two parameter probability distribution with the following log-likelihood function (King 1989):

$$lnL(\lambda_i, \sigma^2 | y_i) = C_i - y_i ln(\sigma^2) + \sum_{j=1}^{y_i} ln[\lambda_i + (\sigma^2 - 1)(j - 1)], \qquad (7.2)$$

where

$$C_i = \begin{cases} -e_i^\lambda & \text{for } \sigma^2 = 1 \\ -e_i^\lambda ln(\sigma^2)(\sigma^2 - 1)^{-1} & \text{for } \sigma^2 > 1 \\ -e_i^\lambda ln(\sigma^2)(\sigma^2 - 1)^{-1} - ln(D_i) & \text{for } 0 < \sigma^2 < 1, \end{cases}$$

$$D_i = \sum_{m=0}^{\left(\frac{-\lambda_i}{\sigma^2-1}+1\right)} \frac{\Gamma\left(\frac{-\lambda_i}{\sigma^2-1}+1\right)}{y_i! \Gamma\left(\frac{-\lambda_i}{\sigma^2-1}-y_i+1\right)} (1-\sigma^2)^{y_i}(\sigma^2)^{\frac{-\lambda_i}{\sigma^2-1}-y_i}.$$

The maximization of this log likelihood function with respect to the two parameters gives estimates of λ and σ^2 without specifying whether the data are over-, under-, or Poisson dispersed. The log-likelihood in (7.2) reduces to a Poisson log-likelihood for $\sigma^2 = 1$, to a negative-binomial for $\sigma^2 > 1$, and to a reparameterized binomial for $0 < \sigma^2 < 1$. Regression parameters, as usual, are estimated by modeling $\lambda_i = exp(x_i'\beta)$.

7.2.2 Tests of Serial Correlation

As indicated in the previous section, in the absence of serial correlation, a static regression with variance adjusted for over- or under-dispersion is adequate for both estimation and inference. Formal hypothesis testing methods are available to ascertain significance of the observed serial correlation. These tests can indicate if any time series corrections are necessary. Let z_t denote the standardized residual from a static Poisson regression model such that $z_t = \frac{y_t - \lambda_t}{\sqrt{w_t}}$, where $\lambda_t = \lambda(\boldsymbol{x}_t, \boldsymbol{\beta}), w_t = (\lambda_t, \alpha)$, and α is a dispersion parameter. The residuals are standardized so that z_t have asymptotically constant variance. Following Box-Jenkins modeling in the continuous case, the estimated autocorrelation $\hat{\rho}_k$ at lag k is given by (Cameron and Trivedi 2013):

$$\hat{\rho}_k = \frac{\sum_{t=k+1}^{T} z_t z_{t-k}}{\sum_{t=1}^{T} z_t^2}. \tag{7.3}$$

The overall test for serial correlation that guards against incorrect standardization is

$$T_k = \frac{\sum_{t=k+1}^{T} z_t z_{t-k}}{\sqrt{\sum_{t=k+1}^{T} z_t^2 z_{t-k}^2}}. \tag{7.4}$$

T_k is asymptotically distributed as $N[0, 1]$ under the null hypothesis that $\rho_j = 0, j = 1, \ldots, k$. The related overall test for serial correlation is based on the sum of the first l squared T_k statistics. The statistic is known as the Box-Pierce portmanteau statistic (T_{BP}).

$$T_{BP} = \sum_{k=1}^{l} (T_k)^2 \tag{7.5}$$

T_{BP} is asymptotically $\chi^2(l)$ under the null hypothesis of no serial correlation up to lag k.

After removing deterministic trend, the test for serial correlation at lag $k = 2$ for opioid drug poisoning mortality data shows a statistically nonsignificant result ($T_k = 1.59, p = 0.44$). Therefore, static regression allowing for over-dispersion is sufficient for further inferential analysis.

7.2.3 Parameter-driven Generalized Linear Model

The model described in the previous section can help solve the problem of over-dispersion in ecological count data. The explicit assumption in those models is that the observations are independent. The presence of significant serial correlation violates the independence assumption. Zeger (1988) presented a parameter-driven model in which autocorrelation is introduced through latent process ϵ_t. A sequence of event counts y_t is assumed to be independent conditional on this latent process. The mean and variance of y_t is given by

$$u_t = E(y_t|\epsilon_t) = exp(\boldsymbol{x}_t'\boldsymbol{\beta})\epsilon_t, \quad w_t = var(y_t|\epsilon_t). \tag{7.6}$$

The latent process ϵ_t is assumed to be a stationary process with expected value of 1, variance σ^2 and covariances $cov(\epsilon_t, \epsilon_{t-k}) = \rho_{k\sigma^2}$ for $0 \leq k \leq T-1$. Then the unconditional moments of y_t are given by

$$\mu_t = E(y_t) = exp(\boldsymbol{x}_t'\boldsymbol{\beta}), \quad var(y_t) = \mu_t + \sigma^2 \mu_t^2. \tag{7.7}$$

An estimating equation based on quasi-likelihood is used to obtain the consistent estimates of β. For independent data, the estimate of β is the root of the following estimating equation Zeger et al. (1988):

$$U(\beta) = \frac{\partial \mu'}{\partial \beta} V^{-1}(y - \mu) = 0. \tag{7.8}$$

The V is a $T \times T$ diagonal matrix. However, for time series data, V will include off-diagonal elements such that $V = A + \sigma^2 A R_\epsilon A$, where

$$A = \begin{pmatrix} \mu_1 & 0 & \cdots & 0 \\ 0 & \mu_2 & \cdots & 0 \\ \vdots & \vdots & \ddots & \vdots \\ 0 & 0 & \cdots & \mu_T \end{pmatrix},$$

and

$$R_\epsilon = \begin{pmatrix} 1 & \rho_\epsilon(1) & \rho_\epsilon(2) & \cdots & \rho_\epsilon(T-1) \\ \rho_\epsilon(1) & 1 & \rho_\epsilon(1) & \cdots & \rho_\epsilon(T-2) \\ \vdots & \vdots & \vdots & \ddots & \vdots \\ \rho_\epsilon(T-1) & \rho_\epsilon(T-2) & \rho_\epsilon(T-3) & \cdots & 1 \end{pmatrix}.$$

The solution of (7.8) requires the inversion of V which is a $T \times T$ matrix. To simplify the computation, Zeger (1988) proposed a modification in which the actual autocorrelation matrix R_ϵ is approximated by a band diagonal matrix of a finite autoregressive process of a given order. If $S = diag(\mu_t + \sigma^2 \mu_t)$, then V is approximately $V_R = S^{1/2} R(\rho) S^{1/2}$. The inverse of V_R is easily obtained by decomposing $R(\rho)$, such that

$$V_R^{-1} \approx S^{-1/2} L' L S^{-1/2},$$

where L is a matrix that applies a linear filter to the data. For example, in the case of pth-order autoregressive process

$$L_t y_t = y_t - \rho_1 y_{t-1} - \ldots - \rho_k y_{t-k} \quad \text{for } k < t.$$

Thus, L is a $(T-k) \times T$ matrix. To further illustrate the form of L, suppose $k = 2$. Then

$$L = \begin{pmatrix} -\rho_2 & -\rho_1 & 1 & 0 & \cdots & 0 \\ 0 & -\rho_2 & -\rho_1 & 1 & \cdots & 0 \\ \vdots & \vdots & \vdots & \vdots & \ddots & \vdots \\ 0 & 0 & \cdots & -\rho_2 & -\rho_1 & 1 \end{pmatrix}.$$

The estimate of β is obtained using an iterative algorithm. Following the iterative least-squares procedure, estimates of β at the $(p+1)th$ iteration of the process are given by

$$\beta_{p+1} = \left\{ \left(\mathbf{LS}^{-1/2} \frac{\partial \mu}{\partial \beta'} \right)' \left(\mathbf{LS}^{-1/2} \frac{\partial \mu}{\partial \beta'} \right) \right\}^{-1} \left(\mathbf{LS}^{-1/2} \frac{\partial \mu}{\partial \beta'} \right)' \left(\mathbf{LS}^{-1/2} \mathbf{Z} \right),$$

(7.9)

where $\mathbf{Z} = \left(\frac{\partial \mu}{\partial \beta'} \right) \beta + (\mathbf{y} - \mu)$ and the right-hand side is evaluated using $\hat{\beta}_p$ for β. Then, the asymptotic variance-covariance matrix of $\hat{\beta}$ is given by Zeger (1988) as:

$$\mathbf{V}_{\hat{\beta}_R} = \mathbf{I}_0^{-1} \mathbf{I}_1 \mathbf{I}_0^{-1},$$

(7.10)

where $\mathbf{I}_0 = \lim_{n \to \infty} \left(\frac{\partial \mu'}{\partial \beta} \mathbf{V}_R^{-1} \frac{\partial \mu}{\partial \beta} / n \right)$ and $\mathbf{I}_1 = \lim_{n \to \infty} \left(\frac{\partial \mu'}{\partial \beta} \mathbf{V}_R^{-1} \mathbf{V} \mathbf{V}_R^{-1} \frac{\partial \mu}{\partial \beta} / n \right)$.

The marginal mean μ_t of the generalized log-linear parameter-driven model in this section does not depend on the latent process. Therefore, the interpretation of regression coefficients do not depend on assumptions about the unobservable process, ϵ_t. The variance function of the model has the negative-binomial form which allows over-dispersion relative to the Poisson. The degree of over-dispersion depends on the marginal mean μ_t.

7.2.4   Autoregressive Model

The serially correlated error model is a special case of an autoregressive moving average model. The serial correlation in errors implies that y_t has a moving average representation. A straightforward way of specifying a time series model is to specify lagged dependent variable in a log-linear model where the conditional mean is $exp(x_t'\beta + \rho y_{t-1})$. The model, however, is explosive for $\rho > 0$ (Cameron and Trivedi 2013). Zeger and Qaqish (1988) introduced the following more natural multiplicative model

$$\mu_{t|t-1} = exp(x_t'\beta + \rho \, lny_{t-1}^*)$$

(7.11)

without specifying any distributional assumption. Assumptions are made only on first and second conditional moments. The y_{t-1}^* is a transformation of y_{t-1} defined as either

$$y_{t-1}^* = max(c, y_{t-1}), \quad 0 < c < 1$$

or

$$y_{t-1}^* = y_{t-1} + c, \quad c > 0$$

so that $y_{t-1} = 0$ is not an absorbing state. The model can be broadened by considering an AR(1) error model

$$\begin{aligned} \mu_{t|t-1} &= exp\left(x_t'\beta + \rho(ln \, y_{t-1}^* - x_{t-1}'\beta) \right) \\ &= exp(x_t'\beta) \left(\frac{y_{t-1}^*}{x_{t-1}'\beta} \right)^{\rho}. \end{aligned}$$

(7.12)

Further, the conditional variance of the response is assumed to be

$$Var(y_t|t-1) = v_t = \phi V(\mu_{t|t-1}), \tag{7.13}$$

where ϕ is an unknown dispersion parameter, and $V(\mu_{t|t-1})$ is a variance function. The model (7.12) can be further generalized as follows (Zeger and Qaqish 1988) :

$$\mu_{t|t-1} = exp\left(x_t'\beta + \sum_{i=1}^{q} \theta_i\{ln\ y_{t-1}^* - x_{t-1}'\beta\}\right). \tag{7.14}$$

Let $\gamma' = (\beta', \theta')$ and assume that c is known. The parameters of model (7.14) can be estimated by a quasi-likelihood approach (McCullagh and Nelder 1989). The estimate $\hat{\gamma}$ is the root of the log-QL estimating equation

$$
\begin{aligned}
U(\gamma) &= \sum_{t=1}^{T} \frac{\partial \mu_{t|t-1}}{\partial \gamma} v_t^{-1}(y_t - \mu_{t|t-1}) \\
&= \sum_{t=1}^{T} Z_t(y_t - \mu_{t|t-1})
\end{aligned}
\tag{7.15}
$$

where $Z_t' = \left(x_t', (ln\ y_{t-1}^* - x_{t-1}'\beta), \ldots, (ln\ y_{t-q}^* - x_{t-q}'\beta)\right)$. Equation (7.15) has the form of generalized linear model score function. The difference is that Z_t' depends on unknown parameters. Consequently, a second level of iteration is necessary to solve (7.15) using an iteratively re-weighted least-squares approach. Note that $\mu_{t|t-1}$ can be expressed as follows:

$$\mu_{t|t-1} = exp\left(\tilde{x}_t'\beta + \sum_{i=1}^{q} \theta_i\{ln\ y_{t-1}^*\}\right),$$

where $\tilde{x}_t = x_t - \sum_{i=1}^{q} \theta_i x_{t-q}$ is a time-filtered version of x_t. Hence, the model parameters can be estimated by regressing y_t on $\tilde{x}_t$ and $ln\ y_{t-1}^*$. The following iteration is suggested by Zeger and Qaqish (1988):

1. Given $\hat{\theta}^{(k)}$, calculate $\tilde{x}_t$ and let $D_t = (ln\ y_{t-1}^*, \ldots, ln\ y_{t-q}^*)$.

2. Estimate $\hat{\beta}^{(k+1)}$, the coefficients for calculating $\tilde{x}_t^{(k)}$, and $\hat{\theta}^{(k+1)}$, the coefficients for D_t, using iteratively re-weighted least squares.

3. Repeat steps 1 and 2 to convergence of parameter estimates (or deviance).

If c is unknown, then it can be considered as an additional parameter to be estimated. The previous algorithm requires an additional step to solve for c. After step 2 the following estimating equation is solved for $\hat{c}^{(k+1)}$ given $\hat{\beta}^{(k+1)}$ and $\hat{\theta}^{(k+1)}$.

$$U(\gamma) = \sum_{t=1}^{T} w_t(c)[y_t - \mu_{t|t-1}] = 0, \tag{7.16}$$

where $\gamma = (\beta', \theta', c)$, $w_t(c) = \sum_{i=1}^{q} \theta_i I(y_{t-i} < c)$ and $I(.)$ is the indicator function. Under regularity conditions for the conditional density of $y_t | D_t$ and conditional on D_t

$$\sqrt{T}(\hat{\gamma} - \gamma) \stackrel{T \to \infty}{\Rightarrow} N(0, V^{-1}),$$

where

$$V = \lim_{n \to \infty} \frac{1}{n} \sum_{i=1}^{T} Z_t Z_t' v_t.$$

The scale parameter ϕ appearing in (7.13) can be estimated consistently by

$$\hat{\phi} = \frac{\sum_{i=1}^{T} r_t^2}{T - p},$$

where p is a number of elements in γ, and r_t denotes Pearson residuals, which are defined by

$$r_t = \frac{y_t - \hat{\mu}_{t|t-1}}{\sqrt{V(\mu_{t|t-1})}},$$

for $t = 1, \ldots, T$. Held et al. (2005) have argued that the introduction of parameter c and the regularization of past counts y_{t-1} through their expected values in the model equation (7.12) is slightly unnatural. They proposed a different approach where previous counts act directly on the conditional mean $\mu_{t|t-1}$. Thus, the new model is now

$$\mu_{t|t-1} = exp(x_t'\beta) + \rho y_{t-1}. \tag{7.17}$$

The model can be easily reformulated to include seasonality and temporal trend as follows:

$$\mu_{t|t-1} = exp(\beta_0 + \beta_1 t + \sum_{s=1}^{S} (\beta_s sin(\omega_s t) + \gamma_s cos(\omega_s t)) + \rho y_{t-1}, \tag{7.18}$$

where the Fourier frequencies ω_s are $\omega_s = 2s\pi/S$. The model parameters can be easily estimated by maximum likelihood method using generic optimizing routines, e.g., the optim() function in the R software. The Poisson model can be replaced with negative-binomial model to allow for over-dispersion. The mean structure of negative-binomial model remains the same as in (7.17) but the variance σ_t increases to

$$\sigma_t = \mu_t + \mu_t/\psi,$$

with the additional parameter $\psi > 0$.

7.3 State Space Model

A state space representation of time series specifies a measurement and transition equation. State space methods offer a unified approach to a wide range of models and techniques. It relates observations $y_t, t = 1, 2, \ldots$, on a response variable Y to unobserved "states" or "parameters" α_t by an observation model for y_t given α_t. For event counts, the measurement equation is an event-count distribution, while the transition equation describes how the dynamics of the event count distribution parameters evolves. A number of state space models have been proposed for count data. These models have been limited by unavailability of software for easy implementation and difficulty in interpretation of the model coefficients. A variant of state space model called the Poisson Exponentially Weighted Moving Average Model (PEWMA) is a simple and fast method for modeling persistent event count time series (Brandt et al. 2000). The measurement equation in PEWMA describes how the observed number of events arises as a function of a mean number of events in the past. The state equation describes the importance of past events for predicting the number of events in the current period. After specifying a model in state space form, the Kalman filter is used to estimate the model parameters.

PEWMA assumes that the observed counts at time t are drawn from a Poisson marginal distribution, i.e.,

$$\Pr(y_t|\mu_t) = \left[\frac{\mu_t^{y_t} exp(-\mu_t)}{y_t!} \right]. \tag{7.19}$$

The unobserved mean μ_t is parameterized by the multiplicative equation

$$\mu_t = \mu_{t-1}^* exp(x_t'\beta), \tag{7.20}$$

where β is a $K \times 1$ vector of coefficients and x_t' a $1 \times K$ vector of covariates. A time varying component μ_{t-1}^* is a smoothed mean of the previous observations and is estimated by the Kalman filter. The covariate vector x_t' does not include a constant. Including a constant allows for the introduction of a deterministic trend in the model. The stochastic mechanism for the transition from μ_{t-1} to μ_t is described by following multiplicative transition equation (Brandt et al. 2000):

$$\mu_t = exp(r_t)\mu_{t-1}\eta_t, \tag{7.21}$$

where $\eta_t \sim Beta\left(\omega a_{t-1}, (1-\omega)a_{t-1}\right)$ with $E(\eta_t) = \omega$ for $0 < \omega < 1$. The parameter ω captures discounting in the conditional mean function for the event counts. The parameter r_t describes the growth in the series and insures that $\mu_t > 0$. To identify the model, a gamma prior distribution is specified for μ_{t-1}, such that

$$\Pr(\mu_{t-1}^*; a_{t-1}, b_{t-1}) = \frac{exp(-b_{t-1}\mu_{t-1}^*)\mu_{t-1}^{*\,a_{t-1}-1}b_{t-1}^{a_{t-1}}}{\Gamma(a_{t-1})}. \tag{7.22}$$

Using these assumptions, the joint predictive density, conditional on Y_τ for observations $y_{\tau+1}, \ldots, Y_T$ is (see Brandt et al. 2000):

$$\Pr(y_{\tau+1}, \ldots, Y_T) = \prod_{t=\tau+1}^{T} \Pr(y_t | Y_{t-1})$$

$$= \prod_{t=\tau+1}^{T} \int_0^\infty \Pr(Y_t | \mu_t) \Pr(\mu_t | Y_{t-1}). \qquad (7.23)$$

It is a negative-binomial distribution of the form $Pr(k, r, p) = \frac{\Gamma(k+r)}{k!\Gamma(r)} p^k (1-p)^r$ with $k = y_t$, $r = \omega a_{t-1}$, and $p = (1 + \omega b_{t-1} e^{-x'_t \beta - r_t})^{-1}$. The log-likelihood function for unknown parameters based on predictive density in (7.23) is

$$\begin{aligned}
\ln\; & L(\omega, \beta | a_{t-1}, b_{t-1}, y_t, X_t) \\
= & \sum_{\tau+1}^{T} \ln \Gamma(y_t + \omega a_{t-1}) - \ln(y_t!) \\
& - \ln \Gamma(\omega a_{t-1}) + \omega a_{t-1} \ln \; (\omega b_{t-1} exp(-x'_t \beta - r_t)) \\
& - (\omega a_{t-1} + y_t) \ln \; (1 + \omega b_{t-1} exp(-x'_t \beta - r_t)). \qquad (7.24)
\end{aligned}$$

The estimates of parameters and hyper-parameter is obtained by maximizing (7.24) with respect to ω and β. The maximization require analytical expression of a_{t-1}, b_{t-1} and r_t which are calculated using the Kalman filter. The Kalman filter for PEWMA is defined by following recursive system beginning with starting values of a_{t-1} and β.

$$r_t = \Psi(a_{t-1}) - \Psi(\omega a_{t-1}), \text{where } \Psi \text{ is the digamma function}$$
$$a_{t|t-1} = \omega a_{t-1} \text{ and } b_{t|t-1} = \omega b_{t-1} exp(-x'_t \beta - r_t)$$
$$a_t = a_{t|t-1} + y_t \text{ and } b_t = b_{t|t-1} + 1.$$

7.4   Change-point Analysis

The goal of pharmacovigilance is to identify the change in the incidence of adverse drug reaction in a timely manner. The change-point analysis is the process of detecting distributional changes within time-ordered observations of adverse event rates. In the simplest case of a single change-point, the problem is to determine the unknown location of time point τ where the change has occurred. More formally, an ordered sequence of observations $y_1, \ldots, y_\tau$ and

$y_{\tau+1}, \ldots, y_T$ are assumed to follow two distinct models. The change-point analysis can determine whether the rate of adverse events has changed (elevated) during the life span of the drug. If such change has occurred, the change-point analysis identifies the approximate time of increase in incidence rate. In more complex situations, change may occur in multiple locations and/or multiple parameters during a long period of observation. A change-point analysis is performed only after all the data have been collected. Therefore, some way to identify that the change has occurred is needed. Traditionally, control charts are used to detect changes. Recently, sequential testing methods have been used for vaccine surveillance. We begin by describing a Shewhart type control chart known as u-chart.

7.4.1 The u-chart

A u-chart is an attribute control chart used for monitoring the percent of samples having the condition, relative to either a fixed or varying sample size. U-charts show how the process, measured by number of ADRs among population at risk per observation period, changes over time. This chart plots the rate of ADR for each period as a point on a line. The horizontal lines are drawn at the mean number of ADRs and at the upper and lower control limits. However, for ADR monitoring the lower limit is usually set to 0. The distribution of the number of ADRs is assumed to be Poisson with mean equal to λ. This assumption is the basis for calculating the upper and lower control limits. The control limits are calculated as:

$$
\begin{aligned}
UCL &= \lambda + 3\sqrt{\lambda} \\
CL &= \lambda \\
LCL &= \lambda - 3\sqrt{\lambda},
\end{aligned}
$$

where UCL, CL, and LCL denote the upper control limit, control limit, and the lower control limit. In doing so, the adequacy of the normal approximation to the Poisson distribution is assumed. Additionally, it is assumed that a standard value for λ is available. In absence of standard λ, it may be estimated from the set of baseline observations. Let Y be the number of ADRs in the population at risk of n before the drug exposure. Then, the parameters of u charts are:

$$
\begin{aligned}
UCL &= \bar{y} + 3\sqrt{\frac{\bar{y}}{n}} \\
CL &= \bar{y} \\
LCL &= \bar{y} - 3\sqrt{\frac{\bar{y}}{n}},
\end{aligned}
$$

where $\bar{y}$ represents the observed average rate of ADRs in the baseline data. To improve the performance of the u-chart, modification of the above parameters based on Cornish-Fisher expansion has been suggested. However, improvement achieved by such modification has not been substantiated especially for the increase in rate parameter.

We illustrate the u-chart by using Paulozzi et. al (2006) data. The authors commented that various states reported up to three fold increase in opiate deaths from 1990 to 2001. They linked the increase in reported opioid deaths to change that occurred in the way US health professionals managed chronic pain during roughly the same time. The general belief among professionals that the risk of addiction should not prevent the use of prescription opioid analgesics to manage chronic, non-malignant pain led them to acknowledge that opioid analgesics had a legitimate and important role in managing chronic pain. The authors speculated that this change in thinking probably contributed to the dramatic increase in prescriptions written for opioid analgesics from 1990 to 2002. We chart the opioid mortality data from 1979 to 2001 to see when the u-chart raises the alarm signaling "out of control" death rate. Figure 7.3 shows that the u-statistics exceed the UCL around 1992.

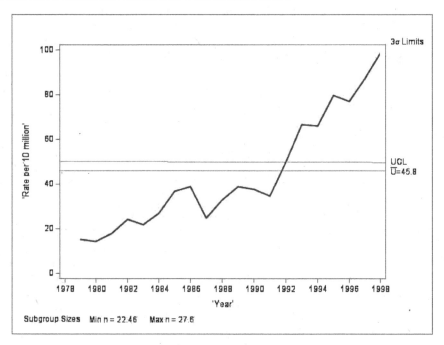

FIGURE 7.3: Unintentional opiate drug poisoning mortality rate.

The u-chart is plotted based on only the current observation, which makes it insensitive to small changes. Therefore, alternatives like the exponentially weighted moving average (EWMA) control chart have been proposed that consider past information. In addition, the observations in time series are often serially correlated. In order to address these issues, Weiss proposed variation of EWMA chart (Weiss and Testik 2009, Weiss 2011) and CUSUM chart for a Poisson INAR(1) process.

7.4.2 Estimation of a Change-point

Let $y_1, \ldots, y_T$ be a sequence of independent observations following a Poisson distribution with means λ_t for $t = 1, 2, \ldots, T$. Here, T is either the time when the "out of control" signal has been given or the monitoring has been terminated for some other reason. The detection of a step change-point is equivalent to testing the following hypothesis:

$$H_0 : \lambda_1 = \lambda_2 = \ldots = \lambda_\tau = \lambda; \text{ vs. } H_1 : \lambda_{\tau+1} = \lambda_2 = \ldots = \lambda_T = \lambda'. \quad (7.25)$$

Chen and Gupta (2011) describe an intuitive method to estimate change-point τ by treating the problem of testing the change-point hypothesis as a model selection problem. They described their method as follows. Under the H_0, the maximum likelihood function is given by

$$L_0(\hat{\lambda}) = \frac{exp(-\tau\hat{\lambda})\hat{\lambda}^{\Sigma_{t=1}^{\tau} y_t}}{\prod_{t=1}^{\tau} y_t!},$$

where $\hat{\lambda} = \frac{M}{T}$, with $M = \sum_{t=1}^{T} y_t$. Therefore, the Schwartz information criterion under H_0 (SIC_0) is given by

$$
\begin{aligned}
SIC_0 &= -2logL_0(\hat{\lambda}) + log\,T \\
&= 2M - 2M\,log\left(\frac{M}{c}\right) + 2log\prod_{t=1}^{T} y_t! + logT.
\end{aligned}
$$

Under H_1, the maximum likelihood function is given by

$$
\begin{aligned}
L_1(\hat{\lambda}, \hat{\lambda}') &= \prod_{t=1}^{\tau} \frac{exp(-\hat{\lambda})\hat{\lambda}^{y_t}}{y_t!} \prod_{t=\tau+1}^{T} \frac{exp(-\hat{\lambda}')\hat{\lambda}'^{y_t}}{y_t!} \\
&= \frac{exp(-\tau\hat{\lambda})\hat{\lambda}^{\Sigma_{t=1}^{\tau} y_t}}{\prod_{t=1}^{\tau} y_t!} \frac{exp(-(T-\tau)\hat{\lambda}')\hat{\lambda}'^{\Sigma_{t=\tau+1}^{T} y_t}}{\prod_{t=\tau+1}^{T} y_t!},
\end{aligned}
$$

where $\hat{\lambda} = \frac{M_\tau}{\tau}$ and $\hat{\lambda}' = \frac{M'_\tau}{T-\tau}$ with M'_τ with $M_\tau = \sum_{t=1}^{\tau} y_t$ and $M'_\tau = \sum_{t=\tau+1}^{T} y_t$. Therefore, the Schwartz information criterion under $H_1(SIC_1)$ is given by

$$
\begin{aligned}
SIC_1 &= -2logL_1(\hat{\lambda}, \hat{\lambda}') + 2log\,T \\
&= 2M_\tau - M_\tau log\frac{M_\tau}{\tau} + 2M'_\tau - M'_\tau log\frac{M'_\tau}{T-\tau} \times 2log\prod_{t=1}^{T} y_t! + 2log\,T.
\end{aligned}
$$

According to Schwarz criterion, the model with the lower value of SIC is preferred. Based on this principle, we reject H_0 if

$$SIC_0 > \min_{1 \leq \tau \leq T-1} SIC_1(\tau)$$

or

$$\min_{1 \leq \tau \leq T-1} \left[M\log\frac{M}{T} - M_\tau\log\frac{M_\tau}{\tau} - M'_\tau\log\frac{M'_\tau}{T-\tau} \right] < \frac{1}{2}\log\frac{1}{T}.$$

The resulting estimate of change-point location $\hat{\tau}$ is

$$\boxed{\hat{\tau} = \arg\min_{1 \leq \tau \leq T-1} SIC_1(\tau).} \tag{7.26}$$

For the time sequence with multiple change-points, a method known as binary segmentation procedure is widely used to determine the number and location of change-points. A general description of the binary segmentation techniques is summarized in Chen and Gupta (2011). The steps involved in this iterative process are as follows:

1. Test for a single change-point hypothesis as in 7.25. If H_0 is not rejected then stop as there is no change-point. Otherwise, go to the next step.

2. Divide the sequence of observations at $y_1, y_2, \ldots, y_T$ into two subsequences where change-point $\hat{\tau}$ is detected in 1. The two subsequences are $y_1, y_2, \ldots, y_\tau$ and $y_{\tau+1}, y_2, \ldots, y_T$.

3. Test for a single change-point hypothesis within each subsequence.

4. Repeat the process until no further subsequences have change-points.

5. The collection of change-point locations found by 1–4 are denoted by $\{\hat{\tau}_1, \hat{\tau}_2, \ldots, \hat{\tau}_q\}$, where q is the estimated number of change-points.

The binary segmentation procedure identifies three change-point locations in the opioid death data. The detected change-points are at 1991, 1993 and 1994. The change-point detection method presented so far does not allow serial dependence and assumes step change in the rate parameter. These methods may not be sufficient when observations are correlated or there is a change in trend.

7.4.3 Change-point Estimator for the INAR(1) Model

The INAR(1) model is defined as

$$Y_t = \alpha \circ Y_{t-1} + \epsilon_t,$$

where ϵ_t are i.i.d according to Poisson(λ) and $Y_0 \approx$ Poisson($\lambda/(1-\alpha)$). Based on the model, the Y_t comprise a stationary Markov chain with marginal distribution Poisson($\lambda/(1-\alpha)$) whose conditional distribution can be written as (see Al-Osh and Alzaid 1987):

$$f(y_t|y_{t-1}) = exp(-\lambda)(y_{t-1}!)C(y_{t-1}, y_t), \qquad (7.27)$$

where $C(x_{t-1}, x_t) = \sum_m^{k=0} \frac{\alpha^k (1-\alpha)^{x_{t-1}-k}\lambda^{x_t-k}}{k!(x_t-k)!(x_{t-1}-k)!}$ and $m = min(x_t, x_{t-1})$. The likelihood function of an INAR(1) model in terms of conditional distributions of each observation is expressed as

$$f_{y_0,\ldots,y_T}(y_t,\ldots,y_T|\alpha,\lambda) = f_{y_0}(y_0)f_{y_1|y_0}(y_1|y_0)\prod_{t=2}^{T} f_{y_t|y_{t-1}}(y_t|y_{t-1}). \qquad (7.28)$$

The INAR(1) model depends on the rate parameter λ and the dependence parameter α. A change can occur on either parameters during the course of observation. Torkamani et al. (2014) have developed a method to estimate change-point in each of these two parameters. It is assumed that the change occurs as a step function at the $(\tau + 1)^{th}$ observation.

7.4.3.1 Change-point Estimator for the Rate Parameter

Torkamani et al. (2014) suggested estimating the rate parameter assuming the same α before and after the change-point. The baseline ADR rate λ_0 and dependence parameter α are assumed to be known quantities. A new value of the rate parameter is denoted by λ_1. Then, the log-likelihood function of this process with a change-point at τ is obtained as (see Torkamani et al. 2014)

$$\begin{aligned}
l(\lambda_1, \tau|y) &= \frac{-\lambda_0}{(1-\alpha)} + ln\left[\frac{(\lambda_0/(1-\alpha))^{y_0}}{y_0!}\right] + \sum_{t=1}^{\tau} ln(y_{t-1}!) - \tau(\lambda_0) \\
&+ \sum_{t=1}^{\tau} ln\left[C_{\lambda_0}(y_{t-1}, y_t)\right] + \sum_{t=\tau+1}^{T} ln(y_{t-1}!) - (T-\tau)(\lambda_1) \\
&+ \sum_{t=\tau+1}^{T} ln\left[C_{\lambda_1}(y_{t-1}, y_t)\right].
\end{aligned} \qquad (7.29)$$

The unknown parameters λ_1 and τ can be estimated by maximizing the log-likelihood function in equation (7.29). As, τ is a discrete variable with known finite values, a maximum log-likelihood can be calculated for each possible value of τ. Thus, for a given value of τ, the first derivative of the log-likelihood with respective to λ is

$$\frac{\partial l(\lambda_1, \tau|y)}{\partial \lambda_1} = -(T-\tau) + \sum_{t=\tau+1}^{T} \frac{C_{\lambda_1}(y_{t-1}, y_t - 1)}{C_{\lambda_1}(y_{t-1}, y_t)}. \qquad (7.30)$$

A closed-form solution does not exist for the equation in (7.30). Therefore, an estimate of λ_1 is obtained using the Newton-Raphson method, which requires expression for second derivative. The expression for second derivative is given in Torkamani et al. (2014) as follows:

$$\frac{\partial^2 l(\lambda_1, \tau | y)}{\partial \lambda_1^2} = \sum_{t=\tau+1}^{T} \frac{C_{\lambda_1}(y_{t-1}, y_t - 2)C_{\lambda_1}(y_{t-1}, y_t) - C_{\lambda_1}(y_{t-1}, y_t - 1)^2}{C_{\lambda_1}(y_{t-1}, y_t)^2}.$$

(7.31)

An estimate of λ_1 is obtained by iteratively solving

$$\hat{\lambda}_1^{k+1} = \hat{\lambda}_1^k - \frac{\partial l(\lambda_1, \tau | y)}{\partial \lambda_1} \left[\frac{\partial^2 l(\lambda_1, \tau | y)}{\partial \lambda_1^2} \right]^{-1}.$$

The procedure starts with initial value $\hat{\lambda}_1^0 = \lambda_0$ and is terminated when $|\hat{\lambda}_1^{k+1} - \hat{\lambda}_1^k| < \nu$, where ν is a pre-specified convergence criterion.

TABLE 7.1: Example to Estimate the Change-Point in Opioid Mortality Data When $\lambda_0 = 15.0$

year	y_t	t	$\hat{\lambda}_1(t)$	loglik
1979	15			
1980	14	1	16.303	-109.568
1981	18	2	17.110	-108.565
1982	24	3	17.749	-107.592
1983	22	4	18.230	-106.851
1984	27	5	19.155	-105.068
1985	36	6	19.787	-103.944
1986	39	7	20.039	-103.853
1987	25	8	20.599	-103.039
1988	33	9	22.426	-98.9434
1989	39	10	23.255	-97.8728
1990	37	11	24.184	-96.7696
1991	34	12	26.054	-93.3635
1992	50	**13**	28.726	-88.3369
1993	66	14	29.258	-90.7369
1994	66	15	28.902	-95.1854
1995	80	16	31.208	-94.2249
1996	77	17	30.346	-99.6884
1997	87	18	34.845	-98.7467
1998	98	19	36.867	-103.497

Table 7.1 shows the result of applying this method to the opioid mortality data. The estimate of new rate parameter at each potential change-point is shown on the $\hat{\lambda}_1(t)$ column and the corresponding value of the likelihood function is shown in the next column. The value of t that maximizes the log-likelihood (-88.33) indicates the estimated time of change at 13*th* (year 1991) observation.

7.4.3.2 Change-point Estimator for the Dependence Parameter

The dependence parameter can be estimated by following a similar procedure. The time-ordered sequence of observations is assumed to have baseline dependence parameter value of α_0. The rate parameter is assumed to remain constant at λ. Assuming that the dependence parameter changes at the $(\tau + 1)$th observation, the log-likelihood function can be written as (Torkamani et al. 2014, see):

$$
\begin{aligned}
l(\alpha_1, \tau | y) &= \frac{-\lambda}{(1 - \alpha_0)} + ln\left[\frac{(\lambda/(1 - \alpha_0))^{y_0}}{y_0!}\right] + \sum_{t=1}^{\tau} ln(y_{t-1}!) - \tau(\lambda) \\
&+ \sum_{t=1}^{\tau} ln\left[C_{\alpha_0}(y_{t-1}, y_t)\right] + \sum_{t=\tau+1}^{T} ln(y_{t-1}!) - (T - \tau)(\lambda) \\
&+ \sum_{t=\tau+1}^{T} ln\left[C_{\alpha_1}(y_{t-1}, y_t)\right].
\end{aligned}
\tag{7.32}
$$

The partial derivative of the log-likelihood function with respect to α_1 is

$$
\frac{\partial l(\alpha_1, \tau | y)}{\partial \alpha_1} = \sum_{t=\tau+1}^{T} \frac{(x_t - \alpha_1 x_{t-1}) - \lambda[C_{\alpha_1}(y_{t-1}, y_t - 1)/C_{\alpha_1}(y_{t-1}, y_t)]}{\alpha_1(\alpha_1 - 1)}.
\tag{7.33}
$$

A closed-form solution does not exist for the equation 7.33. A second partial derivative is needed to implement the Newton-Raphson method to obtain the MLE. Torkamani et al. (2014) provided an expression of the second partial derivative as follows:

$$
\begin{aligned}
\frac{\partial^2 l(\alpha_1, \tau | y)}{\partial \alpha_1^2} &= \sum_{\tau+1}^{T} \frac{-y_{t-1}[\alpha_1(1 - \alpha_1)] - (1 - 2\alpha_1)(y_t - \alpha_1 y_{t-1})}{[\alpha_1(1 - \alpha_1)]^2} \\
&+ \frac{(1 - 2\alpha_1)\lambda}{[\alpha_1(1 - \alpha_1)]^2} \times \frac{C_{\alpha_1}(y_{t-1}, y_t - 1)}{C_{\alpha_1}(y_{t-1}, y_t)} - \frac{\lambda}{\alpha_1(1 - \lambda_1)} \\
&\times \frac{C'_{\alpha_1}(y_{t-1}, y_t - 1)C_{\alpha_1}(y_{t-1}, y_t) - C'_{\alpha_1}(y_{t-1}, y_t)C_{\alpha_1}(y_{t-1}, y_t - 1)}{[C_{\alpha_1}(y_{t-1}, y_t)]^2},
\end{aligned}
$$

where

$$
C'_{\alpha_1}(y_{t-1}, y_t) = \sum_{k=0}^{m} \frac{\alpha^k(1 - \alpha)^{x_{t-1}-k}\lambda^{x_t-k}}{k!(x_t - k)!(x_{t-1} - k)!}\left[\frac{k}{\alpha_1} + \frac{y_{t-k} - k}{1 - \alpha_1}\right].
$$

As stated previously, these methods are used in combination with a control chart (e.g., c-EWMA). Therefore, weaknesses inherent in such control charts also apply to the change-point analysis described in this section. For small

TABLE 7.2: Change-Point Estimate for Dependence Parameter

year	y_t	t	$\hat{\alpha}_1(t)$	loglik
1979	15			
1980	14	1	0.504	-131.817
1981	18	2	0.519	-131.655
1982	24	3	0.529	-131.423
1983	22	4	0.538	-131.134
1984	27	5	0.556	-130.359
1985	36	6	0.567	-129.767
1986	39	7	0.573	-129.41
1987	25	8	0.585	-128.728
1988	33	9	0.629	-125.187
1989	39	10	0.640	-124.203
1990	37	11	0.653	-123.086
1991	34	12	0.681	-120.323
1992	50	**13**	**0.716**	**-116.391**
1993	66	14	0.719	-116.736
1994	66	15	0.714	-118.736
1995	80	16	0.742	-117.877
1996	77	17	0.730	-121.613
1997	87	18	0.794	-120.932
1998	98	19	0.811	-125.163

changes, simulation results have shown that number of observation elapsed between real change and the alert signal from a control chart can be high. The same simulation study has also indicated that the maximum difference between the real change time and its estimate is less than 2 in most of the situations.

For the opioid mortality data, assuming an event rate of 27 death per 10,000,000 and baseline $\alpha_0 = 0.5$, the change-point of dependence parameter is once again estimated to be at 13th observation. The new value of the dependence parameter is estimated to be 0.716.

7.4.4   Change-point of a Poisson Rate Parameter with Linear Trend Disturbance

The change-point estimating procedure presented so far are designed primarily for a step change in the parameter of interest. Perry et al. (2006) proposed an estimator for the change-point of a Poisson rate parameter where the type of change is a linear trend. A linear trend occurs when the rate begins to change linearly from its baseline value over time. Assume that the ADR count of a particular type is initially distributed as Poisson with known rate $\lambda = \lambda_0$. After an unknown point in time τ the rate parameter changes to unknown value $\lambda = \lambda_t$ for $t = \tau + 1, ...,$ where $\lambda_i > \lambda_0$ and the functional form of λ_i is specified as

$$\lambda_i = \lambda_0 + \beta(t - \tau). \tag{7.34}$$

The β in the equation (7.34) is the slope of the linear trend disturbance. Assuming an ADR rate change occurred at τ, the likelihood function is given by

$$L(\tau, \beta) = \prod_{t=1}^{\tau} \frac{exp(-\lambda_0)\lambda_0^{y_t}}{y_t!} \prod_{t=\tau+1}^{T} \frac{exp[-\{\lambda_0 + \beta(t-\tau)\}][\lambda_0 + \beta(t-\tau)]^{y_t}}{y_t!},$$

$$\tag{7.35}$$

where, y_t is the event count at the tth time point. The MLE of the τ is the value of τ that maximizes the likelihood in (7.35). The log-likelihood equation is obtained by taking the logarithm of that in (7.35). The log-likelihood function reduces to the following expression:

$$logL(\tau, \beta) = K - \frac{1}{2}\beta(T-\tau)(T+1-\tau) + log(\lambda_0)\sum_{t=1}^{\tau} y_t + \sum_{t=\tau+1}^{T} y_t log(\lambda_0 + \beta(t-\tau)),$$

$$\tag{7.36}$$

where K is a constant. The partial derivative of (7.36) with respect to β yields

$$\frac{\partial logL(\tau, \beta)}{\partial \beta} = -\frac{1}{2}(T-\tau)(T+1-\tau) + \sum_{t=\tau+1}^{\tau} \frac{y_t(t-\tau)}{\lambda_0 + \beta(t-\tau)}. \tag{7.37}$$

There is no closed form solution for β in equation (7.37). Hence, for a known value of τ, an estimate of β is obtained using Newton's method. The updating equation (see Perry et al. 2006) for implementing Newton's method is

$$\hat{\beta}_{\tau,k+1} = \hat{\beta}_{\tau,k} - \frac{F_1}{F_2} \tag{7.38}$$

where $\hat{\beta}_{\tau,0} = 0$,

$$F_1 = -\frac{1}{2}(T-\tau)(T+1-\tau) + \sum_{\tau+1}^{\tau} \frac{y_t(t-\tau)}{\lambda_0 + \hat{\beta}_{\tau,k}(t-\tau)},$$

and

$$F_2 = -\sum_{t=1}^{\tau} \frac{y_t(t-\tau)}{\lambda_0 + \hat{\beta}_{\tau,k}(t-\tau)}.$$

This provides an estimate of β at each τ without requiring an explicit closed-form expression. Denote such an estimate by $\hat{\beta}_{\tau}$. A profile likelihood estimate of τ is obtained by substituting $\hat{\beta}_{\tau}$, for β in (7.36) over all possible change-points. Hence,

$$\hat{\tau} = \arg\max_{1 \le \tau \le T} \left[-\frac{1}{2}\beta(T - \tau)(T + 1 - \tau) + log(\lambda_0) \sum_{t=1}^{\tau} y_t + \sum_{t=\tau+1}^{T} y_t log(\lambda_0 + \beta(t - \tau)) \right].$$

$$(7.39)$$

Figure 7.4 is a plot of profile log-likelihood for the example data. The baseline event rate is specified as $\lambda_0 = 26$, which is approximately the average of the first 10 data points. A change-point is detected at $\hat{\tau} = 10$. The example data exhibit strong positive trend in rate parameter from the beginning. Therefore, the change-point location is highly dependent on the value of the baseline rate parameter.

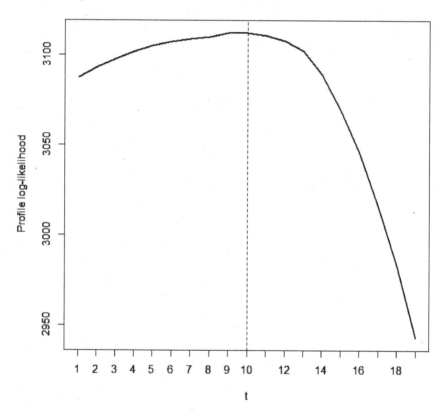

FIGURE 7.4: change-point model with trend disturbance for opiate drug poisoning mortality rate, $\lambda_0 = 26$.

7.4.5 Change-point of a Poisson Rate Parameter with Level and Linear Trend Disturbance

The model can be generalized further to include changes in level as well as the trend of the rate parameter. The mean function $\mu(t) = N(t)\lambda(t)$ is assumed to be a piecewise continuous function of the index variable t (Pawitan 2014), with unknown regression parameters $\beta = (\beta_1, \beta_2)$ and the change-point τ according to

$$\mu(t) = \begin{cases} \mu_1(t)(t, \beta_1) & \text{for } t < \tau \\ \mu_2(t)(t, \beta_2) & \text{for } t \geq \tau. \end{cases} \quad (7.40)$$

For Poisson regression with jump discontinuity between μ_1 and μ_2, the rate parameters can be modeled as

$$log\,(\lambda(t)) = \begin{cases} \beta_{01} + \beta_{11}t & \text{for } t < \tau \\ \beta_{02} + \beta_{12}(t - \tau) & \text{for } t \geq \tau. \end{cases} \quad (7.41)$$

On the other hand, if we want a continuous function of $\lambda(t)$, then rate parameters can be modeled as

$$log\,(\lambda(t)) = \begin{cases} \beta_{01} + \beta_{11}t & \text{for } t < \tau \\ \beta_{01} + \beta_{11}\tau + \beta_{12}(t - \tau) & \text{for } t \geq \tau. \end{cases} \quad (7.42)$$

Regardless of the model for $\lambda(t)$, the likelihood function for Poisson model is given by

$$L(\tau, \beta) = \prod_{t=1}^{\tau} \frac{exp(-\mu_1(t, \beta_1))\mu_1(t, \beta_1)^{y_t}}{y_t!} \prod_{t=\tau+1}^{T} \frac{exp(-\mu_2(t, \beta_2))\mu_2(t, \beta_2)^{y_t}}{y_t!}.$$

$$(7.43)$$

The log-likelihood equation is obtained by taking the logarithm of that in equation (7.43).

$$logL(\tau, \beta) = K + \sum_{t=1}^{\tau} y_t\,log\,\mu_1(t, \beta_1) - \mu_1(t, \beta_1) + \sum_{t=\tau+1}^{T} y_t\,log\,\mu_2(t, \beta_2) - \mu_2(t, \beta_2),$$

$$(7.44)$$

where K is a constant. The partial derivative of (7.44) with respect to β yields

$$\begin{aligned} \frac{\partial logL(\tau, \beta)}{\partial \beta} &= \sum_{t=1}^{\tau} \left(\frac{y_t}{\mu_1(t, \beta_1)} - 1 \right) \frac{\partial \mu_1(t, \beta_1)}{\partial \beta_1} \\ &+ \sum_{t=\tau+1}^{T} \left(\frac{y_t}{\mu_1(t, \beta_2)} - 1 \right) \frac{\partial \mu_1(t, \beta_2)}{\partial \beta_2}. \end{aligned} \quad (7.45)$$

The equation (7.45) is solved for each value of τ and the likelihood equation is evaluated at the estimated value of β. Since equation (7.45) does not have a close-form solution, the Newton-Raphson method is commonly used to solve it iteratively. A profile likelihood estimate $\hat{\tau}$ is obtained by choosing

$$\hat{\tau} = \underset{1 \leq \tau \leq T}{\arg\max} \left[\sum_{t=1}^{\tau} y_t \, log \, \mu_1(t, \hat{\boldsymbol{\beta}}_1) - \mu_1(t, \hat{\boldsymbol{\beta}}_1) + \sum_{t=\tau+1}^{T} y_t \, log \, \mu_2(t, \boldsymbol{\beta}_2) - \mu_2(t, \hat{\boldsymbol{\beta}}_2) \right].$$
(7.46)

Figure 7.5 shows the profile log-likelihood for the example data based on model 7.42, with a maximum at $\hat{\tau} = 13$. The estimated parameters are:

$$\beta_{01} = -13.38 \; (se = 0.025)$$
$$\beta_{11} = 0.08 \; (se = 0.0025)$$
$$\beta_{12} = 0.12 \; (se = 0.003).$$

7.4.6   Discussion

The analytic methods discussed in this chapter are complicated due to the non-linear nature of the count data. Software for implementing these methods are either available as a stand alone program or as freely available R packages. For example, Brandt provides a stand alone R program for the PEWMA model. The Comprehensive R Archive Network has several software packages for change-point analysis. The one that is most relevant to this discussion is the Surveillance package. It provides functions for the modeling and detecting change-point in time series of counts, proportions and categorical data, as well as for the modeling of continuous-time epidemic phenomena. Similarly, the Changepoint package implements various mainstream and specialized change-point methods for finding single and multiple change-points within data. The MCMCpack package provides a suite of functions including a Bayesian Poisson change-point model. The time series analysis procedures specific to non-continuous data are not available in frequently used commercial software such as SAS or SPSS.

Sequential analysis techniques are gaining popularity in the early detection of the adverse events, especially, in the area of vaccine safety. These techniques are usually based on the generalized likelihood ratio test which requires some form of MCMC simulation to determine the critical value of the test statistic (or stopping rule). Sequential analysis methods have shown to shorten the study length by allowing periodic reviews of patients accrued.

Finally, most of the methods described up to this point assume stationary time series data. The example opioid mortality data do not strictly conform to this property. Therefore, the results pertaining to the data may not be valid for inference. Nonetheless, the data adequately illustrate the use of the relevant analytic methods.

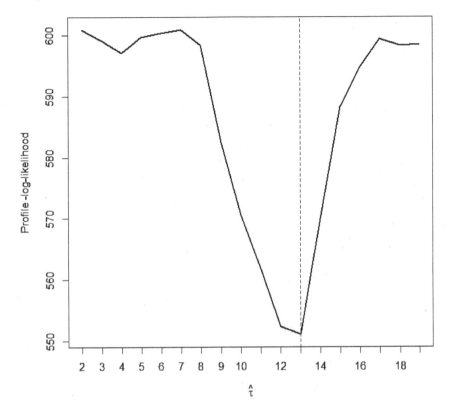

FIGURE 7.5: Profile log-likelihood of the change parameter τ.

7.5 Mixed-effects Poisson Regression Model

The theoretical basis of mixed-effect Poisson regression model is formulated in chapter 5. This model is suitable for rare event data in which the observed number of events in a given region may be small (including zero), and the number at risk (i.e., population size) may vary from region to region. The model estimates overall event rate conditional on a set of covariates, and can also be used to estimate covariate adjusted region-specific estimates of event rates.

We illustrate an application of a mixed-effects Poisson regression model to examine the association between antidepressant medication prescription rate and suicide rate in children aged 5-14, by analyzing associations at the county level across the United States. The National Center for Health Statistics of the CDC maintains the National Vital Statistics including suicide rate data. suicide rates for 1996-1998 were obtained from the CDC for each US county by sex, race, and age. County-level antidepressant prescription rate data [IMS Health (Plymouth Meeting, PA)] came from a random sample of 20,000 pharmacies (stratified by type, size, and region) from the 36,000 pharmacies in the IMS database, representing over half of all retail pharmacies in the continental U.S. The data do not include hospital prescriptions. For each county, prescription rates (number of pills per county) were obtained for SSRIs (citalopram, paroxetine, fluoxetine, fluvoxamine, and sertraline).

The relation between SSRI antidepressant prescriptions and suicide rate adjusted for county-specific case-mix (sex, race, and income) is examined by a mixed-effects Poisson regression model. This model is suitable because the observed number of suicides in a given county may be small (including zero), and the number at risk (i.e., population size) may vary from county to county. The model estimates overall suicide rate conditional on sex, race, income, and antidepressant prescription, and can also be used to estimate covariate adjusted county-specific estimates of suicide rates. In terms of antidepressant drug prescription, the natural logarithm of number of pills per person per year is used to adjust for differential population size of counties, and to eliminate excessive influence of counties with extremely high or low antidepressant prescription rates. In the model, sex, race, and income were considered fixed-effects and the intercept and antidepressant SSRI prescription effects were treated as random effects. This model specification allows the suicide rate and the relationship between antidepressants and suicide to vary across counties. As such, county-specific changes in suicide rates attributable to changes in SSRI prescriptions can be estimated, adjusted for the sex and race composition of each county. The effect of policy changes (e.g., adding or eliminating SSRIs) can be estimated by accumulating the county-specific estimates over all counties. To test the possibility that the observed associations are simply due to access to quality health care, median county-level income, and number of psychiatrists and child psychiatrists in the county were included as covariates. To decompose the overall relationship into intra-county and inter-county components, a model was fitted using the county mean SSRI prescription and yearly deviation from the mean (hybrid model described in Chapter 10).

The observed number of childhood (ages 4-15) suicides from 1996-1998 was 933 and the estimated rate (based on actual SSRI use) was 836, a difference of 32 suicides per year (10%). Maximum marginal likelihood estimates(MMLE), standard errors (SE), and associated probabilities are presented in Table 7.3.

Empirical Bayes estimates of county-level suicide rates adjusted for effects of race and sex were obtained (see Figure 7.6). An empirical Bayes estimate of 1.0 represents an adjusted rate equal to the national rate, an empirical Bayes estimate of 2.0 represents a doubling of the national rate, and an empirical Bayes estimate of 0.5 represents half of the national rate. Similar to the adult population, highest adjusted rates are typically found in some of the

TABLE 7.3: Maximum Marginal Likelihood Estimates, Standard Errors, and Probability Values for the Clustered Poisson Regression Model

Effect	MMLE	SE	p-value
Intercept	-3.82279	0.23437	0.00001
Log (SSRI)	-0.17238	0.05836	0.00314
Sex	-1.05543	0.08076	0.00001
Race	-0.35843	0.11892	0.00258
Sex by Race	0.07412	0.235	0.75244
Year	0.04334	0.04067	0.28656
County Variance	0.26602	0.18475	0.07496
SSRI Variance	0.11508	0.0062	0.00001

less densely populated areas of the western U.S., such as Arizona, Utah, and Montana, many of which include areas with American Indian reservations (Figure 7.6). For example, Apache County in Arizona include Hopi Indian reservations, Uintah County in Utah includes Ouray, Rosebud, and Yellow Stone counties in Montana include Northern Cheyenne. By contrast, adjusted suicide rates are lowest in the large cities such as Chicago, New York, Boston, Los Angeles, San Diego, Seattle, Miami, and the eastern seaboard in general. There are a few exceptions, for example, Laredo Texas that has a low adjusted suicide rate. The overall relationship between prescribed SSRIs and suicide rate was statistically significant (MMLE$=-0.17, p < .003$). The negative MMLE indicates that SSRI prescriptions are associated with a decrease in suicide rate.

The average population of children aged 5-14 in 1996-1998 was 38,812,743, and the number of suicides over this three-year period was 933, (0.8 per 100,000 per year). If there were no SSRI prescriptions, the model estimates 253 more suicides per year (an 81% increase). These effects are apparent in the raw data (see Figure 7.7). For the lowest deciles (low SSRI prescription rate) the overall observed suicide rate is as high as 1.7 per 100,000, whereas for the highest deciles (high SSRI prescription rate) the suicide rate is as low as 0.7 per 100,000.

To control for access to quality mental health care, two additional analyses were performed. First, median income for each county from the 2000 U.S. Census was included as a predictor in the model. While income is inversely related to suicide rate (MMLE$= -0.01, p < 0.0006$), the SSRI effect remained significant (MMLE$= -0.12, p < 0.04$). Second, we adjusted for access to mental health care by including the number of psychiatrists and child psychiatrists per county in the model. Again, the SSRI effect remained significant (MMLE$= -.14, p < .02$).

Finally, the SSRI effect was decomposed into between and within-county effects. A significant between-county effect was observed as before: namely a negative association between SSRI prescriptions and suicide (MMLE$=-0.15, p < 0.007$). within-county effects were not significant indi-

cating that fluctuations in SSRI prescriptions for children over the three year
time interval within counties was not associated with either increases or decreases in suicide rate.

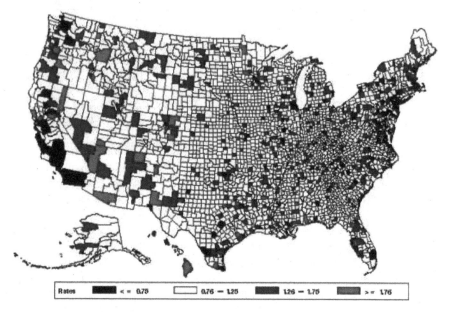

FIGURE 7.6: Statistical (empirical Bayes) estimates of county-specific adjusted annual suicide rates in the United States. An empirical Bayes estimate
of 1.0 indicates that the rate for the county was equal to the national rate of
0.8 per 100,000 in 5-14 year olds. An empirical Bayes estimate of 2.0 represents a doubling of the national rate, and an empirical Bayes estimate of 0.5
represents half of the national rate. The estimates are based on all data from
1996-1998, adjusted for age, sex, and race.

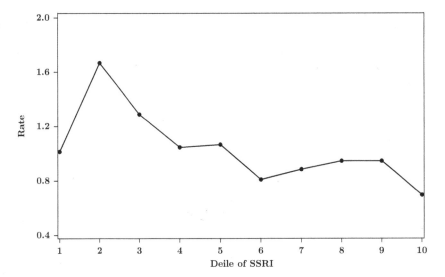

FIGURE 7.7: The relationship between SSRI prescriptions and observed suicide rate per 100,000, in the United States 1996-1998.

8

Discrete-time Survival Models

"In the name of Hippocrates, doctors have invented the most exquisite form
of torture ever known to man: survival."
(Louis Bunuel (1900-1983), Spanish Film-maker)

8.1 Introduction

A fundamental tool in pharmacoepidemiology is understanding the determinants of time to the first adverse event. While there is often interest in the number of events during the period of measurement, time to the first event is the purest measure of the safety (or lack there of) of a drug. A major advantage of time to event analysis or survival analysis is that it provides a natural solution to the problem of censoring. In time to event models a subject can either experience the event during the observation period, be measured throughout the entire observation period but fail to experience the event, or have a more limited window of observation due to factors such as change or discontinuation of insurance coverage, loss to follow-up or death. Subjects who are terminated from study without experiencing the event of interest are termed censored. The ability to accommodate censoring in statistical analysis is fundamental in pharmacoepidemiology. Of course an entire book could be devoted to the topic of survival analysis, and indeed many books have been written on the subject (e.g., Kalbfleisch and Prentice 2011, Elandt-Johnson and Johnson 1999, Miller 2011, Hosmer et al. 2008, Fleming and Harrington 2011). In this text we discuss so called "discrete-time survival models" because they can easily accommodate many of the features of time to event data that are characteristic of drug safety studies.

Efron (1988) first noted the connection between survival analysis and logistic regression for analysis of survival data that are discrete or grouped within time intervals. While the Kaplan-Meier estimator and associated life-table methods including the proportional hazard general linear model or so called "Cox regression" model (Cox 1972) are considered nonparametric because the hazard function need not be specified, they can be inefficient compared to the parametric survival models to be described in this chapter. Furthermore, as noted by Hedeker and Gibbons (2006), the parametric versions of these models based on the original idea of Efron (1988) allow them to quite easily accommodate time-varying covariates, non-proportional hazards, random-effects due to clustering or so called frailty models, and competing risks, either individually or in combination (see Hedeker et al. (2000) and Gibbons et al. (2003)).

To fix ideas, it is useful to begin with Efron's original characterization of the problem. Efron showed that parametric survival models could be fitted by what he termed "partial logistic regression" a name he selected based on Cox (1975) theory of partial-likelihood. Note that these models of course can be fitted using full-likelihood methods as well. He showed that by discretizing the data into a number of small time intervals the method is quite similar to the Kaplan-Meier estimator, which it reduces to when the number of parameters used to describe the survival function becomes large (for example when time is treated as a categorical data and "dummy-coded" contrasts to baseline are used. When the number of time-points is large (e.g., greater than 10), a low degree polynomial is often sufficient to characterize the time function.

To illustrate the method, he used data from the now famous head and neck cancer study which compared radiation therapy alone to radiation therapy plus chemotherapy, the data for the radiation arm only are displayed below in Table 8.1.

In Table 8.1, n_i represents the number of patients at risk at the beginning of month i, s_i the number of patients who died during month i, and s_i' the number of patients lost to follow-up during month i. As an example, in the tenth month, there were $n_{10} = 19$ patients at risk in the beginning of the month, $s_{10} = 2$ who died, and $s_{10}' = 1$ patient lost to follow-up. The estimated Kaplan-Meier survival curves are displayed in Figure 8.1. The combined treatment (Arm B) has significant benefit over radiation alone (p=0.01).

Following Efron (1988) we assume that the number of deaths s_i is binomially distributed given $n_i \mid s_i \approx B_i(n_i, h_i)$, independently for $i = 1, 2, \ldots, N$. It follows that s_i has the discrete density

$$\binom{n_i}{s_i} h_i^{s_i} (1 - h_i)^{n_i - s_i}, s_i = 0, 1, 2, \ldots, n_i. \tag{8.1}$$

Here h_i represents the probability that the patient died in the ith time interval conditional on surviving to the beginning of the ith interval (i.e., the discrete hazard rate). The corresponding survival function is therefore

$$G_i = \prod_{1 \leq j < i} (1 - h_j), \tag{8.2}$$

which is the probability that the patient did not die during the first $i - 1$ time intervals and therefore survived to at least the beginning of the ith interval. The life-table method simply estimates h_i by $\hat{h}_i = s_i / n_i$ and then substitutes $\hat{h}_i$ for h_i to compute the life-table survival estimate

TABLE 8.1: Data for Arm A of the Head-and-Neck-Cancer Study Discretized by Month

Month	n	s	s'	Month	n	s	s'
1	51	1	0	25	7	0	0
2	50	2	0	26	7	0	0
3	48	5	1	27	7	0	0
4	42	2	0	28	7	0	0
5	40	8	0	29	7	0	0
6	32	7	0	30	7	0	0
7	25	0	1	31	7	0	0
8	24	3	0	32	7	0	0
9	21	2	0	33	7	0	0
10	19	2	1	34	7	0	0
11	16	0	1	35	7	0	0
12	15	0	0	36	7	0	0
13	15	0	0	37	7	1	1
14	15	3	0	38	5	1	0
15	12	1	0	39	4	0	0
16	11	0	0	40	4	0	0
17	11	0	0	41	4	0	1
18	11	1	1	42	3	0	0
19	9	0	0	43	3	0	0
20	9	2	0	44	3	0	0
21	7	0	0	45	3	0	1
22	7	0	0	46	2	0	0
23	7	0	0	47	2	1	1
24	7	0	0				
Total					628	42	9

$$\hat{G}_i = \prod_{1 \le j < i} (1 - \hat{h}_j). \tag{8.3}$$

However, Efron suggested that instead, we estimate h_i by logistic regression, where

$$\lambda_i = log[h_i/(1 - h_i)] \tag{8.4}$$

and

$$h_i = \frac{1}{1 + exp(-\lambda_i)}. \tag{8.5}$$

The logistic regression model specifies

$$\lambda_i = \boldsymbol{x}_i \boldsymbol{\beta} \tag{8.6}$$

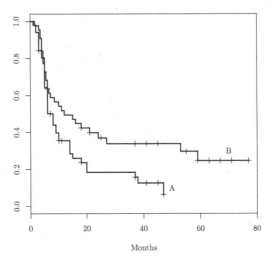

FIGURE 8.1: Kaplan-Meier estimated survival curves (A=Radiation, B=Radiation+Chemotherapy)

where β is a $p \times 1$ vector of unknown parameters and x is a $1 \times p$ covariate vector which at a minimum contains the time interval midpoints; for example,

$$x_i = (1, t_i, t_i^2, t_i^3), i = 1, 2, \ldots, N. \tag{8.7}$$

Efron compared the standard life-table estimate to the cubic time model above and a cubic-linear spline model (cubic before 11 months and linear thereafter). Figure 8.2 compares the parametric versus nonparametric survival curves for Arm A (radiation only). In Figure 8.2, the triangles are based on the cubic time function and the filled circles represent the cubic-linear spline. It is clear that both models do an excellent job of reproducing the life-table.

Figure 8.3 shows an almost perfect fit of the cubic-linear spline to the life-table for Arm B (radiation plus chemotherapy).

8.2 Discrete-time Ordinal Regression Model

When the number of time-intervals is relatively small (e.g., < 10), the parametric survival model can be estimated using an ordinal logistic regression model (see Hedeker and Gibbons (2006) for a review). For this, assume that time is represented by the positive values $c = 1, 2, \ldots, C$. For each subject,

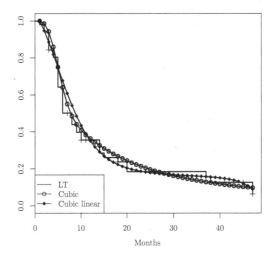

FIGURE 8.2: Comparison of parametric versus nonparametric survival curves (arm A=radiation only)

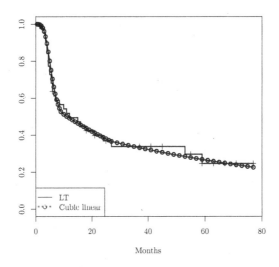

FIGURE 8.3: Comparison of parametric (cubic-linear spline)versus nonparametric survival curves (arm B=Radiation+Chemotherapy)

observation continues until time Y_{ij} at which point either an event occurs ($d_{ij} = 1$) or the observation is censored ($d_{ij} = 0$), where censoring indicates being observed at c but not at $c+1$. Define P_{ijc} as the probability of death (or some other relevant outcome such as the first experience of an adverse event), up to and including time interval c, that is,

$$P_{ijc} = Pr[Y_{ij} = c] \qquad (8.8)$$

and so the probability of survival beyond time interval c is simply $1 - P_{ijc}$, which is the "survivor function." McCullagh (1980) proposed the following grouped-time version of the continuous-time proportional hazards model using the complementary log-log link function to provide interpretation of the estimated model parameters in terms of hazard ratios instead of odds ratios as is traditional in logistic regression using a logistic link function:

$$log[-log(1 - P_{ijc)}] = \lambda_c \boldsymbol{x}'_{ij}\boldsymbol{\beta}. \qquad (8.9)$$

The corresponding cumulative failure probability is therefore

$$P_{ijc} = 1 - exp(-exp(\lambda_c + \boldsymbol{x}'_{ij}\boldsymbol{\beta})). \qquad (8.10)$$

In this model, $\boldsymbol{x}_{ij}$ can only include covariates that do not vary with time (also see Prentice and Gloeckler 1978). The threshold terms λ_c represent the logarithm of the integrated baseline hazard (i.e., when $\boldsymbol{x} = 0$). While the above model is the same as that described in McCullagh (1980), it is written so that the covariate effects are of the same sign as the Cox proportional hazard model. A positive coefficient for a regressor then reflects increasing hazard (i.e., lower values of Y) with greater values of the regressor.

8.3   Discrete-time Ordinal Regression Frailty Model

The idea of frailty dates back to Greenwood and Yule (1920) on accident proneness, and represents a convenient way of adding random-effects which explain unobserved heterogeneity into survival models. If certain individuals were really prone to having accidents, and "accident proneness" was observable, then among individuals with the same level of proneness, accidents would be independent within individuals (i.e., conditional independence). This is the basic idea of a random-effect model; namely, the correlation between members of a defined cluster such as a hospital, county, or state, having similar characteristics which produce correlation among their responses. In general, many of these characteristics are unobserved and by adding a random effect to the model we are essentially computing a unit-specific residual that describes how the sum of the effects of these unmeasured characteristics produces a systematic deviation from the overall response. In longitudinal data, random-effect models permit unobserved characteristics to modify the rate of change over time for a given individual. In survival analysis, a frailty is an unobserved random proportionality factor that modifies the hazard function of an individual or of related individuals. There are two classes of frailty models, univariate and multivariate. In the univariate case, the variability of the survival data is segmented into a part that depends on observed risk factors and is therefore predictable and a part that is initially unpredictable because it is based on unmeasured characteristics. By contrast, in the multivariate case, the data are clustered in some way (e.g., within research centers in a multi-center RCT) or in cases where recurrence of the disease in the same individual is of interest. Here we can add random-effects to the model in an attempt to accommodate the dependence within observed clusters. This cluster-specific random effect is the frailty.

To explore these models in connection with discrete-time survival models, we follow the approach taken by Hedeker and Gibbons (2006). Adding (standardized) random-effects to the fixed-effects discrete time survival model of McCullagh (1980),

$$log[-log(1 - P_{ijt})] = \lambda_c + x'_{ij}\beta + z'_{ij}T\theta_i, \tag{8.11}$$

where z_{ij} is the design matrix for the r random-effects for the jth time period nested within the ith subject. This is a mixed-effects ordinal regression model with complementary log-log link function instead of the logistic. Though the logistic model was originally proposed by Efron (1988) in the present context, its regression coefficients are not invariant to time interval length, requiring the intervals to be of equal length. This is not true for the complementary log-log link function, which has the added advantage of providing coefficients interpretable as hazard ratios rather than odds ratios.

In the ordinal treatment, survival time is represented by the ordered outcome Y_{ij}, which is designated as being censored or not. Alternatively, each survival time can be represented as a set of dichotomous dummy codes indicating whether or not the observation failed in each time interval that was experienced (Allison 1982, D'Agostino et al. 1990, Singer and Willett 1993). Specifically, each survival time Y_{ij} is represented as a vector with all zeros except for its last element, which is equal to d_{ij} (i.e., =0 if censored and −1 for an event). The length of the vector for observation ij equals the observed value of Y_{ij} (assuming that the survival times are coded as $1, 2, ..., C$). These multiple time indicators are then treated as distinct observations in a logistic regression model. In the multivariate case, a given cluster's response vector Y_i is then of size $\sum_{j=1}^{n_i} Y_{ij} \times 1$. This latter approach is particularly useful for handling time-dependent covariates and fitting non-proportional hazards models because the covariate values can change across time.

For this approach, define p_{ijc} to be the probability of failure in time interval c, conditional on survival prior to c:

$$p_{ijc} = Pr\left[Y_{ij} = c \mid Y_{ij} \geq c\right]. \tag{8.12}$$

Similarly, $1 - p_{ijc}$ is the probability of survival beyond time interval c, conditional on survival prior to c. The discrete-time proportional hazards frailty model is then written as

$$log[-log(1 - p_{ijc})] = x'_{ijc}\beta + z'_{ij}T\theta_i \qquad (8.13)$$

where now the covariates x can vary across time and so are denoted as x_{ijc}. The first elements of x are usually time-point dummy codes. Because the covariate vector x now varies with c, this approach automatically allows for time-dependent covariates, and relaxing the proportional hazards assumption only involves including interactions of covariates with the time-point dummy codes, or continuous polynomial time trends.

Under the complementary log-log link function, the two approaches (ordinal and binary) yield identical results for the parameters that do not depend on c. Comparing these two approaches, notice that for the ordinal approach each observation consists of only two pieces of data: the (ordinal) time of the event and whether it was censored or not. Alternatively, in the dichotomous approach each survival time is represented as a vector of dichotomous indicators, where the size of the vector depends upon the timing of the event (or censoring). Thus, the ordinal approach can be easier to implement and offers savings in terms of the dataset size, while the dichotomous approach is superior in its treatment of time-dependent covariates and relaxing of the proportional hazards assumption.

Hedeker and Gibbons (2006) prepared the following table to help compare the two approaches.

TABLE 8.2: Ordinal and Dichotomous Representations of Discrete-Time Survival Data.

| Outcome | Ordinal | | Binary |
	Dependent Variable	Event Indicator	Dependent Variable
censor at t_1	$y = 1$	$d = 0$	$y_1 = 0$
event at t_1	$y = 1$	$d = 1$	$y_1 = 1$
censor at t_2	$y = 2$	$d = 0$	$y_1 = 0$
			$y_2 = 0$
event at t_2	$y = 2$	$d = 1$	$y_1 = 0$
			$y_2 = 1$
censor at t_3	$y = 3$	$d = 0$	$y_1 = 0$
			$y_2 = 0$
			$y_3 = 0$
event at t_3	$y = 3$	$d = 1$	$y_1 = 0$
			$y_2 = 0$
			$y_3 = 1$

Note that for the binary model experiencing the event is coded 1 so that lower coefficient values indicate decreased risk of experiencing the event and therefore increased survival time.

8.4   Illustration

Gibbons et al. (2007) studied a cohort of 226,866 veterans who had a new diagnosis of major depressive disorder (MDD) without a history of MDD or antidepressant treatment in the previous 2 years. The sample was restricted to patients aged 19 and older, and was weighted towards patients over 25 years of age. Comparisons of suicide attempt rates were made both within patients (before and after initiation of treatment) and between individuals (i.e., comparison of those taking and not taking antidepressant medication). The suicide attempt rate was significantly lower for patients treated with an SSRI only (monotherapy) compared with those without antidepressant treatment (123/100,000 for SSRIs vs 335/100,000 for no antidepressant; OR=0.37; p<0.0001). In patients treated with an SSRI only, the rate of suicide attempts was significantly lower after treatment (123/100,000) than before treatment (221/100,000) (relative risk 0.56; p < 0.0001). Analyses stratified by age did not confirm the FDA's findings of increased suicidality for 18-24 year-olds. Comparison of suicide attempt rates for depressed patients not treated with antidepressants, versus those patients treated with SSRIs only, yielded consistent estimates of decreased risk with treatment for patients aged 18 to 25 years (OR=0.35; 95%CI 0.14, 0.85; p < 0.021), 26 to 45 years (OR=0.44; 95% CI 0.29, 0.65; p < 0.0001), 46 to 65 years (OR=0.42; 95% CI 0.30, 0.59; p < 0.0001) and >65 years (OR=0.38; 95%CI 0.16, 0.91; p < 0.036). Differences in suicide attempt rates before and after treatment initiation were also unrelated to age. The difference between the VA data and the FDA data in young adults is not due to differences in active treatment suicide attempt rates (477/100,000 VA vs 551/100,000 FDA), but rather the difference in suicide attempt rates in untreated patients versus placebo controls 1368/100,000 VA vs 268/100,000 FDA. Lack of treatment in an observational study, and receiving placebo in an RCT appear to be associated with quite different suicide attempt rates. There are several possible explanations. First, it may be that patients in RCTs are not representative of the patients seen in routine practice, and that patients selected for RCTs are less suicidal. By contrast, in routine practice, the most suicidal patients may not be offered antidepressant treatment for fear of exacerbating their suicidal tendencies based on the recent regulatory attention to this issue. Second, patients receiving placebo in RCTs may still receive supportive clinical contact, which may decrease their suicidal tendencies, whereas the patients in the VA who do not receive medication may not be receiving any other form of supportive care. Any of these potential sources of selection can lead to bias in observational studies. The VA data have been reanalyzed using a discrete-time survival model (Gibbons and Mann 2011). Their analysis revealing a significant decrease in suicide attempt rate during months with SSRI (monotherapy) treatment (hazard ratio [HR]=0.17; 95% CI 0.10, 0.28; $p < 0.0001$). This compares favorably with the observed data, for which the monthly suicide attempt rate was 207/805,525 (0.026%) for untreated months and 17/328,648 (0.005%) for treated months, yielding a raw HR of 0.19. Overall, the suicide attempt rate decreased with time from the index episode (see Figure 8.4). The top panel of Figure 8.4 is the estimated hazard function under the proportional hazards assumption, whereas the bottom panel relaxes that assumption (i.e., non-proportional hazards model where hazard ratio is not constant over time). Figure 8.4 (bottom panel) reveals that the difference in suicide attempt rate is largest early in treatment (favoring SSRI treatment) but hazard rates are essentially equivalent by approximately nine months following the index depression episode.

8.5   Competing Risk Models

A distinct advantage of the discrete-time parametric representation of the more traditional Cox proportional hazard model is the ability to easily extend the model to include random-effects, time-varying covariates, non-proportional hazards, and competing risks. The use of these models in competing risk survival models is perhaps least well known, yet is a direct generalization of the models for a single risk presented to this point. The basic idea is to use the binary representation and replace the logistic regression model for a binary outcome with a multinomial logistic regression for a nominal outcome. As an example, if we are interested in the effects of a drug exposure on stroke, death by other causes than stroke is a competing risk, because once experienced one is no longer at risk for stroke. We could simply censor the observation at the time of death, however, death is an important outcome in and of itself and quite different than simply being lost to follow-up. In this example, there are $C = 3$ unique events (death not due to stroke, stroke, and censored). When the data are clustered, perhaps within ecological units or subjects are repeatedly measured on multiple episodes for repeatable events, mixed-effects versions of the multinomial regression model can be used. In the following sections we describe the general model and present an interesting application.

8.5.1   Multinomial Regression Model

When the subjects are not clustered within higher order units (e.g., clinics, counties, ...) and there is a single outcome for each subject, then a simple multinomial regression model will suffice (Cox 1970, Bock 1970, Nerlove and

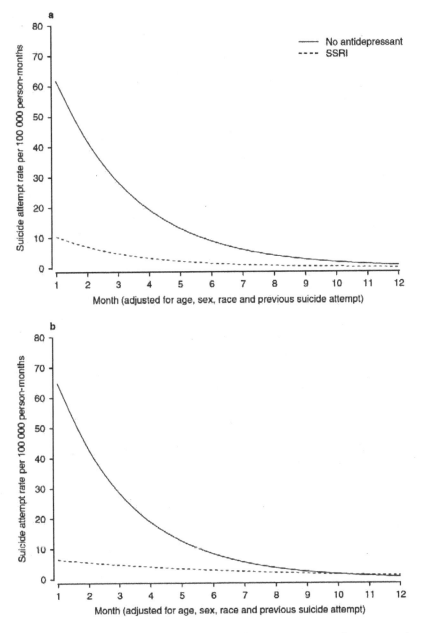

FIGURE 8.4: The effect of SSRIs on suicide attempt rate (a: proportional hazards; b: non-proportional hazards)

Press 1973, Plackett 1974, Agresti 1990). This is, in fact the traditional competing risk drug safety problem described above. For subject i, the probability that $y_i = c$ (i.e., the response occurs for subject i in category c) is given by

$$P_{ic} = P(y_i = c \mid \beta) = \frac{\exp(z_{ijc})}{1 + \sum_{h=1}^{C} \exp(z_{ih})} \quad \text{for } c = 1, 2, \ldots C \quad (8.14)$$

$$P_{i0} = P(y_i = 0 \mid \beta) = \frac{1}{1 + \sum_{h=1}^{C} \exp(z_{ih})}. \quad (8.15)$$

Estimation is achieved via maximum likelihood similar to logistic regression for binary outcomes. The fundamental difference is that we now have $C - 1$ regression functions, corresponding to contrasts between the C categories. Using this model in place of a standard logistic regression in a discrete-time survival model produces a competing risk discrete-time survival model with one category for censoring (i.e., subjects who experienced none of the $C - 1$ events) and $C - 1$ categories for the competing events of interest. During each discrete-time interval (e.g., month) a subject may have any of the $C - 1$ events of interest; however, once an event occurs the subject's record ends. A subject who never experiences the event will have $y_{it} = 0$ for all t.

8.5.2   Mixed-Effects Multinomial Regression Model

Hedeker (2003) developed a general mixed-effects multinomial logistic regression model extending earlier work by Daniels and Gatsonis (1997), Revelt and Train (1998), and Hartzel et al. (2001), also see Hedeker and Gibbons (2006). This model can be used when the data are either clustered or longitudinal (repeatable events within individuals). Let i denote the level-2 units (e.g., hospitals), and let j denote the level-1 units (e.g., patients within hospitals). Assume that there are $i = 1, \ldots N$ level-2 units and $j = 1, \ldots, n_i$ (subjects within each level 2 unit). In the discrete-time survival model, the n_i units include the set of all available time intervals (e.g. months) for all subjects in unit i. Let y_{ij} be the value of the nominal outcome variable. Adding random-effects to the multinomial logistic regression model gives the probability for subject j in unit i, responding in category $y_{ij} = c$ conditional on β and α as:

$$P_{ijc} = P(y_{ij} = c \mid \beta, \alpha) = \frac{\exp(z_{ijc})}{1 + \sum_{h=1}^{C} \exp(z_{ijh})} \quad (8.16)$$

$$P_{ij0} = P(y_{ij} = 0 \mid \beta, \alpha) = \frac{1}{1 + \sum_{h=1}^{C} \exp(z_{ijh})}. \quad (8.17)$$

for $c = 1, 2, \ldots, C$, where $z_{ijc} = x'_{ij}\beta_{ic} + w'_{ij}\alpha_c$. Here, w_{ij} is the $p \times 1$ covariate vector, and x_{ij} is the design vector for the r random-effects, both vectors being for the jth subject nested within unit i. Correspondingly, α_c is a $p \times 1$ vector of unknown fixed regression parameters, and $\boldsymbol{\beta}_{ik}$ is a $r \times 1$ vector of unknown random-effects for level-2 unit i. For the general case of multiple random-effects, their distribution is assumed to be multivariate normal with mean vector $\boldsymbol{\mu}_c$ and covariance matrix $\boldsymbol{\Sigma}_c$. Notice, that the regression coefficient vectors $\boldsymbol{\beta}$ and $\boldsymbol{\alpha}$ carry the c subscript. Thus, for each of the p covariates and r random-effects, there will be C parameters to be estimated. Additionally, the random effect variance-covariance matrix $\boldsymbol{\Sigma}_c$ is allowed to vary with c.

It is convenient to standardize the random-effects by letting $\boldsymbol{\beta}_{ic} = \boldsymbol{T}_c\boldsymbol{\theta}_i + \boldsymbol{\mu}_c$, where $\boldsymbol{T}_c\boldsymbol{T}'_c = \boldsymbol{\Sigma}_c$ is the Cholesky decomposition of $\boldsymbol{\Sigma}_c$. The model is now given as

$$z_{ijc} = \boldsymbol{x}'_{ij}(\boldsymbol{T}_c\boldsymbol{\theta}_i + \boldsymbol{\mu}_c) + \boldsymbol{w}'_{ij}\boldsymbol{\alpha}_c , \tag{8.18}$$

where $\boldsymbol{\theta}_i$ are mutually independent $N(0,1)$ variates.

Parameter estimation is described in detail by Hedeker (2003) and Hedeker and Gibbons (2006). Note that in the case of a discrete-time survival model, the n_i level-1 units represent the total number of person-time-intervals (e.g., person-months) for the subjects in cluster i.

Hazard Rates and Cumulative Survival:

Once we have estimated the model parameters, we may also wish to display the hazard rates (e.g., over time) for different exposure patterns. In addition, we may want to also display the cumulative survival curves for different exposures. Consider a model with two random-effects (e.g., one for stroke and one for death from any other cause). We can estimate the probability of each outcome conditional on a particular covariate vector (e.g., exposure pattern) as

$$P_{ij2} = \frac{\exp(\sigma_2\theta_i + \mu_2 + \boldsymbol{w}'_{ij}\boldsymbol{\alpha}_2)}{1 + \exp(\sigma_1\theta_i + \mu_1 + \boldsymbol{w}'_{ij}\boldsymbol{\alpha}_1) + \exp(\sigma_2\theta_i + \mu_2 + \boldsymbol{w}'_{ij}\boldsymbol{\alpha}_2)} \tag{8.19}$$

$$P_{ij1} = \frac{\exp(\sigma_1\theta_i + \mu_1 + \boldsymbol{w}'_{ij}\boldsymbol{\alpha}_1)}{1 + \exp(\sigma_1\theta_i + \mu_1 + \boldsymbol{w}'_{ij}\boldsymbol{\alpha}_1) + \exp(\sigma_2\theta_i + \mu_2 + \boldsymbol{w}'_{ij}\boldsymbol{\alpha}_2)} \tag{8.20}$$

$$P_{ij0} = \frac{1}{1 + \exp(\sigma_1\theta_i + \mu_1 + \boldsymbol{w}'_{ij}\boldsymbol{\alpha}_1) + \exp(\sigma_2\theta_i + \mu_2 + \boldsymbol{w}'_{ij}\boldsymbol{\alpha}_2)} \tag{8.21}$$

These are referred to as "unit-specific" probabilities because they indicate response probabilities for particular values of the random unit effect θ_i (Neuhaus et al. 1991, Zeger et al. 1988). Replacing the parameters with their estimates and denoting the resulting unit-specific probabilities as $\hat{P}_{ss}$, marginal probabilities $\hat{P}_m$ are then obtained by integrating over the random-effect distribution, namely $\hat{P}_m = \int_\theta \hat{P}_{ss}\, g(\theta)\, d\theta$. Numerical quadrature can be used for this integration as well. These marginal probabilities represent the hazard rate for a particular competing risk of interest (e.g., mortality or stroke) expressed as a rate per unit time. The cumulative survival rate is then computed by summing the time-specific risks over time, adjusting for the changing number of subjects at risk at that time point.

Intra-class Correlation

The intra-class or intra-cluster correlation is a useful method of expressing the magnitude of the level-2 variance component. For the random-intercept model, we denote the underlying response tendency associated with category c for person-time j in level-2 unit i as Y_{ijc}. The random-intercept model for the latent variable Y_{ijc} is therefore,

$$Y_{ijc} = \boldsymbol{w}'_{ij}\boldsymbol{\alpha}_c + \sigma_c\theta_i + \varepsilon_{ijc} \quad c = 0, \ldots, C. \tag{8.22}$$

Assuming $c = 0$ as the reference category, $\boldsymbol{\alpha}_0 = \sigma_0 = 0$, the model can be rewritten as

$$Y_{ijc} = \boldsymbol{w}'_{ij}\boldsymbol{\alpha}_c + \sigma_c\theta_i + (\varepsilon_{ijk} - \varepsilon_{ij0}) \quad c = 1, \ldots, C, \tag{8.23}$$

(see Hedeker, 2003). The level-1 residuals ε_{ijc} are distributed according to a type I extreme-value distribution (Maddala 1983, page 60). Furthermore, the standard logistic distribution is obtained as the difference of two independent type I extreme-value variates (McCullagh and Nelder 1989). As a result, the level-1 variance is given by $\pi^2/3$, which is the variance of the standard logistic distribution. The intra-class correlation is therefore estimated as $r_c = \hat{\sigma}_c^2/(\pi^2/3 + \hat{\sigma}_c^2)$, where $\hat{\sigma}_c^2$ is the estimated level-2 variance for category c assuming a normally distributed random-effect distribution.

8.6 Illustration

In 1998, then Secretary of the Department of Health and Human Services Donna Shalala noticed geographic inequities in median waiting time for liver transplantation of 30 versus 300 days within adjacent organ allocation areas. Dr. Shalala was concerned that life and death outcomes were "accidents of geography." In the fall of 1998, Congress requested that the Institute of Medicine (IOM) conduct a study to evaluate the potential impact of pending regulations developed by the Department of Health and Human Services on a set of important specific issues related to organ procurement and transplantation. A large part of the IOM committee's work focused on a review and analysis of approximately 68,000 liver transplant waiting list records that describe every change in status made by every patient on the Organ Procurement and Transplantation Network (OPTN) waiting list for liver transplants from 1995 through the first quarter of 1999. The methodology and results of the analysis are described in the original IOM (1999) of Medicine (1999) report and in Gibbons et al. (2003).

The objective of the analysis was to determine the degree to which there was geographic heterogeneity in liver transplantation rates and to identify possible inefficiencies in the system that would account for the large observed differences in waiting times across geographic units. At the time, there were 62 organ procurement organizations (OPOs) which were responsible for organ allocation within discrete geographic areas in the United States. The OPOs covered quite different population sizes ranging from 1 million or less to approximately 10 million lives. The system was local in nature, such that if an organ was donated in OPO 10 it would have to be transplanted or at least offered to all patients on the waiting list in OPO 10 prior to sharing the organ with a different OPO. At the time, patients where classified in status categories of 1, 2A, 2B, and 3, where status 1 represented the most severely ill patients with approximately a week to live, followed by status 2A and 2B who's life expectancy was measured in weeks or months, followed by status 3 patients who were currently in no eminent danger of death if not transplanted. However, prioritization for transplantation was based on waiting time and not on severity of illness or likelihood of death. As such, an organ could be allocated to a less severely ill patient who had been waiting longer than a more severely ill patient who was in greater need of the transplant. In addition, the local nature of the allocation system led to cases in which a status 3 patient was transplanted in an OPO when a status 1 patient in the adjacent OPO died. By a simple examination of the actual transplant data, it became immediately apparent that the large geographic discrepancies in transplant rates were produced by differences across the OPOs in when to list patients in terms of the progression of their illness. Some OPOs listed patients early, when they were in status 3 to maximize their time on the list and likelihood of transplantation once their illness progressed. Other OPOs only listed more severely ill patients. Since approximately 70% of the patients on the wait-list were status 3, the median waiting time was for a status 3 patient, the more listed in a specific OPO, the longer the median waiting time. OPOs that restricted their list to status 1 and 2 either transplanted the patients or they died, leading to a much shorter waiting time. To model the more subtle determinants of the allocation system, the committee realized that they would need to (a) accommodate competing risks of death while waiting and transplantation, and (b) random OPO effects to examine geographic variability (inequity). To this end, they used a discrete time competing risk frailty model to simultaneously evaluate the competing risks of wait-list mortality and transplantation. In the following, we describe the model parameterization and some of the key results of the IOM committee's analyses.

8.6.1 Model Parameterization

Stratified analyses were performed separately for the time spent in each status level, with the exception of 2A for which there were too few subjects. For status 1, time refers to days, whereas for status 2B and 3, time refers to months. In all analyses, the outcome measure is the nominal measure of transplant, wait-list death, or other. Other can be shifting to another status level and never returning to the status level in question, being too sick to transplant, being delisted, being transplanted at another center, or still waiting. In terms of covariates, there were age (0-5, 6-17, 18 and over), sex (female=0, male=1), race (black=1 else 0), blood type (O or B = 1 else 0) and OPO transplant volume (small, medium, and large based on number of transplanted patients in 1995-1999). For blood type, a contrast between types O and B versus A and AB was used because the former two can only receive donation from a subset of donors whereas the latter can receive donation from almost all potential donors.

8.6.2   Results

A summary of several statistics of interest that help characterize the sample and waiting time distributions is presented in Table 8.3. Maximum marginal likelihood estimates, standard errors, and corresponding probabilities for Wald test statistics are presented in Table 8.4, separately for status levels 1, 2B, and 3, respectively. In the following we provide an overview of the most important findings.

Geographic Inequity:

In terms of geographic inequity, systematic OPO-specific effects accounted for less than 5% of the total variance (i.e., intra-cluster correlation of 0.045) in transplantation rates for status 1 patients (see Table 8.3). The geographic distribution for the most severely ill patients is therefore reasonably equitable with mean waiting time of 4.8 days (see Table 8.3). In contrast, OPO-specific effects accounted for 13% of the variability in transplantation rates for status 2B patients (see Table 8.4) and 35% of the variability for status 3 patients (see Table 8.4). This implies that the systematic variation in waiting time across OPOs is almost completely determined by variations in waiting times for the less severely ill patients, with little variation for the most severely ill patients. This finding is further illustrated in Figure 8.5 where the empirical Bayes (EB) estimates of the OPO-specific adjusted transplantation effects are displayed.

The interpretation of the EB estimate is OPO i's deviation from the population rate, adjusted for covariates. As such, the y axis in Figure 8.5 is in a log-odds scale, where values of 1, 2, and 3 represents increases in the likelihood of transplantation by factors of 2.7, 7.4, and 20.1, respectively. Negative values represent corresponding decreases in probability of transplantation relative to the overall population rate.

Moreover, while transplantation rates of these less severely ill patients vary significantly, they have little relationship to mortality. In all cases, systematic OPO differences in pre-transplantation mortality rates accounted for less than

TABLE 8.3: Characteristics of Liver Transplant Patients by Status, 1995–1999

	Totals	Status 1	Status 2	Status 3
Total patients, 1995–1999	33,286	5,294	14,264	26,907
Percentage receiving a transplant	47.1	52.4	50.2	21.3
Percentage dying prior to transplantation	8.3	9.2	6.1	5.2
Percentage post-transplant mortality	5.4	11.1	5.0	1.9
Percentage male	58.7	54.1	59.9	58.7
Percentage with A or AB blood type	16.0	15.3	15.4	15.8
Percentage African American	7.7	11.2	8.3	6.9
Mean age (years)	45.0	36.3	44.9	46.1
Mean waiting time (days)	255.6	4.8	56.8	285.1

1% of the variation in overall adjusted mortality rates. No significant effects of race or gender were observed indicating that the system is equitable for women and minorities once they are listed.

OPO Volume and Size:

Smaller OPOs are more likely than larger OPOs to transplant status 2B and 3 patients (see Table 8.4). For status 1 patients, OPO size played no role in transplantation or mortality rates. In contrast, for status 2B and 3 patients, OPO size was significantly related to transplantation rates. For large OPOs (9+ million) the initial one month transplantation rates were 5% for status 2B patients and 3% for status 3 patients. By contrast in the smaller OPOs (4 million or less), initial one-month transplantation rates were as high as 17% for status 2B patients and 9% for status 3 patients. Based on these results the committee recommended that at least 9 million people be included in an organ allocation region to maximize the chance of transplantation for the most severely ill patients.

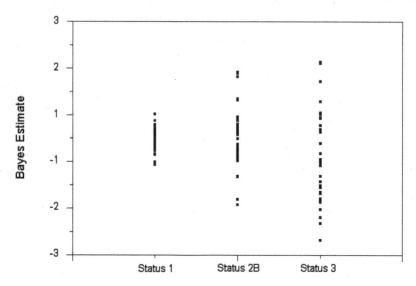

FIGURE 8.5: OPO-specific Bayes estimates $(\sigma_1\theta_i)$ of transplantation rates by status category adjusted for competing risk of mortality and model covariates (e.g., sex, race, blood type).

The Effect of Sharing:

Further evidence in support of the committee's broader sharing recommendation was drawn from several regional and state-wide sharing arrangements among two or more OPOs, most typically for status 1 patients. The results of these "natural experiments" revealed that sharing significantly increased the status 1 transplantation rate from 42% without sharing to 52% with sharing, lowered average status 1 waiting times from 4 to 3 days, and decreased status 1 pre-transplantation mortality from 9% to 7%. Not surprisingly, sharing significantly decreased the rate of transplantation for less severely ill patients. For example, among small OPOs that served a population of 2 million or less, the status 3 transplantation rate decreased from 31% for those OPOs that did not share to 6% for those that did share, making more organs available for more severely ill patients. Though sharing decreased status 3 transplantation rates, there was no concomitant increase in pre-transplantation mortality of status 3 patients.

Waiting Times and Need for Transplant:

The committee also studied the relationship of transplantation and pre-transplantation mortality to waiting time, since this was a major factor in the original allocation system. For status 1 patients, the rates were constant over the first 12 days of listing at approximately 15% for transplantation per day and 3% for mortality (see Figure 8.6 panel A), but for status 2B and 3 patients both rates decreased rapidly over time (see Figure 8.6 panels B and C). For status 2B, transplantation rates decreased from 12% to 5% per month over a 12 month period while pre-transplant mortality rates decreased from 3% to 0.3% per month. For status 3 patients, transplantation rates decreased from 4% to 0.05% per month over a 12 month period and pre-transplant mortality rates decreased from 2% to 0.2% per month.

Figure 8.7 displays estimated cumulative time-to-event distributions for status 1 (panel A), status 2B (panel B), and status 3 (panel C). Inspection of Figure 8.7 reveals that after 12 days 80% of the status 1 patients at risk are transplanted whereas 10% die while waiting. For status 2B, 60% of patients at risk through 12 months are transplanted and 7% die while waiting. For status 3, 20% of patients at risk through 12 months are transplanted and 8% die while waiting. These estimates differ somewhat from the observed rates in Table 8.3 because subjects were not always observed for these period of times due to becoming too ill to transplant (and removed from the list) or changing status category.

TABLE 8.4: Mixed-Effects Competing Risk Survival Models for Patient Time in Status Levels 1, 2B, and 3—Maximum Likelihood Estimates (Standard Errors)

	Status 1	Status 2B	Status 3
Transplant versus Other			
Intercept	-1.829 (0.276)	-2.077 (0.129)	-3.593 (0.210)
Day (1), month (2B, 3)	0.016 (0.015)	-0.092 (0.016) ***	-0.220 (0.030) ***
Age 0-5 vs. ≥ 18	-0.907 (0.188) ***	0.470 (0.103) ***	1.156 (0.154) ***
Age 6-17 vs. ≥ 18	-0.362 (0.234)	0.135 (0.243)	0.844 (0.268) **
Gender (1 = male)	-0.098 (0.198)	0.126 (0.087)	0.054 (0.186)
Race (1 = black)	-0.275 (0.268)	0.134 (0.222)	0.158 (0.304)
Blood type (1 = B or O)	-0.076 (0.196)	-0.577 (0.062) ***	-0.477 (0.098) ***
OPO volume (M vs. L)	-0.054 (0.319)	0.590 (0.157) ***	1.179 (0.149) ***
OPO volume (S vs. L)	0.261 (0.336)	0.560 (0.187) **	0.757 (0.228) ***
Random OPO effect SD	0.393 (0.144) **	0.689 (0.064) ***	1.335 (0.162) ***
Mortality versus Other			
Intercept	-3.685 (0.482)	-3.313 (0.227)	-3.654 (0.172)
Day (1), month (2B, 3)	0.023 (0.047)	-0.213 (0.039) ***	-0.216 (0.041) ***
Age 0-5 vs. Adult	-0.968 (0.378) **	-0.195 (0.381)	-2.119 (2.099)
Age 6-17 vs. Adult	-1.001 (0.551)	-0.516 (0.641)	-1.193 (2.000)
Gender (1 = male)	0.077 (0.371)	0.014 (0.191)	-0.063 (0.268)
Race (1 = black)	0.162 (0.448)	-0.082 (0.359)	0.027 (0.544)
Blood type (1 = B or O)	0.003 (0.433)	-0.005 (0.164)	-0.017 (0.231)
OPO volume (M vs. L)	0.203 (0.491)	0.202 (0.126)	-0.526 (0.300)
OPO volume (S vs. L)	-0.230 (0.930)	0.355 (0.151) **	-0.658 (0.358)
Random OPO effect SD	0.042 (0.298)	0.116 (0.049) **	0.137 (0.157)

$*p < .05$, $**p < .01$, $***p < .001$.

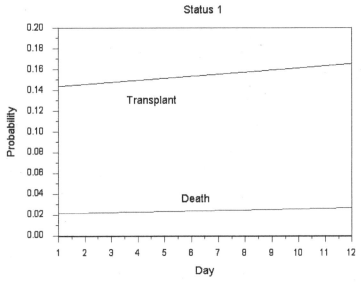

(a) Estimated hazard rates for status 1

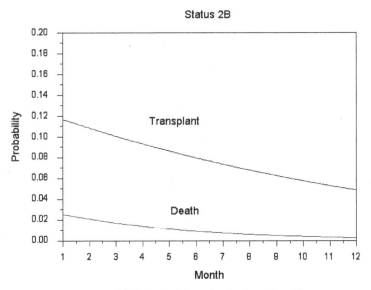

(b) Estimated hazard rates for status 2B

FIGURE 8.6: Continued on next page

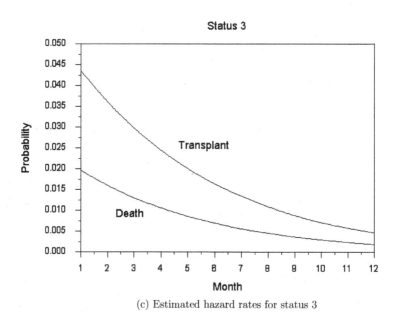

(c) Estimated hazard rates for status 3

FIGURE 8.6: Estimated hazard rates for (a) status 1, (b) status 2B, and (c) status 3 patients awaiting liver transplantation. The hazard rate describes the likelihood of transplantation or mortality at a given point in time (using one whole day (status 1) or one whole month (status 2B and 3) as the unit) adjusted for the competing risks(i.e., transplantation or mortality) and the model covariates (e.g., sex, race, blood type).

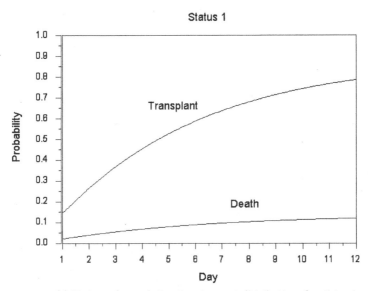

(a) Estimated cumulative time-to-event distributions for status 1

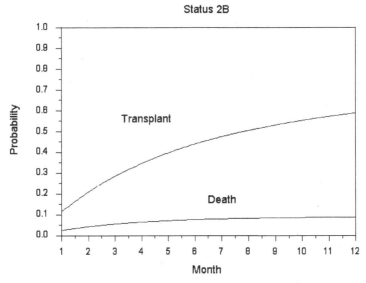

(b) Estimated cumulative time-to-event distributions for status 2B

FIGURE 8.7: Continued on next page

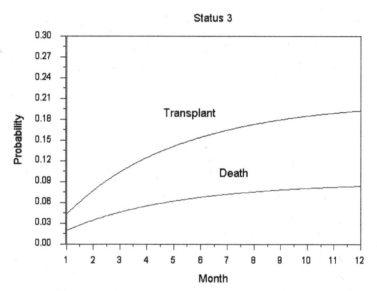

(c) Estimated cumulative time-to-event distributions for status 3

FIGURE 8.7: Estimated cumulative time-to-event distributions for (a) status 1, (b) status 2B, and (c) status 3 patients awaiting liver transplantation. The cumulative time-to-event distribution describes the overall adjusted likelihood of transplantation or mortality up to a particular point in time.

8.6.3 Discussion

From a statistical perspective, this case study is useful in that it illustrates the important role that statisticians play in the development of public policy. Clearly, without the analysis of these data, the IOM committee would not have reached these conclusions, and the life-saving changes in the regulations would not have occurred. This example also illustrates that relatively complex statistical methods can, in fact, be used to evaluate important public policy questions and to communicate the results to a largely non-statistical audience, including the U.S. Congress. The notion, that complex statistical methods will hinder the dissemination of research findings to policy makers and the public, was not borne out.

The analysis revealed that the rate of liver transplantation of the most severely ill (status 1) patients is relatively homogeneous across OPOs. However, the allocation of organs is not efficient because many organs that could be used for transplantation of status 1 patients are being transplanted into less severely ill patients, especially in smaller OPOs due to the local nature of the original allocation system. The IOM analysis revealed that this inefficiency resulting from small OPOs is minimized when allocation areas comprise a minimum population of 9 million people. Their analysis of existing broader sharing arrangements confirmed this result by demonstrating that broader sharing of organs led to an overall increase in the rate at which the most severely ill patients were transplanted and a concomitant decrease in the excess transplantation of the least severely ill patients, without increasing pre-transplantation mortality.

9

Research Synthesis

"Philosophy, like medicine, has plenty of drugs, few good remedies, and hardly any specific cures."
(Sbastien-Roch Nicolas De Chamfort (1741 - 1794), French writer)

9.1 Introduction

Meta-analysis is useful for the combination of effect sizes which may be measured using a variety of different metrics. By contrast, research synthesis involves a reanalysis of the complete original data commonly measured and collected from a number of different studies. The advantage of research synthesis over meta-analysis is that we can use all available data from each subject and each study even if the timeframes are not identical (e.g., weekly versus monthly assessments) as long as the overall timeframe is comparable. The analysis of longitudinal data is generally not possible in meta-analysis where the unit of analysis is a statistic which summarizes the results of each study. For example, in meta-analysis we might combine information on average change in treated and control subjects where sample size and both measures of mean change and its variability (e.g., standard deviation of change scores) are available from each study. This requirement raises issues related to the treatment of missing data, where we must choose a method of imputation of the endpoint of interest. For example, we can use *last observation carried forward* (LOCF) in which the last available measurement is used as a proxy for the measurement that would have been obtained had the subject completed the study. In many cases, however, all that may be available are the summary statistics for those subjects that completed the study. These statistics may be quite biased in that they have little to do with the totality of subjects that were randomized to the treated and control conditions of interest. In many cases, a mixture of both types of data are present, leading to pooled estimates with questionable validity. The same is not true for research synthesis where all available data from each subject are available and form the basis of the pooled analysis. Here we can model the within person and within study components of variance which produce both person-specific and study-specific deviations from the overall response process. This approach to research synthesis is more firmly grounded in statistical theory in that it is much more robust to the presence of missing data. The usual models operate under the "missing at random" assumption (Rubin 1976) and even models for "not missing at random" (Rubin 1976) are possible if data regarding the missing data process are also available. As used here, the term research synthesis implies a reanalysis of the data preserving the nesting of subjects within studies and allowing the trajectories and even the effect of treatment to vary from subject to subject and study to study.

Statistically, research synthesis is based on three-level linear or non-linear mixed-effects regression models. Gibbons et al. (2012a,b) have illustrated the methodology for both the benefits and safety of the antidepressants fluoxetine and venlafaxine, where they synthesized the complete longitudinal data from all randomized patients enrolled in 41 such studies. They examined rates of change in both efficacy as measured by the Hamilton Depression Rating Scale (HAM-D) or Child Depression Rating Scale (CDRS) and safety as measured by the rate of change in suicidal thoughts and behavior based on both spontaneous reports of attempts and prospective clinician measurements of ideation and behavior. These rates of change were allowed to vary from patient to patient and study to study. Separate analyses were performed for youth, adults, and the elderly so that the same outcome measure would be available for each analysis. A combined analysis of all adult data was also conducted since both adult and the elderly samples both used the same outcome measure. These data are used to illustrate the general methodology that will now be presented.

9.2 Three-level Mixed-effects Regression Models

Research synthesis involves the nesting of repeated measurements within individuals and the nesting of individuals within studies. In general we use data from RCTs as the basis for the analysis so that biases associated with observational studies are for the most part eliminated. However, study to study variability can be produced by indications for treatment and differences in design of the studies, so the statistical combination of the complete data from multiple studies does not support the same level of causal inference had all of the subjects been enrolled in a single large well controlled RCT.

9.2.1 Three-level Linear Mixed Model

As noted above, consider a research synthesis of all available longitudinal data from each subject from N studies comparing a treatment versus relevant control condition. Following Hedeker and Gibbons (2006) we have $i = 1 \ldots N$ studies, $j = 1 \ldots n_i$ subjects in study i, and $k = 1 \ldots n_{ij}$ observations for subject j in study i. Further denote $N_i = \sum_{j=1}^{n_i} n_{ij}$, which is the total number of observations within study i. Suppose that we wanted to fit a model with a single random study effect (i.e., intercept) and two random subject effects (i.e., intercept and trend). In terms of the random effects, this model could be written as follows:

$$
\begin{bmatrix} y_{i1} \\ y_{i2} \\ y_{i3} \\ \dots \\ \dots \\ \dots \\ y_{in_i} \end{bmatrix}
=
\begin{bmatrix}
1 & Z_{i1} & 0 & 0 & \dots & 0 \\
1 & 0 & Z_{i2} & 0 & \dots & 0 \\
1 & 0 & 0 & Z_{i3} & \dots & 0 \\
\dots & \dots & \dots & \dots & \dots & \dots \\
\dots & \dots & \dots & \dots & \dots & \dots \\
\dots & \dots & \dots & \dots & \dots & \dots \\
1 & 0 & 0 & 0 & \dots & Z_{in_i}
\end{bmatrix}
\begin{bmatrix} \gamma_i \\ v_{i1} \\ v_{i2} \\ v_{i3} \\ \dots \\ \dots \\ v_{in_i} \end{bmatrix}
+
\begin{bmatrix} \varepsilon_{i1} \\ \varepsilon_{i2} \\ \varepsilon_{i3} \\ \dots \\ \dots \\ \dots \\ \varepsilon_{in_i} \end{bmatrix}
$$

or,

$$ y_i = Z_i v_i^* + \varepsilon_i $$

where $\gamma_i \sim \mathcal{N}(0, \sigma_\gamma^2)$, $v_{ij} \sim \mathcal{N}(0, \Sigma_\beta)$, and $\varepsilon_{ijk} \sim \mathcal{N}(0, \sigma_\varepsilon^2)$. With a single random study effect, the number of random-effects equals $r+1$, where r is the number of random subject effects. However, for a given study i the dimension of v^* equals $n_i \times r + 1$, which we denote as R_i, the i subscript indicates that this value varies depending on the size of the study. Adding covariates to this model yields

$$ y_i = X_i \beta + Z_i v_i^* + \varepsilon_i, \tag{9.1} $$

where X_i is a known $N_i \times p$ design matrix for the fixed-effects, β is the $p \times 1$ vector of unknown fixed regression parameters, Z_i is a known $N_i \times R_i$ design matrix for the random-effects, v_i^* is the $R_i \times 1$ vector of unknown random-effects, and ε_i is the $N_i \times 1$ error vector.

As a result, the observations y and random coefficients v^* have the joint multivariate normal distribution:

$$
\begin{bmatrix} y_i \\ v_i^* \end{bmatrix} \sim \mathcal{N} \left(\begin{bmatrix} X_i \beta \\ 0 \end{bmatrix}, \begin{bmatrix} Z_i \Sigma_i Z_i' + \sigma_\varepsilon^2 I_i & Z_i \Sigma_i \\ \Sigma_i Z_i' & \Sigma_i \end{bmatrix} \right)
$$

where the random coefficients v_i^* and variance-covariance matrix Σ_i are given as:

$$
\begin{bmatrix} \gamma_i \\ v_{i1} \\ v_{i2} \\ \dots \\ v_{in_i} \end{bmatrix} \sim \mathcal{N} \left(\begin{bmatrix} 0 \\ 0 \\ 0 \\ \dots \\ 0 \end{bmatrix} \begin{bmatrix} \sigma_\gamma^2 & 0 & 0 & \dots & 0 \\ 0 & \Sigma_v & 0 & \dots & 0 \\ 0 & 0 & \Sigma_v & \dots & 0 \\ \dots & \dots & \dots & \dots & \dots \\ 0 & 0 & 0 & \dots & \Sigma_v \end{bmatrix} \right).
$$

The i subscript for the variance covariance matrix Σ_i merely reflects the number of observations within the study, not the number of parameters which is the same for all studies.

The mean of the posterior distribution of $\boldsymbol{v}^*$, given $\boldsymbol{y}_i$, yields the EAP estimator ("Expected A Posteriori") of the study effects and individual trend parameters:

$$\tilde{\boldsymbol{v}}_{ii}^* = \left[\boldsymbol{Z}_i'(\sigma_\varepsilon^2 \boldsymbol{I}_i)^{-1} \boldsymbol{Z}_i + \boldsymbol{\Sigma}_i^{-1} \right]^{-1} \boldsymbol{Z}_i'(\sigma_\varepsilon^2 \boldsymbol{I}_i)^{-1} (\boldsymbol{y}_i - \boldsymbol{X}_i \boldsymbol{\beta})$$

with covariance matrix

$$\boldsymbol{\Sigma}_{\theta|y_j} = \left[\boldsymbol{Z}_j'(\sigma_\varepsilon^2 \boldsymbol{I}_j)^{-1} \boldsymbol{Z}_j + \boldsymbol{\Sigma}_j^{-1} \right]^{-1}.$$

Differentiating the log-likelihood, $\log L = \sum_{i=1}^{N} \log h(\boldsymbol{y}_i)$, yields:

$$\frac{\partial \log L}{\partial \boldsymbol{\beta}} = \sigma_\varepsilon^2 \sum_{i=1}^{N} \boldsymbol{X}_i' \boldsymbol{u}_i$$

$$\frac{\partial \log L}{\partial \boldsymbol{\Sigma}^*} = \frac{1}{2} \sum_{i=1}^{N} \boldsymbol{D}_i' \boldsymbol{G}_i' \mathrm{vec} \left[\boldsymbol{\Sigma}_i^{-1} (\boldsymbol{\Sigma}_{\theta|y_j} + \tilde{\boldsymbol{v}}_{ii}^* (\tilde{\boldsymbol{v}}_{ii}^*)' - \boldsymbol{\Sigma}_i) \boldsymbol{\Sigma}_i^{-1} \right]$$

$$\frac{\partial \log L}{\partial \sigma_\varepsilon^2} = \frac{1}{2} \sigma_\varepsilon^{-4} \sum_{i=1}^{N} -n_i \sigma^2 + \boldsymbol{u}_i' \boldsymbol{u}_i + \mathrm{tr} \left[\boldsymbol{\Sigma}_{\theta|y_j} \boldsymbol{Z}_i' \boldsymbol{Z}_i \right]$$

where $\boldsymbol{u}_i = \boldsymbol{y}_i - \boldsymbol{Z}_i \tilde{\boldsymbol{v}}_{ii}^* - \boldsymbol{X}_i \boldsymbol{\beta}$, and $\mathrm{vech}\boldsymbol{\Sigma}_i = \boldsymbol{D}_i \boldsymbol{\Sigma}^*$. In this notation, $\boldsymbol{\Sigma}^*$ represents the vector with only the unique variance-covariance parameters, and $\boldsymbol{D}_i$ is a matrix of ones and zeros that is necessary to pick off only the correct terms.

9.2.1.1 Illustration: Efficacy of Antidepressants

Concerns have been raised that the efficacy of antidepressant treatment has been overstated (Turner et al. 2008). They found that among 74 FDA registered RCTs that were published, 94% were positive but only 51% of all registered trials were positive. Meta-analyses have suggested that antidepressants are only effective in the most severely ill patients (Kirsch et al. 2008). While provocative, these finding raise as many questions as they attempt to answer. The first is a so-called "vote-counting method" consisting of a simple tally of the significance dichotomized at the 5% level of each study. For example it could be that the larger studies were published and those studies were the only studies that had sufficient statistical power to detect a significant difference between treated and control conditions. One could imagine a situation

in which none of the individual studies yielded a statistically significant finding, but the true effect in the population was significant and of public health
importance. With respect to the moderation by severity of depression at baseline, it is hard to imagine how this could even be analyzed using meta-analysis
in which all that is available is the average severity level for each study. The
relationship between severity of illness and efficacy of treatment exists at the
level of the individual and is not reliably assessed using study-level aggregated
information.

To study this question more rigorously, Gibbons et al. (2012a) obtained
complete person-level longitudinal data from 12 adult (2,635 patients and
14,048 measurements), 4 geriatric (960 patients and 5,209 measurements),
and 4 youth (708 patients and 2,536 measurements) RCTs of fluoxetine and
21 adult trials of venlafaxine (immediate release (IR) 11 adult studies with
2,421 patients and 10,634 measurements and for extended release (ER) there
were 10 adult studies with 2,461 patients and 12,481 measurements). Analysis
focused on the CDRS for children and the HAM-D for adults, which were used
to estimate rate of change as well as response and remission rates at 6 weeks.

These data were analyzed using three-level linear mixed-effects regression
models as described above. Level 1 represents the measurement occasion, level
2 the patient, and level 3 the study. An overall analysis was performed for both
drugs (fluoxetine and venlafaxine IR and ER) in adults and geriatrics. Youth
were not included in the combined analysis because they were assessed with
the CDRS. Separate analyses were performed for fluoxetine adult, geriatric,
and youth trials, and venlafaxine IR and ER adult trials. The intercept and
slope of the time trends were random-effects at both patient and study levels, allowing time-trends to vary across patients and studies. Heterogeneity
of treatment effect was tested by including a random treatment by time interaction. Time was number of days from treatment initiation. The primary
effect of interest was change in slope between treatment and control over 6
weeks. Six weeks was selected because it was the minimum trial duration and
therefore study and length of treatment were unconfounded. A variety of parameterizations of time were considered, but the best fitting model was based
on a simple linear function of time through 6 weeks.

Adult Studies

To estimate response and remission rates in the presence of missing data,
empirical Bayes estimates of each subject's trend was used to impute a CDRS
or HAM-D score at day 42, if the actual day 42 score was missing. For adults
and geriatric patients, response was a 50% reduction in HAM-D score at week
six, and remission was HAM-D<8. For youth, response was a 50% reduction
in CDRS score at week six and remission was CDRS-R<28. Number needed
to treat (NNT) was also computed for each endpoint and sample.

To provide an overview of the results, we present the findings for the overall analysis for fluoxetine and venlafaxine IR and ER in adults and geriatrics.

The estimated average rate of change over 6 weeks was -11.82 HAM-D units for drug versus -9.26 HAM-D units for placebo MMLE = -2.55, SE = 0.20, p<0.0001), indicating 28% greater improvement for drug. Estimated linear time trends and observed daily mean scores are presented in Figure 9.1. Variation in the treatment effect over studies was not statistically significant (SD = 0.16, p=0.06).

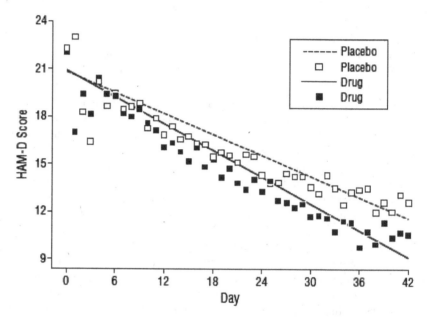

FIGURE 9.1: Overall observed and estimated time-trends for adults.

The estimated response rate for drug was 58.4% versus 39.9% for placebo (OR=2.11, 95% CI 1.93-2.31, p<0.001, NNT=5.41). Remission rates were 43.0% versus 29.3% for drug and placebo respectively (OR=1.82, 95% CI 1.66-2.00, p<0.001, NNT=7.30).

No effect of baseline severity on treatment efficacy was found for either dichotomous (p=0.27) or continuous (p=0.10) baseline severity measures. For patients with low severity, rate of change in symptoms over 6 weeks was -9.40 for drug versus -7.20 for placebo. For high severity patients the rate of change was -12.85 for drug versus -10.07 for placebo. The estimated difference was 2.20, 95% CI 1.65-2.76 for low severity and 2.78, 95% CI 2.26-3.29 for high severity. Estimated response rates were 54.8% vs. 37.3% (difference of 17.5%) for treated vs. placebo low severity patients and 57.7% vs. 40.5% (difference of 17.2%) for high severity patients. Estimated remission rates were 49.9% vs. 36.6% (difference of 13.3%) for treated vs. placebo low severity patients and 37.8% vs. 25.1% (difference of 12.7%) for high severity patients.

Youth Studies

The estimated average rate of change over 6 weeks was -15.96 CDRS units for placebo and -20.58 CDRS units for fluoxetine (MMLE = -4.62, SE = 1.26, p<0.0001), indicating 30% greater improvement for fluoxetine.

The estimated response rate for fluoxetine was 29.8% versus 5.7% for placebo (OR=6.66, 95% CI 3.07-14.48, p<0.001, NNT=4.16). Remission rates were 46.6% versus 16.5% for fluoxetine and placebo respectively (OR=4.23, 95% CI 2.64-6.77, p<0.001, NNT=3.33. The finding of higher remission than response rates questions the validity of the CDRS remission threshold score of 28.

No effect of baseline severity on treatment efficacy was found (p=0.90). For low severity patients, the rate of change in symptoms was -17.60 for fluoxetine versus -12.56 for placebo. For high severity patients the rate of change was -28.86 for fluoxetine versus -24.40 for placebo. The estimated difference was 5.04, 95% CI 2.56-7.52 for low severity and 4.45, 95% CI -0.58-9.49 for high severity. Estimated response rates were 23.0% vs. 3.2% (difference of 19.8%) for treated vs. placebo low severity patients and 40.2% vs. 17.2% (difference of 23.0%) for high severity patients. Estimated remission rates were 54.1% vs. 19.4% (difference of 20.6%) for treated vs. placebo low severity patients and 28.9% vs. 7.5% (difference of 21.4%) for high severity patients.

Discussion

The results of this research synthesis reveal clear efficacy of antidepressant medications across the lifespan which translate into important clinical differences in terms of response and remission rates. Previous findings that the effect is restricted to the most severely ill patients based on meta-analysis using average study-level severity is not confirmed when patient-level data form the basis for the analysis. Interestingly, the largest effect of treatment is seen in children. Although not described here, the efficacy of antidepressants in the elderly was statistically significant, but clinically marginal with NNTs of 17 and 39 for response and remission, respectively. The reanalysis of these data in contrast to the meta-analysis of these data reveal a far more detailed picture of the efficacy of these medications. While the overall mean difference is on the order of only 3 points on a 40 point scale, small differences in the mean response translate to large gains in the tails of the distribution in terms of response and remission rates.

9.2.2 Three-level Non-linear Mixed Model

For a binary, ordinal, count, or time-to-event outcome, the linear mixed-model described above is no longer valid because the link function is no longer the identity. As a result, the integrals in the likelihood function must be evaluated numerically leading to a more computationally complex solution. Nevertheless, this type of problem is easily solved as long as the number of random-effects is relatively small. For example a model with random intercept and trend at both subject and study levels has four random-effects and is computationally tractable despite the number of studies and subjects. Following Hedeker and Gibbons (2006) we present a general derivation using a probit link function; however, the logistic model is a simple extension of the general result.

Stacking the unobservable latent response vectors of each subject within a study $(\boldsymbol{y}_{ij})$, the three-level model for the resulting N_i response vector for the ith study, $i = 1, 2, \ldots, N$, can be written as follows:

$$
\underbrace{\begin{bmatrix} \boldsymbol{y}_{i1} \\ \boldsymbol{y}_{i2} \\ \boldsymbol{y}_{i3} \\ \cdots \\ \cdots \\ \boldsymbol{y}_{in_i} \end{bmatrix}}_{\substack{\boldsymbol{y}_i \\ N_i \times 1}} = \underbrace{\begin{bmatrix} \boldsymbol{1}_{i1} & \boldsymbol{Z}_{i1} & 0 & 0 & \cdots & 0 \\ \boldsymbol{1}_{i2} & 0 & \boldsymbol{Z}_{i2} & 0 & \cdots & 0 \\ \boldsymbol{1}_{i3} & 0 & 0 & \boldsymbol{Z}_{i3} & \cdots & 0 \\ \cdots & \cdots & \cdots & \cdots & \cdots & \cdots \\ \cdots & \cdots & \cdots & \cdots & \cdots & \cdots \\ \boldsymbol{1}_{in_i} & 0 & 0 & 0 & \cdots & \boldsymbol{Z}_{in_i} \end{bmatrix}}_{\substack{\boldsymbol{Z}_i \\ N_i \times ((n_i \times r)+1)}} \underbrace{\begin{bmatrix} \upsilon_{0i} \\ \boldsymbol{v}_{i1} \\ \boldsymbol{v}_{i2} \\ \boldsymbol{v}_{i3} \\ \cdots \\ \boldsymbol{v}_{in_i} \end{bmatrix}}_{\substack{\boldsymbol{v}_i^* \\ ((n_i \times r)+1) \times 1}}
$$

$$
+ \underbrace{\begin{bmatrix} \boldsymbol{1}_{i1} & \boldsymbol{X}_{i1} \\ \boldsymbol{1}_{i2} & \boldsymbol{X}_{i2} \\ \boldsymbol{1}_{i3} & \boldsymbol{X}_{i3} \\ \cdots & \cdots \\ \cdots & \cdots \\ \boldsymbol{1}_{in_i} & \boldsymbol{X}_{in_i} \end{bmatrix}}_{\substack{\boldsymbol{X}_i \\ N_i \times (p+1)}} \underbrace{\begin{bmatrix} \beta_0 \\ \beta_1 \\ \cdots \\ \beta_p \end{bmatrix}}_{\substack{\boldsymbol{\beta} \\ (p+1) \times 1}} + \underbrace{\begin{bmatrix} \boldsymbol{e}_{i1} \\ \boldsymbol{e}_{i2} \\ \boldsymbol{e}_{i3} \\ \cdots \\ \cdots \\ \boldsymbol{e}_{in_i} \end{bmatrix}}_{\substack{\boldsymbol{e}_i \\ N_i \times 1}},
$$

where the following independent components are distributed, $\beta_{0i} \sim \mathcal{N}(0, \sigma_{(3)}^2)$, $\boldsymbol{v}_{ij} \sim \mathcal{N}(0, \boldsymbol{\Sigma}_{(2)})$, and $\boldsymbol{e}_i \sim \mathcal{N}(0, \sigma_\varepsilon^2 \boldsymbol{I}_{n_i})$. Notice, there are n_i subjects in study i and N_i total observations for study i (the sum of all repeated observations for all subjects within the study). The number of random subject-level effects is r, and the number of fixed covariates in the model (excluding the intercept) is p. In the case of binary responses, each person has an $n_{ij} \times 1$ vector $\boldsymbol{y}_{ij}$ of underlying response strengths, an $n_{ij} \times r$ design matrix $\boldsymbol{Z}_{ij}$ for their r random-effects $\boldsymbol{v}_{ij}$, and a $n_{ij} \times p$ matrix of covariates $\boldsymbol{X}_{ij}$. The covariate matrix usually includes the random effect design matrix so that the overall intercept, linear term, etc., is estimated and thus the random-effects represent deviations from these overall terms.

A characteristic of the probit model is the assumption that there is an unobservable latent variable (y_{ijk}) related to the actual binary response through a "threshold concept" (Bock 1975). We assume the underlying latent variable y_{ijk} is continuous and that the binary response $y_{ijk} = 1$ occurs when y_{ijk} exceeds a threshold γ (i.e., $P(y_{ijk} = 1) = P(y_{ijk} > \gamma)$). In terms of the latent response strength for subject j in study i on occasion k (y_{ijk}) we obtain

$$y_{ijk} = \beta_{0i} + \mathbf{z}'_{ijk}\mathbf{v}_{ij} + \mathbf{x}'_{ijk}\boldsymbol{\beta} + \varepsilon_{ijk} \ . \tag{9.2}$$

With the above mixed regression model for the latent variable y_{ijk}, the probability that $y_{ijk} = 1$ (a positive response occurs), conditional on the random-effects $\mathbf{v}^*$, is given by:

$$\Pr(y_{ijk} = 1|\mathbf{v}^*) = (2\pi\sigma_\varepsilon^2)^{-\frac{1}{2}} \int_\gamma^\infty \exp\left[-\frac{1}{2\sigma_\varepsilon^2}(y_{ijk} - v_{0i} - \mathbf{z}'_{ijk}\mathbf{v}_{ij} - \mathbf{x}'_{ijk}\boldsymbol{\beta})^2 \right] dy$$

$$= \ \Phi[-(\gamma - s_{ijk})/\sigma_\varepsilon] \tag{9.3}$$

where $s_{ijk} = \beta_{0i} + \mathbf{z}'_{ijk}\mathbf{v}_{ij} + \mathbf{x}'_{ijk}\boldsymbol{\beta}$, and $\Phi(\cdot)$ represents the cumulative standard normal density function. Without loss of generality, the origin and unit of z may be chosen arbitrarily. For convenience, let $\gamma = 0$, and to insure identifiability let $\sigma_\varepsilon = 1$.

Let $\mathbf{y}_i$ be the vector pattern of binary responses from study i for the n_i individuals examined at the n_{ij} time-points. Assuming independence of the responses conditional on the random-effects, the probability of any pattern $\mathbf{y}_i$, given $\mathbf{v}_i^*$, is equal to the product of the probabilities of the individual responses (both between and within individuals in cluster i):

$$\ell(\mathbf{y}_i \mid \mathbf{v}_i^*) = \prod_{j=1}^{n_i} \prod_{k=1}^{n_{ij}} [\Phi(s_{ijk})]^{y_{ijk}} [1 - \Phi(s_{ijk})]^{1-y_{ijk}} \ . \tag{9.4}$$

Then the marginal probability of $\mathbf{y}_i$ is expressed as the following integral of the likelihood, $\ell(\cdot)$, weighted by the prior density $g(\cdot)$:

$$h(\mathbf{y}_i) = \int_{\mathbf{v}^*} \ell(\mathbf{y}_i \mid \mathbf{v}_i^*) \, g(\mathbf{v}^*) \, d\mathbf{v}^* \ , \tag{9.5}$$

where $g(\mathbf{v}^*)$ represents the distribution of $\mathbf{v}^*$ in the population.

Orthogonalization of the Model Parameters

For numerical solution of the likelihood equations, Gibbons and Bock (1987) orthogonally transform the response model using the Cholesky decomposition of $\boldsymbol{\Sigma}_{\mathbf{v}^*}$ (Bock, 1975). Specifically, let $\mathbf{v}^* = \mathbf{T}^*\boldsymbol{\theta}^*$, where $\mathbf{T}^*\mathbf{T}^{*'} = \boldsymbol{\Sigma}_{\mathbf{v}^*}$ is the Cholesky decomposition of $\boldsymbol{\Sigma}_{\mathbf{v}^*}$. Then $\boldsymbol{\theta}^* = \mathbf{T}^{*-1}\mathbf{v}^*$, and so, $\mathcal{E}(\boldsymbol{\theta}^*) = \mathbf{0}$ and $\mathcal{V}(\boldsymbol{\theta}^*) = \mathbf{T}^{*-1}\boldsymbol{\Sigma}_{\mathbf{v}^*}(\mathbf{T}^{*-1})' = \mathbf{I}$. The reparameterized model is then

$$s_{ijk} = \sigma_{(3)}\theta_{0i} + \mathbf{z}'_{ijk}\mathbf{T}\boldsymbol{\theta}_{ij} + \mathbf{x}'_{ijk}\boldsymbol{\beta} \ , \tag{9.6}$$

where θ_{0i} and $\boldsymbol{\theta}_{ij}$ are the standardized random-effects for cluster i and individual j in cluster i respectively. Notice that since only a single random cluster effect is assumed, $\sigma_{(3)}$ is a scalar while $\mathbf{T}$ is the Cholesky (i.e., square root) factor of the $r \times r$ matrix $\boldsymbol{\Sigma}_{(2)}$. The marginal probability then becomes

$$h(\mathbf{y}_i) = \int_{\boldsymbol{\theta}^*} \ell(\mathbf{y}_i \mid \theta, \boldsymbol{\beta})\, g(\boldsymbol{\theta}^*)\, d\boldsymbol{\theta}^* , \tag{9.7}$$

where $g(\boldsymbol{\theta}^*)$ is the multivariate standard normal density.

The major problem with this representation of the marginal probability is that the dimensionality of $\boldsymbol{\theta}^*$ is $(n_i \times r) + 1$ and numerical integration of equation (9.7) would be exceedingly slow and computationally intractable if $(n_i \times r) + 1$ is greater than 10. Note, however, that conditional on the study-effect $\theta_{(3)}$, the responses from the n_i subjects in study i are independent; therefore, the marginal probability can be rewritten as:

$$h(\mathbf{y}_i) = \int_{\theta_{(3)}} \left\{ \prod_{j=1}^{n_i} \int_{\boldsymbol{\theta}_{(2)}} \left(\prod_{k=1}^{n_{ij}} [\Phi(s_{ijk})]^{1-y_{ijk}} [1 - \Phi(s_{ijk})]^{y_{ijk}} \right) g(\boldsymbol{\theta}_{(2)}) d\boldsymbol{\theta}_{(2)} \right\} g(\theta_{(3)}) d\theta_{(3)} , \tag{9.8}$$

where $\boldsymbol{\theta}_{(2)}$ are the r subject-level random-effects. Here the integration is of dimensionality $r+1$ and is tractable as long as the number of level two random-effects is no greater than three or four. In longitudinal studies, we typically have one or two random-effects at level two (e.g., a random intercept and/or trend for each individual) and one or two random-effects at level three (e.g., random study intercept and linear trend).

Estimation

The estimation of the covariate coefficients $\boldsymbol{\alpha}$ and the population parameters in $\boldsymbol{T}$ requires differentiation of the log likelihood function with respect to these parameters. The log likelihood for the patterns from the N clusters can be written as:

$$\log L = \sum_{i}^{N} \log h(\mathbf{y}_i) . \tag{9.9}$$

Let $\boldsymbol{\eta}$ represent an arbitrary parameter vector; then for $\boldsymbol{\alpha}$, $v(\boldsymbol{T})$ (which denotes the unique elements of the Cholesky factor $\boldsymbol{T}$), and $\sigma_{(3)}$, we get:

$$\frac{\partial \log L}{\partial \boldsymbol{\eta}} = \sum_{i=1}^{N} h^{-1}(\mathbf{y}_i) \int_{\theta_{(3)}} \ell_i(\theta_{(3)}) \tag{9.10}$$

$$\left\{ \sum_{j=1}^{n_i} h^{-1}(\mathbf{y}_{ij}) \int_{\boldsymbol{\theta}_{(2)}} \sum_{k=1}^{n_{ij}} \left(\frac{y_{ijk} - \Phi(s_{ijk})}{\Phi(s_{ijk})[1 - \Phi(s_{ijk})]} \right) \right.$$

$$\left. \ell_{ij}(\boldsymbol{\theta}) \phi(s_{ijk}) \frac{\partial s_{ijk}}{\partial \boldsymbol{\eta}} g(\boldsymbol{\theta}_{(2)}) d\boldsymbol{\theta}_{(2)} \right\} g(\theta_{(3)}) d\theta_{(3)} , \tag{9.11}$$

where

$$\ell_{ij}(\boldsymbol{\theta}) = \ell_{ij}(\boldsymbol{\theta}_{(2)}, \theta_{(3)}) = \prod_{k=1}^{n_{ij}} [\Phi(s_{ijk})]^{1-y_{ijk}} [1 - \Phi(s_{ijk})]^{y_{ijk}} , \qquad (9.12)$$

$$\ell_i(\theta_{(3)}) = \prod_{j=1}^{n_i} \int_{\boldsymbol{\theta}_{(2)}} \ell_{ij}(\boldsymbol{\theta}) g(\boldsymbol{\theta}_{(2)}) d\boldsymbol{\theta}_{(2)} \qquad (9.13)$$

$$= \prod_{j=1}^{n_i} h(\mathbf{y}_{ij}) ,$$

and

$$\frac{\partial s_{ijk}}{\partial \boldsymbol{\beta}} = \mathbf{x}_{ijk} \qquad \frac{\partial s_{ijk}}{\partial \mathrm{v}(\boldsymbol{T})} = \mathbf{J}_r(\boldsymbol{\theta}_{(2)} \otimes \mathbf{z}_{ijk}) \qquad \frac{\partial s_{ijk}}{\partial \sigma_{(3)}} = \theta_{(3)} ,$$

and $\mathbf{J}_r$ is the transformation matrix of Magnus and Neudecker (1995) which eliminates the elements above the main diagonal.

As in the two-level case described by Gibbons and Bock (1987) and Gibbons et al. (1994) the method of scoring can be used to provide MMLEs and numerical integration on the transformed $\boldsymbol{\theta}$ space can be performed (Stroud and Secrest 1966). An advantage of numerical integration is that alternative prior distributions for the random-effects can be considered. Thus, for example, we can compare parameter estimates for a normal versus rectangular prior to determine the degree to which our estimates are robust to deviation from the assumed normality of the distribution for the random-effects.

9.2.3 Three-level Logistic Regression Model for Dichotomous Outcomes

In the previous discussion we have focused on a three-level random-effects probit regression model, however, many researchers are more familiar with the logistic regression model. Fortunately, modification of the response function and associated likelihood equations is trivial as Gibbons et al. (1994) and Hedeker and Gibbons (1994) have shown for two-level logistic regression models. Following Gibbons et al. (1994) we replace the normal response function (i.e., the CDF, or cumulative distribution function) $\Phi(z_{ijk})$ with

$$\Psi(s_{ijk}) = \frac{1}{1 + \exp[-s_{ijk}]} , \qquad (9.14)$$

and the normal density function $\phi(z_{ijk})$ (i.e., the PDF, or probability density function) with the product

$$\Psi(s_{ijk})(1 - \Psi(s_{ijk})) . \qquad (9.15)$$

As in the normal case, we let $\gamma = 0$, however, the residual variance correspond-ing to the standard logistic distribution is $\pi^2/3$. Application of the logistic re-sponse function is attractive in many cases in which the response probability is small because the logistic distribution has greater tail probability than the normal distribution.

9.2.3.1 Illustration: Safety of Antidepressants

In 2004 the FDA issued a black box warning for antidepressants and risk of suicide in children and adolescents. The original warning was based on a meta-analysis of adverse event reports of suicidal thoughts and behaviors from 25 RCTs. These trials were typically short-term and limited to the newer an-tidepressant classes of SSRIs) and SNRIs. Results of the analysis revealed an overall odds ratio of OR=1.78 (95% CI =1.14-2.77) indicating that the rate of suicidal thoughts and behavior was significantly higher in children random-ized to active antidepressant treatment relative to placebo. A similar analysis conducted by FDA on prospectively measured suicidal thoughts and behavior in the youth studies, failed to detect any evidence of increased risk of antide-pressant treatment in these same studies (Hammad 2004). The FDA analysis ignored the timing of the suicidal events and did not adjust for differential time on treatment.

Gibbons et al. (2012b) analyzed both prospective clinician ratings of sui-cidal thoughts and behavior augmented with spontaneous reports of suici-dal behavior from the same 41 RCTs described in the previous illustration. Data were analyzed using a three-level mixed-effects ordinal regression model with categories absent, thoughts, ideation, and behavior. For safety, all data through 12 weeks were used where available. The dichotomous event rates (thoughts, ideation, and attempts combined) for treated and control patients for each drug (fluoxetine and venlafaxine) and age group (youth, adult, el-derly for fluoxetine and IR and ER in adults for venlafaxine) are displayed in Table 9.1. For youth, there is no discernible pattern. On four weeks placebo was higher than treated, on other four weeks treated was higher than placebo, and on one week they had identical rates. Of the 36 other weekly comparisons there were only 7 (19%) in which treated was higher than placebo in terms of the rate of suicidal thoughts and behavior.

TABLE 9.1: Observed Percentage (n) of Suicidal Events Over Time

Week	Fluoxetine						Venlafaxine			
	Youth		Adult		Elderly		IR		ER	
	Placebo	Treatment	Placebo	Treatment	Placebo	Treatment	Placebo	Treatment	Placebo	Treatment
0	20.6 (315)	18.8 (393)	5.4 (1008)	4.7 (1627)	3.2 (470)	2.7 (490)	6.3 (919)	5.5 (1502)	1.6 (994)	1.7 (1467)
1	13.2 (114)	14.4 (139)	3.6 (883)	2.4 (1364)	2.5 (354)	1.6 (368)	4.9 (716)	2.5 (1061)	1.0 (871)	0.9 (1276)
2	14.8 (189)	9.5 (253)	4.5 (904)	2.1 (1382)	1.8 (393)	1.7 (409)	2.8 (719)	1.3 (1096)	1.0 (903)	0.6 (1264)
3	8.8 (148)	8.8 (205)	2.2 (731)	1.7 (1261)	2.2 (360)	0.5 (370)	1.7 (662)	1.2 (1034)	1.1 (819)	0.5 (1145)
4	14.3 (105)	5.8 (139)	2.2 (683)	1.1 (1151)	1.9 (364)	1.4 (360)	1.7 (641)	0.4 (965)	0.7 (807)	0.3 (1182)
5	15.6 (90)	11.5 (96)	1.3 (609)	0.7 (1006)	1.6 (313)	2.1 (339)	1.5 (196)	0.9 (321)	0.5 (199)	1.8 (278)
6	8.4 (167)	10.9 (183)	1.7 (529)	1.2 (910)	1.6 (309)	0.6 (310)	1.3 (397)	1.0 (619)	0.7 (614)	0.6 (900)
7	9.0 (78)	14.6 (96)	1.5 (335)	0.4 (491)	1.3 (160)	2.8 (144)	1.0 (196)	1.1 (357)	1.2 (169)	0.7 (276)
8	4.0 (50)	8.8 (68)	0.7 (297)	1.2 (259)	1.9 (53)	1.5 (66)	0.0 (117)	0.6 (177)	0.2 (448)	0.6 (725)
9+	13.6 (81)	4.8 (105)	0.0 (396)	0.0 (288)	3.7 (108)	0.0 (118)	1.8 (57)	0.0 (116)	0.7 (300)	0.6 (690)

Overall Analysis of Suicidal Events in Adults

In the combined adult population a statistically significant decrease in suicidal events over time was found (MMLE=-0.2091, SE=0.0289, p<0.0001). This finding is displayed graphically in terms of the probability of each suicidal event class in Figure 9.2. The rate of change was 58% faster in treated patients relative to controls, which results in an estimated 78.9% decrease in probability of suicidal events for controls after 8 weeks of study participation and a 90.5% decrease for treated patients. Figure 9.2 displays the estimated probabilities for each of the three ordinal response categories in treated and control patients respectively. The solid lines represent the estimated probabilities for controls, and the dashed lines represent estimated probabilities for treated patients. The top set of curves are for "wishes he were dead or any thoughts of possible death to self" or worse, the middle set are for "suicide ideas or gestures," and the bottom set are for "suicide attempts or suicides." Figure 9.2 reveals that the majority of suicidal events (19% at baseline) was of low severity (thoughts of death), followed by ideation with a baseline rate of 3%, and suicide attempts or completion at 0.1% at baseline. The beneficial effect of treatment on probability of suicidal events is apparent at approximately 2 weeks following treatment initiation.

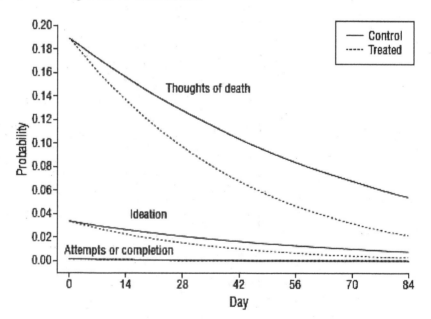

FIGURE 9.2: Probabilities of suicidal events in adult fluoxetine and venlafaxine studies.

Gibbons and colleagues (2012b) then conducted a mediational analysis to determine the extent to which changes in depression severity accounted for the difference in suicidal event rates between treated and control subjects. The mediation model on all adult (including elderly) patients revealed the following. First, there was a significant overall faster reduction in depressive symptoms (excluding suicidal thoughts and behavior) over time for treatment versus control (treatment difference at 12 weeks MMLE=-4.0337, SE=0.2730, p<0.0001). This estimate indicates an average estimated difference in depressive severity of 4.03 HAM-D units between treated and control patients at 12 weeks. Second, they found a statistically significant main effect of depressive severity on contemporaneous suicide risk (MMLE=0.3070, SE=0.0094, p<0.0001) indicating that depressive severity is positively associated with suicidal events. The treatment by depressive severity interaction was not statistically significant, indicating that the relationship between depressive severity and suicidal events was similar for treated and control patients (MMLE=0.0159, SE=0.0127, p=.2085). Following adjustment for depressive severity, the treatment by time interaction was still statistically significant (MMLE=-0.0620, SE=0.0314, p=0.0482); however, it was dramatically reduced from the model that did not adjust for depressive severity (see Figure 9.3). The percentage of the overall treatment effect attributable to mediation was 77%. This finding reveals that the majority of the beneficial effect of antidepressant treatment on suicide risk is mediated through the effect of antidepressant treatment on depressive severity.

To interpret these findings in terms of population-averaged effects, we transformed these individual level effect parameters for models into population average rates of suicide ideation or attempts over time, adjusted for the mediator. Figure 9.3 illustrates this mediational effect by plotting the marginal probability of suicide risk for each threshold in treated and control patients adjusting for depressive severity. In terms of depressive severity, we have selected a hypothetical patient who begins the trial severely depressed (HAM-D = 30) and improves at a rapid rate of 0.35 HAM-D units per day through 12 weeks. In contrast to the clear intervention differences in Figure 9.2, Figure 9.3 reveals that there is essentially no difference in suicide risk attributable to treatment once the effect of depressive severity is controlled.

Analysis of Suicidal Events in Youth

For youth treated with fluoxetine, the treatment by time interaction was not statistically significant (MMLE=0.0809, SE=0.0595, p=0.1739) indicating that we could find no difference between treated and control patients in terms of suicide risk. The marginal odds ratios indicated a 61.3% decrease in probability of suicidal thoughts or behavior for controls after 8 weeks of study participation and a 50.3% decrease for treated patients. Youth patients on fluoxetine decreased their depressive symptoms faster than patients on placebo (treatment difference at 12 weeks MMLE=-3.8976, SE=1.5238, p<0.01). A statistically significant main effect of depressive severity (MMLE=0.1261,

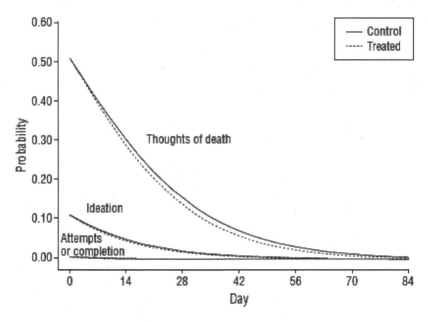

FIGURE 9.3: Probabilities of suicidal events adjusting for depression severity in adult fluoxetine and venlafaxine studies.

SE=0.0116, p<0.0001) on suicidal events was found, indicating that depressive severity is positively associated with suicidal events. The treatment by depressive severity interaction was not statistically significant, indicating that the relationship between depressive severity and suicidal events was the same for treated and control patients (MMLE=-0.0046, SE=0.0141, p=0.7422). Despite a strong association between depressive severity and suicidal events in youth, treatment with fluoxetine was not found to be related to suicide events when compared to placebo.

Discussion

Results of this analysis revealed that in adults, antidepressant treatment is protective in terms of suicidal events relative to placebo. This effect appears to be largely mediated by the reduction in the severity of depressive symptomatology which is significantly larger for treated than control subjects. In youth, antidepressant treatment was also successful in significantly decreasing the severity of depression relative to placebo; however, for youth there was no reduction or increase in suicidal events with active treatment. Apparently suicidal risk in children is driven by other factors than depression, perhaps social in nature.

10

Analysis of Medical Claims Data

"A single death is a tragedy; a million deaths is a statistic."
(Joseph Stalin)

10.1 Introduction

There are several advantages of the use of medical claims data for post-marketing surveillance. First, they represent person-level data, similar to RCTs and spontaneous reports, but unlike spontaneous reports, we know the population at risk. Second, several medical claims databases such as the Veterans Administration (VA) or PharMetrics databases contain longitudinal information on adverse events, concomitant medications, and comorbid diagnoses both before and after the drug exposure. Third, the populations that can be sampled are often large enough to study even the rarest of events such as suicide attempts and completion, whereas meta-analyses of RCTs are often restricted to more distal measures such as suicidal ideation, which may have little to do with suicide completion, the adverse event of interest. The primary limitation of medical claims data is that they are observational, and any association identified may or may not represent a causal link between the drug and the adverse event. The primary objective is to design and analyze an observational study such that many of the benefits of a randomized study are preserved. In the following, we describe some of the experimental strategies relevant to analysis of observational pharmacoepidemiologic data and the associated statistical methods that can be used in conjunction with such designs.

10.2 Administrative Claims

Administrative claims databases have a long history in pharmacoepidemiology (Strom 2006), but as noted by Madigan et al. (2014) their recent use has grown dramatically given advances in computational methods, high speed server technology and the processing and storage of large data streams. These are real-world resources which track utilization and adverse events in patients who are often more representative of routine practice than those patients who enroll in RCTs. These data are longitudinal in nature, reflecting reimbursement claims for both treatment and the filling of prescriptions including the date of service and/or prescription and length of supply. As such, medical or administrative claims data represent event histories where the timing of exposures and adverse events can be reconstructed in a reasonably complete longitudinal record for each subject. The fact that each patient's record varies in length adds complexity to the analytic process. In the United States where insurance reimbursement is dependent on filing a claim that contains diagnostic and treatment information, a cohort can be constructed based on an index diagnosis. It is often useful to restrict the diagnosis to a new episode by requiring no claims for that diagnosis for a fixed period before the index diagnosis (e.g., 1 or 2 years) and no filled prescriptions for medications used to treat the condition of interest (e.g., no previous treatment with antidepressants for a patient with a new diagnosis of depression). These designs have been referred to as "new user" or "incident user" designs (Schneeweiss 2010). The ability to define a cohort in terms of a new index diagnosis is valuable because it helps minimize variability in patient characteristics and even severity of illness at baseline. When defined in this way, the indication for treatment can be reasonably well controlled. In contrast, many other countries that have universal health care (e.g., Sweden) do not require coding of diagnostic information in administrative records. It is for this reason that cohorts in these countries are more frequently defined by the initiation of a new treatment episode. The disadvantage is that patients receiving the medication may do so for a multitude of different indications introducing heterogeneity in background severity levels and potential masking of some drug safety signals. A more subtle difference is that when the cohort is defined by an index diagnosis, some subjects may not be treated for a period of time (if ever) and comparisons before and after initiation of treatment or between-subjects treated and not treated with the same diagnosis are possible. Of course there may be other important differences between patients with the same diagnosis who do and do not receive treatment (e.g., severity of illness). It is for these reasons that it is important to collect data on comorbid diagnoses and concomitant medications in an effort to control for the treatment selection process both statically and dynamically.

There are distinct disadvantages of U.S. administrative databases relative to those in countries with universal health care. First, U.S. claims databases are typically based on insurance claims, and one must therefore have insurance in order to be recorded. This limits generalizability of the results to patients who can afford insurance or to those who are employed and insurance is provided to them. In the U.S. patients often change their insurance provider, and, therefore, it is not uncommon to have longitudinal information which is limited to a few year time window. This is generally not true for administrative records from countries that have universal health care where data across the lifespan of an individual is often available, allowing for the assessment of much longer term risks to be investigated. Furthermore, data collected in these countries do not suffer from selection biases based on economic factors which govern access to health care.

As noted by Madigan et al. (2014) administrative claims data are far from perfect. For example, diagnoses may be recorded to justify maximum reimbursement or to rule out a condition that the patient does not have. Record verification studies have yielded mixed results (Pladevall et al. 1996, Donahue et al. 1997, Tunstall-Pedoe 1997, García Rodríguez and Pérez Gutthann 1998, Strom 2001, Lee et al. 2005, So et al. 2006, Harrold et al. 2007, Lewis et al. 2007, Leonard et al. 2008, Miller et al. 2008, Varas-Lorenzo et al. 2008, Wilchesky et al. 2004, Hennessy et al. 2010, Wahl et al. 2010).

The choice of comparator is also an important consideration. In studies of the smoking cessation drug varenicline, RCTs generally compared varenicline to placebo. However, in administrative claims data, there would generally not be a claim for "cold turkey," and comparison to nicotine replacement therapy is generally conducted. The choice of comparator is important because in some cases, some drugs are reserved for the most severely ill patients or warnings related to the use of the drug in a certain population may limit its use in more severe cases. This is a distinct advantage of within-subject designs where an active comparator is not required, but rather pre versus post drug exposure comparisons are performed or periods of time with and without drug exposure are compared within the same individual.

Perhaps the most worrisome issue with administrative claims data is bias. One of the key sources of bias is confounding by indication. For example, patients with depression are at higher risk of suicide and more likely to take antidepressants than those without depression, hence one will always find an overall positive association between antidepressants and suicide. Similarly, a naive analysis would indicate that minoxidil, a drug for treating baldness, causes baldness since all people taking minoxidil are balding and many may in fact worsen following treatment, particularly if it is initiated later in the course of male pattern baldness and is therefore less effective in either reversing or halting progression of hair loss. While it might appear that within-subject designs are immune from such bias, that is not true at all. The decision to initiate treatment may be associated with the severity of illness and the severity of illness may be associated with an adverse event. Following the black box warning for antidepressants and suicide in youth, the rate of antidepressant treatment decreased (Gibbons et.al. 2009), and it may be that only the most severely ill children also at highest risk of suicide were provided antidepressant treatment, thereby producing confounding by severity of indication (i.e., depressive illness) and suicidal adverse events.

10.3 Observational Data

Randomized clinical trials eliminate bias by ensuring that the probability of being treated does not depend on factors related to the outcome of interest. This is achieved through randomization. When the sample is large enough, randomization insures that all potential confounders, both observed and unobserved, are balanced across the experimental and control conditions of the experiment. If important covariates are either not included or not collected in the experiment, it may decrease precision of our estimate of the treatment effect, but it will not produce bias. The same is not true, however, for observational studies. Bias in our estimate of the treatment versus control difference can easily be produced for numerous reasons and all observational studies regardless of how well controlled and how clever the statistical modeling of the data are subject to such bias. The previous chapter on causal inference highlights several experimental design and statistical analytic approaches to controlling for hidden bias, but none are foolproof and none can truly replace randomization. However, observational studies remain a critically important tool for studying drug safety. They can involve sample sizes of sufficient size to study rare events whose frequency is too small to be studied in RCTs. They also allow us to study the generalizability of findings from RCTs to real-world patient populations who will ultimately take the medication of interest.

Madigan et al. (2014) reviewed statistical approaches to studying observational data with emphasis on drug safety. They reviewed the work of the Observational Medical Outcomes Partnership (Stang et al. 2010) which was designed to examine operating characteristics of various methods for the analysis of observational data. In the following, we review several of the analytic methods used in their study and report their results on each method's ability to identify known drug adverse event relations and negative controls.

10.4 Experimental Strategies

10.4.1 Case-control Studies

Case-control studies can be particularly useful for the analysis of rare adverse events. The basic idea is to identify a sample of cases who have experienced the adverse event of interest and a set of controls who are similar to the cases in terms of a series of observable characteristics, but who have not experienced the adverse event. The goal of the analysis is to then compare the rate of exposure (i.e., a particular drug) between the cases and the controls. If a significant difference is identified (typically based on a conditional logistic regression analysis) then there is evidence that the drug is related to the adverse event. In some cases propensity score matching can be used to identify controls that are matched in probability on a large number of potential confounders to the cases. More often, however, the cases and controls are matched on a smaller set of observable characteristics (e.g., age and sex) and other potential confounders are included as covariates in the analysis (Månsson et al. 2007).

The major limitation of case-control studies in drug surveillance is that the somewhat limited number of observed potential confounders are inadequate for matching the cases and controls in terms of severity of illness. Since the more severely ill patients may have increased likelihood of both taking the drug and experiencing the adverse event, the drug appears to be associated with the adverse event when both are simply related to severity of illness. As an example, consider the tri-variate relationship between depression, suicidality, and treatment with an SSRI. The most severely depressed patients have the highest likelihood of both being treated with a newer antidepressant and exhibiting suicidal behavior. Case-control studies have identified links between antidepressant treatment and suicidality (Olfson and Marcus 2009). However, suicide attempt rate among cases prior to taking antidepressant medication is often considerably higher than among matched controls, leading to confounding by indication that has not been resolved through matching or covariate adjustment. As an example, Gibbons et al. (2009) found that among patients with bipolar depression, those treated with an antiepileptic drug (AED) were five times more likely to make a suicide attempt following the index diagnosis but prior to initiation of treatment than patients who were not treated with an AED or lithium. However, while propensity score matching which included adjustment for suicide attempt in the year prior to the index diagnosis, eliminated bias for many potential confounders such as concomitant medication and comorbid diagnoses, it did not eliminate the difference in suicide attempt rates following the index diagnosis but before initiation of treatment (70.52 per 1000 patient years for treated and 38.07 per 1000 patient years for untreated (OR=1.85; 95% CI, 1.22-2.81; P=.004). These effects have nothing to do with the exposure (which in all of these cases occurred after the suicide attempt, but rather, confounding produced by selection effects which lead one patient down the path of medication, and another not. Interestingly, after initiation of treatment, there was no difference in suicide attempt rates before and after treatment: 12.88 per 1000 patient years for the treated and 10.46 per 1000 patient years for those not treated with an AED or lithium (OR=1.23; 95% CI,0.89-1.71; P=.22).

10.4.2 Cohort Studies

A cohort study is one in which a sample from a well defined population is identified based on a set of pre-specified criteria. In drug surveillance there are two general approaches to conducting a cohort study. The cohort can be defined in terms of an illness (e.g., cardiovascular disease) or based on an exposure; for example all patients taking a statin. In addition to defining the indication for inclusion of patients into the cohort we must also define the timeframe. In some cases we may wish to identify new cases who are defined as not having been diagnosed with the disease of interest or treated with the drug or drugs of interest for a period of k years, and having a minimum of k years or months of observation following initial exposure to the drug. This type of strategy works well for databases with long-term enrollment patterns such as the VA, but may be less ideal for managed care databases where patients are typically continuously enrolled for a shorter period of time. In this case, the cohort study can be designed to have a fixed time window before and after the indication (either diagnostic date or first treatment date), for example a period of one year before and after the indication. The primary advantage of collecting data before and after diagnosis or drug exposure is that we can evaluate the rate of the adverse event both before and after the start of treatment. If the drug is producing the adverse event, then rates should generally be higher following initiation of the drug rather than before it. In some cases, however, the natural course of the disease is related to the decreased likelihood of the adverse event, and the comparison of pre versus post exposure adverse event rates is to some extent confounded with the natural course of the disease. Strategies for disentangling this type of confound are presented in the following sections.

Unlike the case-control study in which we are comparing exposures between those patients with and without the adverse event, the typical cohort study compares adverse event rates between those patients with and without the drug exposure. By having data prior to the exposure, we can often adjust for severity of illness by including whether the patient has a history of the adverse event prior to diagnosis, and then compare post diagnostic adverse event rates between those receiving the drug treatment and those not receiving it.

10.4.3   Within-subject Designs

Within-subject designs are those in which the same patients are repeatedly measured over time, typically before and after initiating drug treatment. The basic idea is to compare the rate of the adverse event before and after the exposure to the drug. Of course, this design strategy cannot be used with fatal adverse events. The strength of the design is that we are comparing the adverse event rate in patients all of whom ultimately will select to use the drug, before and after they ultimately do. As such, the selection effects due to time-stationary confounders (e.g., genetic factors) are eliminated because the analysis is restricted to only those patients who will at some time take the medication. It does not, however, eliminate selection effects due to time varying confounders (e.g., severity of illness). In this case, the natural course of the disease (e.g., decrease in the severity of symptomatology over time) can become confounded with the pre-post nature of the design. In some cases, the emergence of the adverse event may even lead to treatment. For example, a suicide attempt may lead to the identification of the depressive disorder which may in turn lead to treatment. By regression effect alone, we would expect the adverse event to decrease and this decrease could incorrectly be attributed to a protective effect of the drug. Fortunately, it is unlikely that such regression effects would mask a negative effect of the drug; however, when the indication for treatment is positively related to the likelihood of the adverse event, one must take great care in properly adjusting for the natural course of the disease.

Within-subject designs are also useful for understanding the effects of pattern or intensity of exposure on the adverse event rate. For example, breaking the surveillance time into discrete intervals (e.g., months), allows the analyst to explore the temporal association between drug exposure and the adverse event, where drug exposure on month t becomes a time-varying covariate in the model. This type of analysis permits the inclusion of both within-subject and between-subject effects, where patients who never receive the drug have a drug indicator $x_t = 0$ for all values of t, and those that do take the drug have $x_t = 0$ for those months that they did not take the drug and $x_t = 1$ for those months that they did take the drug. Alternatively, for those patients that take the drug, we can set $x_t = 1$ for all values of t following the month of exposure, or following a minimum exposure time (e.g., 30 days or more). This type of within-subject design affords the investigator a finer view of the relationship between drug exposure and the adverse event rate and also allows for adjustment of time since the index episode (e.g., depression) so that the natural course of the illness can be disentangled from the possible effect of the drug.

10.4.3.1   Self-controlled Case Series

Farrington (1995) proposed a special case of a within-subject design, called the SCCS (SCCS) method in the context of vaccine safety. The SCCS uses exposed cases only (i.e., individuals who have experienced the outcome of interest and received the treatment at some point in their data record). The method estimates the strength of association between a time-varying exposure and an outcome of interest. The method was originally developed to study the association between vaccinations and aseptic meningitis (Miller et al. 1993). Data on episodes of aseptic meningitis in children aged 1-2 over a defined calendar period were obtained from laboratory and hospital records and then linked to vaccination records. Inference is derived by computing the ratio of the rate of the event during an exposure period to the rate of events in the absence of the exposure. A similar approach was described by Maclure (1991), the case-crossover method in which exposures immediately preceding the adverse event time are compared to exposures during one or more control periods at times far removed from the appearance of the event of interest. The method assumes stationarity of the exposure distribution which is not required for the case series method. More specifically, the SCCS method assumes that the adverse events arise from a non-homogeneous Poisson process, where drug exposure may influence the time-varying event rate. The model assumes that patient i has an individual unknown event rate e^{ϕ_i} and exposure status $(0,1)$ during each time period (day, week, month), which has a multiplicative effect on the baseline rate e^{β_j}. Patient i is observed for T_i discrete time periods, so the event rate for patient i during period t is

$$\lambda_{it} = e^{\phi_i + x_{it}\beta}, \qquad (10.1)$$

where $x_{it} = 1$ if patient i is exposed to the drug during time interval t, otherwise $x_{it} = 0$. The usual approach to estimation is based on maximum likelihood conditioning on the total number of adverse events experienced by patient i, i.e. conditional maximum likelihood estimation using the total number of events as a sufficient statistic for ϕ_i to eliminate the patient-specific effects in the likelihood. The model parameters can also be estimated using marginal maximum likelihood as described in section 5.5. Here, patient is the clustering variable, and for each patient we have T measurement occasions. The drug exposure is treated as a time-varying covariate and can be expanded to simultaneously evaluate the effect of J drugs. A model with a random intercept allows the baseline risk to vary over individuals making it essentially identical to the traditional SCCS model. However, the drug effect(s) can also take on person-specific values, allowing the effect of the drug(s) to be heterogeneous over individuals. The random-effect approach makes the added assumption that the random-effect is unrelated to the exposure variable and that the random-effect deviations have a parametric form, typically normal, which have limited their use. A more detailed comparison of various random-effect versus fixed-effect solutions to this problem is presented in detail later in this chapter (also see Allison (2009)).

Note that in many ways discrete-time survival models are quite similar to SCCS models. The difference is that discrete-time survival models censor the data at the point of the first event and are not restricted to the analysis of cases only, although there is no reason that they cannot be. Although they are based on logistic regression instead of a Poisson regression, when multiple drugs are considered, there is no reason why SCCS models could not be estimated using a logistic regression model as well, since we would generally only consider a single event during each time interval. Generally discrete-time survival models use a log-log link function to provide estimates that are interpretable as hazard ratios, but again the interpretation of the model parameters between the two models when restricted to the first event are essentially the same. Note that if a single event is considered, then the need for conditional maximum likelihood estimation is obviated and traditional maximum likelihood can be used. When multiple time-to-event episodes are considered for the same subjects, a "stratified Cox regression model" (Allison 1995) can be used to produce a similar fixed-effect solution based on conditional maximum likelihood estimation to the Poisson-based SCCS model. We discuss the stratified Cox model and its random-effect counterparts in greater detail in the following sections.

10.4.4 Between-subject Designs

Between-subject designs involve comparison of patients who took the drug versus those that did not. Often it is most useful to compare monotherapy versus no therapy, at least with respect to the other drugs within the relevant class of drugs. Concomitant drug therapy with related classes of drugs can be included in the statistical model as covariates. For example, the class of drugs of interest may be SSRIs, and we may consider SSRI monotherapy either with respect to all other antidepressants (e.g., other SSRIs, SNRIs, and TCAs) or with respect to the other SSRIs. In the latter case, concomitant use of SNRIs and TCAs as well as antipsychotics and anxiolytics should be included as covariates in the analysis of the relationship between SSRIs and the adverse event of interest. The importance of considering monotherapy is that patients using multiple drugs within the same class may be of greater initial severity and/or treatment resistant and may in general have higher rates of adverse events that are related to the indication of interest (e.g., depression). The goal of the analysis is to compare the effects of taking a particular drug versus not taking that drug, not on the use of several drugs versus no drug.

The primary limitation of between-subject designs is that they are subject to confounding by indication and/or severity of the indication. In general more severely ill patients will be treated with pharmacotherapy; therefore, we would expect them to have a greater incidence of adverse effects that are related to the severity of illness. Various matching strategies, such as propensity score matching are helpful for reducing bias; however, only to the extent that the potential confounders are available and measurable. This is yet another reason that it is so important to obtain data on adverse events, concomitant treatment, and concomitant diagnoses prior to treatment with the drug of interest. While within-subject designs eliminate time-stationary confounding, between-subject designs in and of themselves neither eliminate or even reduce any confounding.

A final complication of between-subject designs is time. If a cohort is defined in terms of an index episode of a particular disorder, and the likelihood of the adverse event decreases or increases with time from the index episode, then time from the index episode may confound the drug effect of interest. To the extent that patients are not treated with the drug at the time of diagnosis, the treated patients will have a period of risk further away from the index episode than the untreated controls and as a consequence may have a lower rate of the adverse event that has nothing to do with the drug. To solve this problem we need to match treated and untreated patients in terms of the timing of treatment in addition to other demographic and prognostic factors. However, the untreated patients do not have a time of treatment. In this case, we can match treated and control patients on other potential confounders, and then match each pair in terms of time of risk based on the treated patient. In this way, confounding between time from index diagnosis and treatment initiation is no longer a factor in the comparison of control and treated patients.

10.5   Statistical Strategies

10.5.1   Fixed-effects Logistic and Poisson Regression

Logistic regression can be used when interest is restricted to the first adverse event, whereas Poisson regression can be used when the focus of analysis is on multiple adverse events within a given time frame. Fixed-effects models are used for between-subject comparisons that consider a single drug and a single adverse event. For simple within-subject comparisons a conditional logistic or Poisson regression model can be used (Allison, 1995), the parameters of which can be estimated using (GEE). Hedeker and Gibbons (2006) provide a general overview of these models. A note of caution, the term "fixed-effects" can be confusing because it is used to refer to quite different things in different disciplines. In economics, fixed-effects models are typically used to analyze longitudinal or clustered data to provide a within-unit inference by conditioning on a sufficient statistic for the clustering variable or simply introducing "fixed-effects" for the clustering unit (e.g., subject or county). The use of fixed-effects for the clusters is the distinguishing feature of the model, even though there typically are other fixed-effects in the model (e.g., other regressors), which is perhaps why economists refer to these as "fixed-effects" models. By contrast, in statistics, fixed-effects are typically the terms in a model which do not vary across clustering units in a mixed-effects model that contains both "fixed-effects" and "random-effects." Similarly, statisticians often refer to a fixed-effects model as a model that has no random-effects in addition to the residual (i.e., the parameter estimates do not have a distribution in the population). In drug safety, SCCS and stratified Cox models are examples of fixed-effects models in the econometric sense as they involve clustered data and use of conditional maximum likelihood estimation, whereas the beta coefficient for sex in a mixed-effects logistic regression for a repeated binary outcome is a fixed-effect in a mixed-effect regression model. Alternatively, a discrete-time survival model for a single time-to-event outcome in a single sample of patients is an example of a fixed-effect model in the statistical sense, but not in the econometric sense.

10.5.2   Mixed-effects Logistic and Poisson Regression

When the data are clustered and/or longitudinal, mixed-effects logistic or Poisson regression models can be used (Hedeker and Gibbons 2006). An example of where mixed-effects models are of particular importance is when multiple drugs and/or adverse events are considered simultaneously. Here, the unit of clustering is the drug-adverse event interaction. We may compare the rate of each adverse event for each drug before and after exposure in an overall analysis, where time (pre versus post exposure) is treated as a random-effect in the model. Empirical Bayes estimates of the random time effect for each drug-adverse event interaction and corresponding posterior variances can be used to construct confidence intervals that can in turn be used to screen large numbers of drug adverse event interactions simultaneously. Similar approaches can be used for between-subject comparisons (nested within drugs and adverse events) and coherence between within-subject and between-subject results can be used as a guide for selecting drug-adverse event interactions that are of concern and in need of further study. As previously noted, "fixed-effects" models (in the econometric sense) such as the SCCS or stratified Cox models can also be used to analyze clustered or longitudinal data (but not both). Three-level mixed-effects models can be used to analyze data that are both clustered and longitudinal (e.g., a multi-center longitudinal randomized controlled clinical trial).

10.5.3   Sequential Testing

Members of the FDA Sentinel Initiative have developed a series of sequential testing strategies for post-marketing surveillance which go far beyond traditional pharmacovigilance methods based on analysis of spontaneous reports. These methods are applied to integrated electronic health-care databases and are based on a between-subject prospective incident user concurrent control cohort design. These methods are particularly useful for a new drug A which is to be compared to an existing drug B early after its entry into the market and sequentially evaluated thereafter. The advantage of the general approach is that it will improve our ability to quickly detect potential safety signals. The limitation of the approach is that it is a between-subject comparison, and it may be difficult to control for differences between patients willing to take a new drug versus a well known alternative, differences which in some cases may be related to severity of illness and may also be related to adverse events of interest. Nevertheless, the methodology may be of considerable use in "signal refinement" which is a preliminary step before conducting a more extensive phase IV observational study or confirmatory randomized clinical trial (Cook et al. 2012). In the following we provide a general overview of the methodology. More details are provided in Cook et al. (2012).

The data to be collected will be analyzed at specific points in time denoted $t = 1, \ldots, T$. Individual i is either exposed to the new drug $D_i = 1$ or to the control drug $D_i = 0$. Each subject either has the adverse event of interest before the end of the analysis t, $Y_i(t) = 1$ or does not $Y_i(t) = 0$. The exposure time $E_i(t)$ denotes the cumulative time prior to analysis t. For a single exposure such as a vaccine, $E_i(t) = 1$ for all subjects. Typically, exposure time is censored at the time that the patient is no longer enrolled in the medical plan, occurrence of the outcome, or the treatment is discontinued and/or switched. Time-varying treatments are not considered in this type of design. We also assume that there is a set of baseline confounders Z_i for each individual. Time-varying confounders are not considered in this type of design. The treatment and control groups can be stratified or matched on the set of baseline confounders Z. Test statistics such as relative risk, hazard ratio, or odds ratio can be used to test the null hypothesis of no difference between treated and control subjects at each analysis point t. If the test statistic exceeds a predefined threshold $c(t)$ we conclude that there is an association between the new drug and the adverse event of interest; otherwise, the study continues to the next analysis time or the pre-defined end of the study (Cook et al. 2012). At each analysis t new exposed subjects can be added as well as additional analysis time for previously enrolled subjects. The critical value $c(t)$ is selected to maintain the overall type I error rate across all analyses taking into account both multiplicity and skewed distribution of the test statistic based on earlier exceedances.

Cook et al. (2012) present a series of different sequential testing procedures based on this general framework. The Lan-Demets method is a group sequential approach that uses error spending (Lan and DeMets 1983), where the error function $\alpha(t)$ can be based on several different boundary functions including Pococks boundary function (Pocock 1982) or the OBrien-Fleming boundary function (O'Brien and Fleming 1979).

The Group Sequential Likelihood Ratio Test (LRT), has been used in vaccine safety studies for a single time exposure. The most common test is the binomial max SPRT (Kulldorff et al. 2011) which is based on matched exposure strata where each exposed subject is matched to one or more unexposed individuals having the same categorical confounders Z.

The Conditional Sequential Sampling Procedure (CSSP) (Li 2009) was designed to handle chronic exposures. Using the entire sample, strata are constructed using categorical confounders and comparisons are performed within these strata at each analysis t and then the test statistics are combined across strata to provide an overall test for that drug and adverse event. The CSSP approach works best for rare events, small number of strata, and analysis times are well separated.

The Group Sequential Estimating Equation Approach controls for confounding using regression and can be applied to both single and chronic exposures. The approach is based on GEE for either logit or Poisson link functions. The generality of the method is based on its use of a regression model to control for confounding; however, if the event is rare this model may be difficult to estimate due to a small number of events.

A comparison of three of the four methods using a fictitious example in which the actual RR=2.0 found similar results for all three methods (Cook et al. 2012). All three methods signaled at the second analysis. These methods hold promise for improving the surveillance of new drugs as they emerge on the market. Comparison of a new drug to existing drug with a better known safety profile raises additional questions which must be considered if this general methodology is to take hold in practice.

10.5.4 Discrete-time Survival Models

Discrete-time survival analysis or person-time logistic regression (Efron 1988, Gibbons et al. 2003) allows us to use drug exposure as a time-varying co-variate in estimating the hazard rate of an adverse event on a month by month (or other discrete time interval) basis. Unlike the previous analyses where exposure was considered constant from the time of treatment initiation through the end of the follow-up period, in this analysis, treatment is evaluated within discrete time intervals and can change from present to absent in any one of 2^t possible patterns. This analysis can combine patients who did not take the drug with non-medication months for patients who did take the drug, and compares them to active treatment months. Discrete-time survival models can determine the effects of duration and pattern of exposure on our overall conclusions. We can also adjust for month, which allows the risk of the adverse event to decrease (or increase) over time. Mixed-effects versions of these models can accommodate clustering of the patients within ecological units such as hospitals, clinics, counties, ..., or the simultaneous analysis of multiple episodes for a given individual. As described in Chapter 8, they can also accommodate competing risks such as experience of the adverse event or death.

10.5.5 Stratified Cox Model

The stratified Cox model (Allison 1995) is a "fixed-effects" solution for the Cox regression model that can be used for analysis of clustered time-to-event data. The data for each individual can be clustered within higher order units such as clinics, studies, or families (e.g., twin studies) or the individual can be the clustering unit and each individual can be repeatedly studied during different time intervals in which the event of interest can occur multiple times over the entire time interval. Similar to the statistical approach taken for SCCS designs based on conditional maximum likelihood, a fixed-effects solution can be implemented here as well. Essentially, we stratify the sample in terms of the clustering variable and the model allows each unit in the analysis (e.g., person or study) to have its own hazard function. As in the SCCS approach, the inference is "within-unit" so that time-stationary confounding is eliminated. This is an extremely useful tool for drug safety because it allows for the experience of multiple treatment episodes or time periods to be combined within an individual or to incorporate the dependence produced by a single time-to-event record from each individual being recorded within higher-order units such as families, clinics, hospitals, or studies. This latter example (clustering within studies) provides a type of research synthesis when interest lies in understanding the effect of an exposure on time to an adverse event. Here the stratified

Cox model provides a way of synthesizing the within-study effect, eliminating the between study differences from the estimate of the within-study exposure effect.

To provide a basic statistical framework, the Cox proportional hazard model for survival time T_j for observation j given exposure x can be written as

$$\lambda(t_j \mid x) = \lambda_0(t_j)\exp(\beta x_j) , \qquad (10.2)$$

where $\lambda(t_j \mid x)$ is the conditional hazard function at time t_j given exposure x_j, and $\lambda_0(t)$ is the baseline hazard. When the data are clustered,

$$\lambda(t_{ij} \mid \boldsymbol{x}_i) = \lambda_{0i}(t_{ij})\exp(\beta x_{ij}) , \qquad (10.3)$$

where $\lambda(t_{ij}\boldsymbol{x}_i)$ is the conditional hazard function at time t_{ij} given exposure vector $\boldsymbol{x}_i$ in cluster i, and $\lambda_{0i}(t)$ is a cluster-specific baseline hazard. For example, in the case of subjects nested within studies, $\boldsymbol{x}_i$ denotes the set of time-invariant exposures of the n_i individuals in study i. By contrast, when the clustering unit is the individual and each individual has multiple follow-up episodes, then $\boldsymbol{x}_i$ represents the time-varying (within-person) exposure status at each point in time (both within and between repeated follow-up intervals).

Sjölander et al. (2013) presents a detailed discussion of these models in the context of methods for the analysis of twin data, where the clustering unit is the family. In terms of estimation they consider several approaches for estimating β. For example, using a frailty model (a random intercept model) the baseline hazard $\lambda_{0i}(t)$ can be factored into $\lambda_{0i}(t) = \lambda_0(t)z_i$, where z_i is the random-effect or frailty term. The limitation of this approach is that it assumes that z and x are independent, which is unlikely in practice. Alternatively, treating z_i as fixed parameters and maximizing the partial-likelihood over β and the z's jointly (dummy-coding the clustering units) is likely to produce inconsistent estimates as the number of clusters becomes large and the number of individuals or observations within the clusters is small (Allison 2009). The method that they do recommend is based on conditional maximum likelihood, similar to the SCCS approach, because it leads to consistent estimates of β even if the cluster-specific baseline hazard is associated with the exposure variable and even if the number of individuals or observations within the cluster is small. This is what is referred to as the stratified Cox model by Allison (1995).

10.5.6   Between and Within Models

An alternative approach to the analysis of dynamic exposure data is the so-called between-within (BW) or "hybrid" model (Neuhaus and Kalbfleisch 1998, Neuhaus and McCulloch 2006). The basic idea is to decompose the between-cluster and within-cluster effects into uniquely estimable components by expressing $\boldsymbol{x}_i$ in terms of its mean $\bar{x}_i$ and the deviations from the mean

$x'_{ij} = x_{ij} - \bar{x}_i$. Random-effects models are then used to uniquely estimate the within and between exposure effects in the following generalized linear model

$$g\{E(Y_{ij} \mid \boldsymbol{x}_i)\} = \alpha_i + \beta_B \bar{x}_i + \beta_W x'_{ij} . \tag{10.4}$$

The advantage of this approach is that it allows the random-effect α_i to be associated with $\boldsymbol{x}_i$ through β_B, which is a measure of shared confounding. As pointed out by Sjölander et al. (2013) β_B provides a test of the independence assumption between α_i and $\boldsymbol{x}_i$. When $\beta_B = 0$ the independence assumption is viable. A distinct advantage of the BW model over the conditional likelihood approach is that the latter is limited to those subjects (or clusters) for which both the exposure and the outcome of interest occurred. This can severely limit statistical power relative to the BW approach which includes all available information from all clustering units. Sjölander et al. (2013) have recently extended the BW idea to survival analysis

$$\lambda(t_{ij} \mid \boldsymbol{x}_i) = \lambda_{0i}(t_{ij})z_i exp(\beta_B \bar{x}_i + \beta_W x'_{ij}) , \tag{10.5}$$

where the independence assumption is restricted to z_i and x'_i. Based on their simulation studies, they find that the BW model is robust against model misspecification and provides a more powerful test of β_W than the stratified Cox model.

An overlooked assumption regarding methods based on conditional likelihood such as the self-selected case series or stratified Cox model is the assumption of no treatment heterogeneity. This is implicit in the assumption that β_W is invariant over the clustering units. A natural extension of the BW method is to include correlated random-effects for both the baseline hazard and β_W as in

$$\lambda(t_{ij} \mid \boldsymbol{x}_i) = \lambda_{0i}(t_{ij})z_i exp(\beta_B \bar{x}_i + \beta_{Wi} x'_{ij}) . \tag{10.6}$$

This is a natural extension of mixed-effects regression models and allows the BW model to incorporate treatment heterogeneity across the clusters. The same idea can be applied to any generalized linear model, including the Poisson regression model used in the SCCS method. Examples of this are discussed in the following sections.

Finally we note that for multi-center or multi-study research synthesis of randomized clinical trials, randomization eliminates confounding such that β_B is zero by design. In this case, a traditional mixed-effects regression model or frailty model will provide unbiased estimates of β_W (also see Sjolander et.al., 2013).

10.5.7 Fixed-effect versus Random-effect Models

The debate over whether to use fixed-effects versus random-effects models has a long history that predates their use in drug safety. Economists and statisticians have had heated debates regarding the use of these models for many of the same reasons discussed in the previous sections. Economists are often uncomfortable with the assumption of joint normality for the distribution of random-effects in the model and the independence assumption between the random-effects and predictors in the mixed-effects models. By contrast, statisticians are often uncomfortable with the reduced statistical power associated with fixed-effects models which are restricted to the subset of case-exposures in the overall dataset. It is important to note that mixed-effects models were initially developed by statisticians for controlled experiments with clustered units (e.g., split-plot designs). Here the independence assumption holds by design, so the mixed-effect model is clearly preferable. However, the problem of independence of the random-effects and predictors arose when these models were transferred from controlled experiments to observational studies where the independence assumption is often violated. In addition, the notion that the sample of subjects is representative of some population of subjects is not a part of the fixed-effects approach, but is key in the mixed model. Although not a typical issue in these debates is the strong assumption of the fixed-effects approach on the absence of treatment heterogeneity across the clustering units, which is probably more the rule than the exception and as previously discussed can be easily added within the mixed-model framework. Furthermore, as shown by several investigators, the assumption of independence between the random-effects and the predictors in the mixed-effects models can be relaxed by decomposing the within-cluster and between-cluster effects into the cluster mean and within-cluster deviations from the mean and uniquely estimating β_B and β_W (Neuhaus and Kalbfleisch 1998, Raudenbush and Bryk 2002, Sjölander et al. 2013).

In an effort to better understand these issues, Hedeker and Gibbons (2015) have conducted an extensive simulation study of the comparison of fixed and random-effect models based on proportional hazard models (stratified Cox model versus mixed-effects discrete-time survival model) where the clustering unit is the individual and each individual has multiple followup periods in which the time to a discrete and repeatable event is measured. More formally they considered the case in which subject i ($i = 1, \ldots, N$) is evaluated on episode j ($j = 1, \ldots, n_i$) in terms of a time-to-event outcome. The event occurs at some discrete time within each episode (e.g., a week or a month). A given episode is of length n_{ij}, and the event y_{ij} can be censored. The main covariate is a time-varying exposure variable x_{ijk}, where k denotes a discrete time point within episode j. They considered the following four models:

- Conditional model (fixed-effect model) with time-varying exposure x_{ijk}.

- Mixed-effects model with time-varying exposure x_{ijk}.

- Mixed-effects model with the between-subject (BS) and within-subject (WS) decomposition: $\bar{x}_i$ and $(x_{ijk} - \bar{x}_i)$.

- Mixed-effects model with only the WS component: $(x_{ijk} - \bar{x}_i)$ (a variation of the adaptive centering approach; Raudenbush (2009)).

The various simulation studies included the following conditions:

- 1000 datasets.

- N=200 subjects, each with 5 repeated survival episodes ($n_i = 5$ for all subjects).

- For each episode, there are 6 discrete time periods.

- The outcome is time of first event considering the 6 time periods ($n_{ij} = 1$ to 6; censoring at time 6 if the event never occurs).

- The covariate is a time-varying exposure x_{ijk} (0 or 1) which can vary across subjects, episodes, and time periods.

The first simulation was a homogeneous exposure hybrid (BW) model. They simulated a latent variable Y_{ijk}^* for subject i, episode j, and period k, with exposure x_{ijk} (0 or 1) based on the following model:

$$Y_{ijk}^* = \beta_0 + \beta_B \bar{x}_i + \beta_W (x_{ijk} - \bar{x}_i) + \upsilon_i + \varepsilon_{ijk} \tag{10.7}$$

where

- $\bar{x}_i$ = the CDF of the random standard normal variate for subject i,

- x_{ijk} = a random Bernoulli variate with $\pi = \bar{x}_i$,

- υ_i = a random normal subject effect with mean 0 and variance σ_υ^2,

- ε_{ijk} = a random standard logistic distribution with mean 0 and variance $\pi^2/3$.

If $Y_{ijk}^* > 0$ then the event occurs in period k. Note that in the definitions provided above, $\bar{x}_i$ is the "true" exposure mean for subject i which is usually not equal to the observed mean which was used in the simulations, since in practice the true mean is unknown. For each subject and (repeated) episode, a subject contributes up to 6 records as in the following examples:

ID	y	BS effect	WS effect	description
1	1	$\bar{x}_1$	$x_{1jk} = 0/1$	event at first period
2	0	$\bar{x}_2$	$x_{2jk} = 0/1$	event at second period
2	1	$\bar{x}_2$	$x_{2jk} = 0/1$	
6	0	$\bar{x}_6$	$x_{6jk} = 0/1$	event at sixth period
6	0	$\bar{x}_6$	$x_{6jk} = 0/1$	
6	0	$\bar{x}_6$	$x_{6jk} = 0/1$	
6	0	$\bar{x}_6$	$x_{6jk} = 0/1$	
6	0	$\bar{x}_6$	$x_{6jk} = 0/1$	
6	1	$\bar{x}_6$	$x_{6jk} = 0/1$	
7	0	$\bar{x}_7$	$x_{7jk} = 0/1$	censored at sixth period
7	0	$\bar{x}_7$	$x_{7jk} = 0/1$	
7	0	$\bar{x}_7$	$x_{7jk} = 0/1$	
7	0	$\bar{x}_7$	$x_{7jk} = 0/1$	
7	0	$\bar{x}_7$	$x_{7jk} = 0/1$	
7	0	$\bar{x}_7$	$x_{7jk} = 0/1$	

The parameter specifications were as follows:

- $\beta_0 = -.5$,

- $\beta_{WS} = -0.4$,

- $\beta_{BS} = -0.4, 0, 0.4$,

- Intra-class correlation (ICC) $= .3$ for repeated survival outcomes across episodes

$$\sigma_v^2 = \pi^2/3 \frac{ICC}{1 - ICC} = 1.41,$$

- Correlations of -0.25, 0, .25 between BS exposure $\bar{x}_i$ and random subject effect v_i (non-zero correlation is a violation of random-effects model assumption).

The following models were compared:

- Conditional model with time-varying exposure x_{ijk},

- Random intercept model with time-varying exposure x_{ijk} (assumes WS=BS effect),

- Random intercept model with subject mean exposure $\bar{x}_i$ (BS effect) and time-varying exposure deviation $(x_{ijk} - \bar{x}_i)$ (WS effect),

- Random intercept model with only the time-varying exposure deviation $(x_{ijk} - \bar{x}_i)$ (WS effect; adaptive centering approach).

The random intercept models also included time-period indicators (baseline hazard). Results of these simulations are described in the following tables.

TABLE 10.1: Homogeneous Exposure Data: Random Intercept Model with Time-varying Exposure $(\beta_{WS} = -0.4)$

Specifications		Conditional with Time-varying Exposure			Random Intercept with Time-varying Exposure		
BS-corr	BS-effect	avg est	coverage	rejection	avg est	coverage	rejection
-0.25	-0.40	-0.404	0.954	0.728	-0.497	0.881	0.972
-0.25	0.00	-0.400	0.958	0.700	-0.455	0.933	0.941
-0.25	0.40	-0.408	0.935	0.714	-0.426	0.950	0.913
0.00	-0.40	-0.411	0.948	0.723	-0.407	0.948	0.870
0.00	0.00	-0.403	0.950	0.686	-0.367	0.942	0.804
0.00	0.40	-0.404	0.954	0.708	-0.327	0.923	0.708
0.25	-0.40	-0.404	0.959	0.718	-0.306	0.895	0.656
0.25	0.00	-0.398	0.954	0.678	-0.267	0.831	0.511
0.25	0.40	-0.402	0.960	0.661	-0.232	0.767	0.396

TABLE 10.2: Homogeneous Exposure Data: Random Intercept Model with WS and BS Exposure Effects $(\beta_{WS} = -0.4)$

Specifications		Conditional with Time-varying Exposure			Random Intercept with WS Deviation & BS Effect		
BS-corr	BS-effect	avg est	coverage	rejection	avg est	coverage	rejection
-0.25	-0.40	-0.404	0.954	0.728	-0.399	0.954	0.834
-0.25	0.00	-0.400	0.958	0.700	-0.397	0.955	0.812
-0.25	0.40	-0.408	0.935	0.714	-0.409	0.955	0.844
0.00	-0.40	-0.411	0.948	0.723	-0.406	0.952	0.829
0.00	0.00	-0.403	0.950	0.686	-0.405	0.958	0.840
0.00	0.40	-0.404	0.954	0.708	-0.404	0.963	0.838
0.25	-0.40	-0.404	0.959	0.718	-0.401	0.945	0.833
0.25	0.00	-0.398	0.954	0.678	-0.401	0.948	0.816
0.25	0.40	-0.402	0.960	0.661	-0.406	0.954	0.823

Results of these simulations reveal that the conditional model (stratified Cox model) yields good estimates, coverage, and power (see Tables 10.1-10.3). The random intercept model with simple time-varying exposure did poorly because of violation of the assumption of independence of the random-effect and the exposure variable, unless BS=WS and there is zero correlation between the random intercept and the exposure variable $\bar{x}_i$. However, the hybrid model

TABLE 10.3: Homogeneous Exposure Data: Random Intercept Model with WS Effect Only ($\beta_{WS} = -0.4$)

Specifications		Conditional with Time-varying Exposure			Random Intercept with WS Deviation Effect Only		
BS-corr	BS-effect	avg est	coverage	rejection	avg est	coverage	rejection
-0.25	-0.40	-0.404	0.954	0.728	-0.396	0.954	0.834
-0.25	0.00	-0.400	0.958	0.700	-0.395	0.955	0.812
-0.25	0.40	-0.408	0.935	0.714	-0.408	0.955	0.843
0.00	-0.40	-0.411	0.948	0.723	-0.405	0.953	0.828
0.00	0.00	-0.403	0.950	0.686	-0.404	0.960	0.840
0.00	0.40	-0.404	0.954	0.708	-0.405	0.963	0.838
0.25	-0.40	-0.404	0.959	0.718	-0.402	0.947	0.835
0.25	0.00	-0.398	0.954	0.678	-0.403	0.947	0.818
0.25	0.40	-0.402	0.960	0.661	-0.409	0.953	0.825

with both BS and WS effects or the model with just the WS effects provided excellent results with improved power over the stratified Cox model. These results assume a constant exposure effect over subjects.

In the second simulation study, the homogeneous exposure assumption was relaxed based on the following model:

$$Y_{ijk}^* = \beta_0 + \beta_{BS}\bar{x}_i + \beta_{WS}(x_{ijk} - \bar{x}_i) + v_{0i} + v_{1i}x_{ijk} + \varepsilon_{ijk}' \qquad (10.8)$$

and parameter specifications:

- $\beta_0 = -.5$,

- $\beta_{WS} = -0.4$,

- $\beta_{BS} = -0.4, 0, 0.4$,

- ICC = .2 and .362, correlation = -.2

$$\Sigma = \begin{bmatrix} .8225 & -.2480 \\ -.2480 & 1.8664 \end{bmatrix},$$

- ICC = .2 and .294, correlation = 0

$$\Sigma = \begin{bmatrix} .8225 & 0 \\ 0 & 1.3708 \end{bmatrix},$$

- ICC = .2 and .234, correlation = .2

$$\Sigma = \begin{bmatrix} .8225 & .1820 \\ .1820 & 1.0068 \end{bmatrix}.$$

TABLE 10.4: Heterogeneous Exposure Hybrid Model: ($\beta_{WS} = -0.4$) Corr = 0 between BS Exposure Effect and Random Intercept

Specifications		Heterogeneous Exposure WS Deviation & BS Effect			Conditional Time-varying Exposure		
BS-effect	RE-corr	avg est	coverage	rejection	avg est	coverage	rejection
-0.40	-0.20	-0.409	0.945	0.555	-0.324	0.876	0.555
-0.40	0.00	-0.408	0.951	0.614	-0.367	0.911	0.624
-0.40	0.20	-0.408	0.949	0.674	-0.400	0.930	0.702
0.00	-0.20	-0.400	0.946	0.539	-0.343	0.877	0.559
0.00	0.00	-0.390	0.952	0.588	-0.376	0.921	0.636
0.00	0.20	-0.402	0.961	0.657	-0.412	0.924	0.709
0.40	-0.20	-0.400	0.960	0.553	-0.364	0.900	0.611
0.40	0.00	-0.406	0.945	0.615	-0.402	0.900	0.704
0.40	0.20	-0.411	0.950	0.643	-0.436	0.916	0.764

TABLE 10.5: Heterogeneous Exposure WS Effect Only: ($\beta_{WS} = -0.4$) Corr = 0 between BS Exposure Effect and Random Intercept

Specifications		Heterogeneous Exposure WS Deviation & BS Effect			Heterogeneous Exposure WS Deviation Only		
BS-effect	RE-corr	avg est	coverage	rejection	avg est	coverage	rejection
-0.40	-0.20	-0.409	0.945	0.555	-0.352	0.942	0.484
-0.40	0.00	-0.408	0.951	0.614	-0.359	0.938	0.539
-0.40	0.20	-0.408	0.949	0.674	-0.365	0.944	0.603
0.00	-0.20	-0.400	0.946	0.539	-0.392	0.946	0.542
0.00	0.00	-0.390	0.952	0.588	-0.381	0.951	0.595
0.00	0.20	-0.402	0.961	0.657	-0.393	0.957	0.662
0.40	-0.20	-0.400	0.960	0.553	-0.428	0.958	0.632
0.40	0.00	-0.406	0.945	0.615	-0.430	0.947	0.681
0.40	0.20	-0.411	0.950	0.643	-0.433	0.945	0.701

TABLE 10.6: Heterogeneous Exposure Data: ($\beta_{WS} = -0.4$) Corr = -0.25 between BS Exposure Effect and Random Intercept

Specifications		Heterogeneous Exposure WS Deviation & BS Effect			Conditional Time-varying Exposure		
BS-effect	RE-corr	avg est	coverage	rejection	avg est	coverage	rejection
-0.40	-0.20	-0.367	0.944	0.468	-0.280	0.813	0.477
-0.40	0.00	-0.392	0.951	0.574	-0.331	0.888	0.555
-0.40	0.20	-0.433	0.951	0.701	-0.398	0.923	0.698
0.00	-0.20	-0.359	0.945	0.444	-0.302	0.859	0.504
0.00	0.00	-0.399	0.956	0.597	-0.364	0.907	0.632
0.00	0.20	-0.434	0.952	0.726	-0.416	0.923	0.745
0.40	-0.20	-0.355	0.943	0.461	-0.310	0.853	0.507
0.40	0.00	-0.393	0.951	0.589	-0.379	0.912	0.675
0.40	0.20	-0.437	0.954	0.728	-0.449	0.920	0.800

TABLE 10.7: Heterogeneous Exposure Data: $(\beta_{WS} = -0.4)$ Corr $= 0.25$ between BS Exposure Effect and Random Intercept

Specifications		Heterogeneous Exposure WS Deviation & BS Effect			Conditional Time-varying Exposure		
BS-effect	RE-corr	avg est	coverage	rejection	avg est	coverage	rejection
-0.40	-0.20	-0.442	0.945	0.649	-0.382	0.901	0.661
-0.40	0.00	-0.409	0.948	0.602	-0.383	0.911	0.663
-0.40	0.20	-0.368	0.944	0.584	-0.378	0.924	0.662
0.00	-0.20	-0.451	0.933	0.625	-0.398	0.899	0.688
0.00	0.00	-0.412	0.953	0.620	-0.402	0.912	0.680
0.00	0.20	-0.366	0.961	0.551	-0.384	0.942	0.653
0.40	-0.20	-0.442	0.952	0.605	-0.404	0.910	0.698
0.40	0.00	-0.406	0.957	0.604	-0.413	0.929	0.697
0.40	0.20	-0.374	0.954	0.567	-0.411	0.925	0.695

Results of the second simulation study (Tables 10.4-10.7) reveal that in the presence of treatment heterogeneity, the conditional model does not yield good estimates or coverage. The random intercept and exposure model with only the WS component gives good results under zero BS effect (and zero correlation between random intercept and exposure) but somewhat biased results in other situations. The random intercept and exposure model with BS and WS components gives good results in general, but exhibits small bias when both random-effects are correlated and correlation exists between the random intercept and exposure, although coverage remains good.

Finally, Hedeker and Gibbons (2015) addressed the question of non-normality of the random effect distribution on parameter estimates of the within-subject exposure effect. To test this, they simulated data based on homogeneous exposure model drawing random-effects from a uniform distribution (-2 to 2), but analyzed the data using a random-effect hybrid model assuming normally distributed random effects.

TABLE 10.8: Homogeneous Exposure Data: Random-effects from a Uniform Distribution $(\beta_{WS} = -0.4)$

Specifications		Conditional with Time-varying Exposure			Random Intercept with WS Deviation & BS Effect		
BS-corr	BS-effect	avg est	coverage	rejection	avg est	coverage	rejection
-0.25	-0.40	-0.404	0.951	0.671	-0.398	0.941	0.780
-0.25	0.00	-0.400	0.955	0.674	-0.396	0.962	0.794
-0.25	0.40	-0.408	0.952	0.705	-0.407	0.960	0.813
0.00	-0.40	-0.412	0.952	0.685	-0.410	0.948	0.808
0.00	0.00	-0.400	0.933	0.653	-0.397	0.941	0.785
0.00	0.40	-0.410	0.951	0.676	-0.407	0.953	0.793
0.25	-0.40	-0.406	0.958	0.650	-0.406	0.959	0.795
0.25	0.00	-0.407	0.961	0.651	-0.404	0.959	0.773
0.25	0.40	-0.404	0.961	0.639	-0.398	0.948	0.760

Table 10.8 reveals that the parameter estimates for the within-subject ex-

posure effect (β_W) are unbiased for both the fixed-effect and random-effect models when the distribution of the random effects is non-normal. As in the other simulations, the random-effect hybrid model has increased statistical power relative to the conditional stratified Cox model.

In summary, blind usage of conditional models can be inefficient (homogeneous exposure effect) or suffer from considerable bias when there is treatment heterogeneity. The hybrid (BW) model performs well under most conditions including correlation between the random-effect and exposure variable and maximizes statistical power because it makes use of all available data. Sjolander et.al. (2013) has identified extreme conditions in which the BW model produced biased results, although these conditions were not realistic. To our knowledge, similar studies for other response types (e.g., Poisson) have not been conducted; however, we would expect that results would be similar for all non-linear mixed-effects models (see Neuhaus and McCulloch (2006) for binary outcomes).

10.6 Illustrations

In the following, we illustrate several of the previously described methods with real data examples.

10.6.1 Antiepileptic Drugs and Suicide

Anticonvulsant medications are life saving in the treatment of seizure disorders and are also extensively used for other indications such as mood disorders and trigeminal neuralgia. In March of 2005, the FDA sent letters to sponsors of 11 antiepileptic drugs (AEDs) requesting the submission of suicidality data from RCTs. The data consisted of suicide-related adverse event reports and a search for suicide-related terms in electronic data bases related to the studies. The 11 AEDs included gabapentin, divalproex, felbamate, lamotrigine, levetiracetam, oxcarbazepine, pregabalin, tiagabine, topiramate, zonisamide, and carbamazepine. FDA conducted a meta-analysis of 199 placebo-controlled trials including 43,892 patients (27,863 in drug treatment groups and 16,029 in placebo). 0.43% of the patients in drug treatment groups reported suicidal behavior or ideation versus 0.22% of the patients in placebo groups. 2.1 per 1000 (95% CI: 0.7, 4.2) more treated patients reported suicidal behavior or ideation than placebo controls. On January 31, 2008, FDA issued an alert to health care providers warning of increased risk of suicidal thoughts and behavior with AEDs. On July 10, 2008 FDA's scientific advisory committee voted that there was a significant association between AEDs and suicidality but voted against a black box warning. Gibbons et al. (2008) studied the association between AEDs and suicidal behavior in a cohort of 47,918 patients with bipolar disorder with a minimum of a one-year window of information before and after the index date of their illness. Patients with bipolar disorder are at the highest risk of suicide among any of the indications for treatment with AEDs. In some cases the AED is prescribed as a treatment for bipolar disorder and in some cases a treatment for a comordid condition such as neuropathic pain or epilepsy.

10.6.2   Description of the Data, Cohort, and Key Design and Outcome Variables

Data for this study came from the PharMetrics Patient Centric Database, the largest national patient-centric database of longitudinal integrated health care claims data commercially available at that time. The PharMetrics data are nationally representative and not statistically different from the 2000 U.S. Census distributions of age, gender, and region. The universe of data are comprised of medical, specialty, facility, and pharmacy paid claims from more than 85 managed care plans nationally, representing more than 47 million covered lives. In the following, the various methodologies described in this chapter are illustrated using this longitudinal cohort study. Many but not all of these analyses are reported in Gibbons et al. (2008).

Data were collected during fiscal years 2000 through 2006. All patients with an ICD-9 diagnosis of bipolar disorder (ICD-9 codes: 296.0x, 296.1x, and 296.4x-296.8x) who were continuously enrolled in the same health care plan for at least one year before and after the index diagnosis date were included in the sample. A total of 47,918 patients met these criteria, and there were 1,226 patients with at least one suicide attempt. The ICD-9 codes used to identify suicide attempts were E950-E959, where subcategories are E950-E952 (self-inflicted poisoning), E953 (self-inflicted injury by hanging), E954 (drowning), E955 (self-inflicted injury by firearms), E956 (self-inflicted injury by cutting), E957 (self-inflicted injury by jumping from high places), E958 (other/unspecified self-inflicted injury), and E959 (late effects of self-inflicted injury). Based on this definition, suicide attempts include deliberate self harm.

To help insulate findings from bias analyses were restricted to AED monotherapy. AED monotherapy was defined for the one-year period following the index episode as taking only one of the 11 AEDs and not taking lithium. Concomitant antidepressant, other anticonvulsant, and antipsychotic medications were included as covariates. Lithium monotherapy was also examined. Comparator groups included (a) patients who received none of the 11 AEDs or lithium following diagnosis, and (b) patients who received no CNS medication.

10.6.3 Statistical Methods

Between-subject comparisons were based on Poisson regression models using the number of patient exposure days as an offset. Poisson regression analysis was used for between-subject comparisons of no medication (i.e., 11 AEDs and lithium) to pre-treatment and post-treatment AED and lithium conditions, respectively. GEE was used for within-subject analyses that compared suicide attempt rates before and after initiation of therapy. Comparing no AED/lithium treatment to the pre-treatment period allows examination of selection effects. The term pre-treatment indicates prior to the initiation of AED or Li+ monotherapy from the time of diagnosis. To adjust for other potential confounders, all models included concomitant other anticonvulsants, antidepressants, antipsychotics, previous suicide attempts (in the year prior to the index diagnosis), age, sex, and year (2000-2006) as covariates. Results were expressed as event rate ratios (ERR) and associated confidence intervals (CI). The ERR is a rate multiplier which reflects the increased rate associated with treatment versus no treatment. An ERR of 2.0 reflects a doubling of the rate whereas an ERR of 0.5 reflects one-half the risk.

A series of sensitivity analyses were performed to examine the robustness of findings to various model parameterizations. These sensitivity analyses included (a) monotherapy defined up to the first suicide attempt or one year, (b) same as (a) but restricted to patients with at least a 30 day supply of an AED, (c) same as (a) but excluding patients with suicide attempts on the day of the index diagnosis. As a further sensitivity analysis (d) a discrete-time survival model was fitted to these data, where AED treatment was modeled as a time-varying covariate, and the hazard rate of suicide attempts was estimated on a month by month basis. Unlike the previous analyses where exposure was considered constant from the time of treatment initiation through the one-year follow-up, in this analysis, treatment was evaluated on a month by month basis. This analysis combines patients who did not take an AED with non-medication months for patients who did take an AED, and compares them to active treatment months. This analysis determines the effects of duration and pattern of exposure on conclusions. This model also adjusted for month, which allowed the risk of suicide attempt to decrease (or increase) over time. An additional sensitivity analysis (e) was the same as (d) but was restricted to those highest risk patients who made a suicide attempt in the year prior to the index episode.

The final sensitivity analysis (f) was conducted in an attempt to provide a causal inference. In this analysis propensity score matching was used to obtain a 1:1 matched sample of patients who took AED monotherapy versus those who did not take an AED or lithium, where potential confounders included the previously described covariates. For each pair (i.e., AED versus no-AED or lithium) the number of days post diagnosis for the treated patient was used to define the exposure period. A simple comparison of rates between the AED and non-AED groups (pre and post-exposure) was then performed using GEE. This analysis provides a causal inference to the extent that the propensity score matching adjusts for confounding between patients treated and not treated, and the matching on date of treatment initiation adjusts for the natural course of suicide attempts over time.

10.6.4   Between-subject Analyses

Table 10.9 presents number of patients at risk, number of suicide attempts, patient years of exposure, and rate of suicide attempts per 1000 patient years (PYs) of exposure before and after initiation of treatment during the year following the index diagnosis. These statistics are provided for each of the AEDs, lithium, the combination of all AEDs, no AEDs or lithium, and no CNS treatment at all. Table 10.9 reveals that there were a total of 13,385 patients who received one of the 11 AEDs and 25,432 patients who did not receive any of the 11 AEDs or lithium. Post-treatment suicide attempt rates for AEDs (13/1000 PY) and lithium (18/1000 PY) were comparable to no treatment rates (13/1000 PY). Of the 25,432 patients who did not receive an AED or lithium, 11,207 (44%) also did not receive any other CNS medication. Their suicide attempt rate was 15/1000 PY. Felbamate, levetiracetam, pregabalin, tiagabine, and zonisamide had insufficient data for drug-level analysis. Figure 10.9 presents a graphical summary of suicide attempt rates by treatment (before and after treatment initiation).

Following treatment there was no overall significant difference in suicide attempt rates for patients treated with an AED (13/1000 PY) versus patients not treated with an AED or lithium (13/1000 PY), ERR = 0.88, (CI: 0.72-1.08), p<0.22. Similar results were seen for the individual AEDs, with the exception of topiramate (27/1000 PY ERR=1.87, (CI: 1.22-2.87), p<0.004) and carbamazepine (29/1000 PY, ERR=2.37, (CI:1.21-4.61), p<0.01) which had significantly greater post-treatment risk relative to no treatment (see Table 10.10). A small but significant post-treatment increase for lithium versus no treatment was also found (ERR=1.46, (CI: 1.04-2.03), p<0.03). Overall, AEDs were associated with lower suicide attempt rates than lithium (13/1000 versus 18/1000, ERR=0.62, (CI: 0.44-0.89), p<0.008); however, pre-treatment suicide attempt rates were not significantly higher for patients treated with lithium (99/1000 PY) relative to AEDs (72/1000 PY; adjusted ERR is 0.80, (0.51-1.25), p = 0.325). While not statistically significant, the increased rate of suicide attempts observed before treatment for lithium might account for the modestly higher post-treatment rate for lithium relative to AEDs (i.e., they were at greater risk to start suggesting a possible selection effect).

The suicide attempt rate for patients treated with no CNS drug (15/1000 PY) was significantly higher (ERR=0.19, (CI: 0.08-0.47), p<0.0003) than patients treated with an AED only (3/1000 PY), i.e., AED monotherapy but no other CNS drug. In the absence of concomitant treatment, AEDs were associated with significantly decreased risk of suicide attempt relative to untreated patients, despite an almost three-fold increased risk prior to

TABLE 10.9: Suicide Attempt Rate per 1,000 Person Years Before and After Treatment by AED, Lithium, and No Treatment

Drug	N	Before Treatment			After Treatment		
		Attempts	Person Years	Rate 1000 PYs	Attempts	Person Years	Rate 1000 PYs
Gabapentin	1,229	13	213	61	13	1,016	13
Divalproex	4,581	40	412	97	38	4,169	9
Felbamate	na						
Lamotrigine	4,412	24	613	39	50	3,799	13
Levetiracetam	42	0	6	0	0	36	0
Oxcarbazepine	1,463	30	164	183	20	1,299	15
Pregabalin	85	0	29	0	0	56	0
Tiagabine	80	0	16	0	0	64	0
Topiramate	1,063	11	184	60	24	879	27
Zonisamide	84	2	11	182	0	73	0
Carbamazepine	346	2	40	50	9	306	29
Any of 11 AEDs	13,385	122	1,688	72	154	11,697	13
11 AEDs only	1,910	9	204	44	5	1,706	3
Lithium	2,518	23	233	99	40	2,285	18
No AED or Li+	25,432		334	25,432	13		
No Medication	11,207		170	11,207	15		

TABLE 10.10: Event Rate Ratios (Confidence Intervals) Comparing Suicide Rates Before and After Treatment with AED and Lithium and Against No Drug

Drug	Post-Drug vs. No Drug			Pre-Drug vs. No Drug			Post-Drug vs. Pre-Drug		
	ERR	95% CI	p	ERR	95% CI	p	ERR	95% CI	p
Gabapentin	1.16	(0.66-2.05)	.60	6.11	(3.46-10.79)	.0001	0.15	(0.05-0.47)	.001
Divalproex	0.72	(0.51-1.02)	.06	7.27	(5.16-10.25)	.0001	0.10	(0.05-0.19)	.0001
Lamotrigine	0.85	(0.62-1.16)	.31	2.49	(1.63-3.81)	.0001	0.33	(0.19-0.59)	.0001
Oxcarbazepine	0.98	(0.62-1.56)	.94	10.78	(7.31-15.86)	.0001	0.09	(0.04-0.24)	.0001
Topiramate	1.87	(1.22-2.87)	.004	3.96	(2.15-7.29)	.0001	0.52	(0.18-1.48)	.22
Carbamazepine	2.37	(1.21-4.61)	.01	3.21	(0.80-12.94)	.10	0.76	(0.10-6.01)	.80
Lithium	1.46	(1.04-2.03)	.03	7.19	(4.65-11.11)	.0001	0.23	(0.11-0.49)	.0001
Any AED	0.88	(0.72-1.08)	.22	4.88	(3.91-6.09)	.0001	0.19	(0.11-0.26)	.0001
AED only	0.19	(0.08-0.47)	.0003	2.85	(1.46-5.57)	.002	0.05	(0.02-0.18)	.0001

ERR Event Rate Ratio ERR=2.0 indicates a doubling, ERR=0.5 indicates a halving.
Adjusted for other AEDs, antidepressants, antipsychotics, suicide attempts in prior year, age, sex, and year.

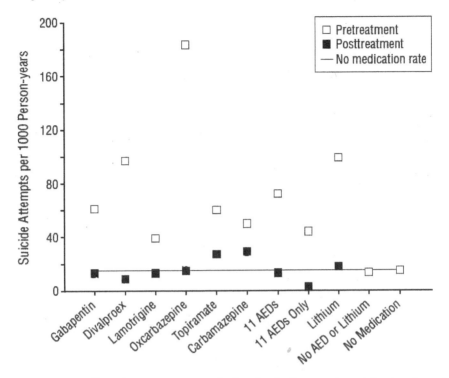

FIGURE 10.1: Suicide attempt rates before and after treatment by treatment type. AED indicates antiepileptic drug.

treatment (44/1000 versus 15/1000, ERR=2.85, (CI: 1.46-5.57), p<0.002, see Tables 10.9 and 10.10), and exhibited significant reduction with treatment. The post-treatment adjusted suicide attempt rate was one twentieth of the pre-treatment rate (44/1000 versus 3/1000, ERR=0.05, (CI: 0.02-0.18), p<0.0001), see Table 10.10.

The sensitivity analyses reported here are for all AEDs combined. Similar results were found for the individual AEDs, but they have less statistical power because of reduced sample size. All of the sensitivity analyses were restricted to a single suicide attempt per individual. The first sensitivity analysis defined monotherapy prior to the first suicide attempt if present (see Table 10.11). The odds ratio for any AED versus no AED or lithium was OR=0.58, CI=0.48-0.71, p<0.0001 (12.6/1000 PY versus 15.3/1000 PY). The second sensitivity analysis only considered the AED to be present if the cumulative prescription(s) consisted of a 30 day or more supply (see Table 10.12), and revealed quite similar results OR=0.58, CI=0.47-0.71, p<0.0001 (12.5/1000 PY versus 15.3/1000 PY). The third sensitivity analysis excluded suicide attempts made on the index episode date (see Table 10.13) and revealed no significant treatment related differences (OR=0.91, CI=0.73-1.12, p<0.37).

TABLE 10.11: Suicide Attempt Rate per 1,000 Persons by AED Drug

Drug	Monotherapy	# of Attempts	Rate 1000 PYs	Rate 1000	OR OR	95% CI 95% CI
Gabapentin	1,225	13	12.8	10.6	0.70	0.39-1.24
Valproate	4,568	40	9.6	8.8	0.48	0.34-0.67
Felbamate	na	na	na	na	na	na
Lamotrigine	4,404	50	13.2	11.4	0.62	0.46-0.85
Levetiracetam	42	0	0.0	0.0	na	na
Oxcarbazepine	1,455	22	17.0	15.1	0.66	0.42-1.04
Pregabalin	85	0	0.0	0.0	na	na
Tiagabine	80	0	0.0	0.0	na	na
Topiramate	1,059	15	17.1	14.2	0.73	0.42-1.24
Zonisamide	82	0	0.0	0.0	na	na
Carbamazepine	346	7	22.9	20.2	1.33	0.62-2.87
Any AED	13,346	147	12.6	11.0	0.58	0.48-0.71
Lithium	2,507	34	14.9	13.6	0.77	0.54-1.11
No-Med	25,579	392	15.3	15.3		

Odds ratio (OR) from logistic model adjusted for medications, age, sex, and previous attempt.

TABLE 10.12: Suicide Attempt Rate per 1,000 Persons by AED Drug - Logistic Regression Model - Only Those Patients with at Least a 30 day Supply of Drug

Drug	Monotherapy	# of Attempts	Rate 1000 PYs	Rate 1000	OR OR	95% CI 95% CI
Gabapentin	1,200	13	13.1	10.8	0.71	0.40-1.27
Valproate	4,487	39	9.5	8.7	0.47	0.34-0.66
Felbamate	na	na	na	na	na	na
Lamotrigine	4,343	50	13.4	11.5	0.63	0.46-0.86
Levetiracetam	41	0	0.0	0.0	na	na
Oxcarbazepine	1,428	20	15.7	14.0	0.61	0.38-0.97
Pregabalin	85	0	0.0	0.0	na	na
Tiagabine	78	0	0.0	0.0	na	na
Topiramate	1,043	15	17.4	14.4	0.73	0.43-1.26
Zonisamide	79	0	0.0	0.0	na	na
Carbamazepine	337	7	23.4	20.8	1.36	0.63-2.94
Any AED	13,121	144	12.5	11.0	0.58	0.47-0.71
Lithium	2,448	32	14.4	13.1	0.74	0.51-1.09
No-Med	25,579	392	15.3	15.3		

Odds ratio (OR) from logistic model adjusted for medications, age, sex, and previous attempt.

10.6.5 Within-subject Analysis

The rate of suicide attempts was significantly greater prior to any AED treatment (72/1000 PY) than after treatment (13/1000 PY), ERR=0.19, (CI: 0.11-0.26), p<.0001. Similar reductions in suicide attempt rates were seen for the individual drugs and lithium, although the results for topiramate (60/1000 vs. 27/1000, ERR=0.52, (CI: 0.18-1.48), p<0.22) and carbamazepine (50/1000 vs. 29/1000, ERR=0.76, (CI: 0.10-6.01), p<0.80) were not statistically significant (see Table 10.10). The pre-treatment rate of suicide attempts in patients who

TABLE 10.13: Suicide Attempt Rate per 1,000 Persons by AED Drug - Logistic Regression Model - Excluding Suicide Date = Index Date

Drug	Monotherapy	# of Attempts	Rate 1000 PYs	Rate 1000	OR OR	95% CI 95% CI
Gabapentin	1,225	13	12.8	10.6	1.13	0.63-2.03
Valproate	4,568	40	9.6	8.8	0.74	0.53-1.05
Felbamate	na	na	na	na	na	na
Lamotrigine	4,404	50	13.2	11.4	0.98	0.71-1.35
Levetiracetam	42	0	0.0	0.0	na	na
Oxcarbazepine	1,455	22	17.0	15.1	1.05	0.67-1.64
Pregabalin	85	0	0.0	0.0	na	na
Tiagabine	80	0	0.0	0.0	na	na
Topiramate	1,059	15	17.1	14.2	1.18	0.69-2.03
Zonisamide	82	0	0.0	0.0	na	na
Carbamazepine	346	7	22.9	20.2	1.99	0.92-4.30
Any AED	13,346	147	12.6	11.0	0.91	0.73-1.12
Lithium	2,507	34	14.9	13.6	1.22	0.84-1.77
No-Med	25,579	255	10.0	10.0		

Odds ratio (OR) from logistic model adjusted for medications, age, sex, and previous attempt.

ultimately received AED treatment was significantly higher than the no treatment suicide attempt rate (ERR=4.88, (CI: 3.91-6.09), p<0.0001) suggesting that patients who receive AED treatment were more severely impaired and therefore at greater risk of suicide. A similar result was found for lithium (see Table 10.10).

10.6.6 Discrete-time Analysis

A discrete-time survival model was used to examine the association between treatment defined on a monthly basis to the first suicide attempt. A significant decrease in suicide attempt rate associated with AED treatment (OR=0.59, CI=0.47-0.75, p<0.0001) was found. Figure 10.2 presents the estimated hazard functions (post-diagnosis) for treated and untreated patients. Overall the suicide attempt rate decreases with time; however, the rates are lower in AED treated patients throughout. Restricting the analysis to only those patients (n=662) that made a suicide attempt in the year prior to the index diagnosis revealed an even larger decrease in suicide attempt rate associated with treatment (OR=0.35, CI=0.17-0.74, p<0.005).

10.6.7 Propensity Score Matching

To further control for possible treatment selection, patients were matched on both a 1:1 propensity score (i.e., matching of patients that did and did not take an AED on a series of potential confounders including prior suicide attempts and other anticonvulsant, antidepressant, and antipsychotic use before and after AED treatment initiation, and initial exposure date assignment (i.e., time from diagnosis of bipolar disorder to initiation of AED treatment) for each pair based on the patient who took the AED. Table 10.14 presents the covariate distributions for AED and no-AED groups before and after match-

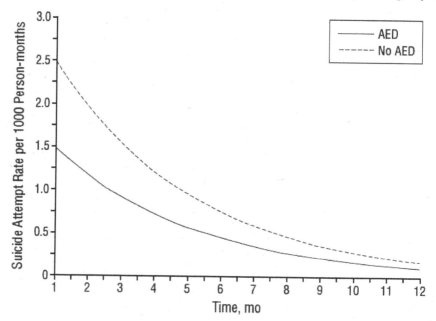

FIGURE 10.2: Hazard functions for suicide rates over time. Comparisons of patients treated with an AED vs patients not treated with an AED were adjusted for age, sex, concomitant treatment, previous suicide attempt, and year.

ing. Table 10.14 presents differences in means for age, and proportions (all other variables), and standardized differences (mean or proportion difference divided by pooled standard deviation). As a rule of thumb, standardized differences of 10% or less are considered well matched (Austin 2007). Table 10.14 reveals large imbalances prior to matching, which disappear in the matched sample. Comparison of the AED and no-AED groups revealed that prior to treatment, the rate of suicide attempts was 70.52/1000 PY for treated and 38.07/1000 PY for untreated (OR=1.85, 95% CI=(1.22-2.81), p<0.0037). Following treatment the suicide attempt rate was 12.88/1000 PY for the treated and 10.46/1000 for untreated (OR=1.23, CI=(0.89-1.71), p<0.22). These results reveal that even after matching, the pre-treatment suicide attempt rate is significantly elevated; however, following treatment there is no significant difference in suicide attempt rates between those who did and did not receive AED treatment.

TABLE 10.14: Comparison of Patient Characteristic Distributions in Original and Propensity Score Matched Samples

	Original Dataset (n=38,817)			Matched Dataset (n=25,574)		
	No-Med	AED	STD Diff	No-Med	AED	STD Diff
Male	40.2	40.0	0.5	40.3	40.1	0.5
Previous suicide attempt	1.1	1.6	4.0	1.4	1.6	1.4
Anticonvulsant before index date	5.2	11.8	23.9	9.1	10.5	4.8
Anticonvulsant after index date	6.0	14.9	29.6	10.9	13.0	6.7
Antidepressant before index date	39.4	66.9	57.5	67.3	65.5	3.9
Antidepressant after index date	42.4	70.6	59.4	71.9	69.3	5.8
Antipsychotic before index date	13.1	23.6	27.4	21.4	22.5	2.6
Antipsychotic after index date	19.9	41.1	47.3	36.1	38.7	5.4
Age	35.4 (15.9)	34.6 (15.2)	4.9	34.6 (15.5)	34.7 (15.3)	0.7
Percentage or mean and standard deviation						

10.6.8 Self-controlled Case Series and Poisson Hybrid Models

To this point in the analysis, we have restricted our attention to AED monotherapy over a one year period. To provide a more general framework we now consider a six month window from the index episode and permit any combination of AED therapy across the 11 AEDs that led to the FDA warning. Furthermore, in the analyses presented in this section we only adjust the relationship between time-varying AED exposure and suicide attempt for potentially time-varying confounders (lithium, other anticonvulsants, antidepressants, and antipsychotic medications). Since these are within-person comparisons, we further restrict the analysis to the 17,370 subjects who took at least one AED during the 6 month period from diagnosis of bipolar illness. This included 104,220 monthly observations and 217 suicide attempts in 187 individuals. The hybrid model that we consider here decomposes the AED exposure into the average of exposed months and the deviation of each month from that average. For example, if a patient was prescribed an AED on 3 of the 6 months the average is 0.5 and the months off AED therapy have a deviation of -0.5 and those on AED therapy 0.5. The Poisson model is fitted with random intercept and deviation effects to accommodate both person-specific variation in the base-rate and treatment heterogeneity. To adjust for concomitant medications, terms in the model were included for treatment with lithium, other anticonvulsants, antidepressants, and antipsychotic medications at each point in time. As a comparison, we also fit a conditional model (SCCS) to the same data.

Results of the analysis of the SCCS analysis revealed a significant effect of AED exposure on suicide attempts, RR=1.60 95% CI=(1.13, 2.28). Results of the analysis for the hybrid model reveal significant confounding for the BS effect RR=0.30 95% CI=(0.17, 0.51) but a non-significant WS exposure effect RR=1.33 95% CI=(0.43, 4.14). While the BS effect reflects differences between individuals which may be confounded with other unmeasured characteristics, it is interesting to note that those subjects receiving more consistent AED treatment have significantly lower probability of making a suicide attempt. Within individuals, there is a greater likelihood of making a suicide attempt on treated months but this effect was not statistically significant using the hybrid mixed-effects model. Of course, this effect could be produced by dynamic confounding where risk of suicide attempt and treatment are correlated with changes in severity of illness. Note that the SCCS is restricted to the analysis of subjects who both took an AED and made a suicide attempt. This ignores information on subjects who took an AED and did not make a suicide attempt which is incorporated in the hybrid model. If we similarly restrict the hybrid model to the case-exposure subsample, the within-subject effect is estimated as RR=1.50 95% CI=(1.07, 2.11), which is slightly smaller than the conditional estimator, but larger than the exposure only cohort. Restricting the sample to the case-exposure subset may increase dynamic confounding with severity of illness.

10.6.9 Marginal Structural Models

To examine the possibility of dynamic confounding, we used a marginal structural model for time to first suicide attempt to analyze the dataset used in the previous section (i.e., six months of follow-up not restricted to AED monotherapy). All 47,918 patients with a new index episode of bipolar disorder were used in this analysis whether or not they took an AED. Discrete-time survival models were used to analyze these data. The simple unweighted analysis without covariate adjustment yielded a significantly increased risk of suicide attempt with any AED treatment OR=1.77 95% CI=(1.42, 2.20). Statistical adjustment for age, sex, prior suicide attempt, concomitant medications (antidepressants, other anticonvulsants, antipsychotics and lithium) and co-morbid disorders (ADHD, anxiety spectrum disorders, psychotic disorders, seizure disorders, and conduct disorders) had little effect on the estimated association OR=1.72 95% CI=(1.38, 2.15). By contrast, the MSM weighted analysis revealed evidence of a protective effect of AED treatment both with OR=0.78 95% CI=(0.62, 0.98) and without OR=0.80 95% CI=(0.63, 1.01) covariate adjustment. These findings reveal that simple covariate adjustment may be insufficient to remove the dynamic confounding in the treatment selection process.

The previous analyses represent a mixture of between-subject and within-subject effects. It should be noted that a hybrid model can also be used for these analyses, where the dynamic AED treatment effect can be decomposed into between and within components as the mean and deviation of the monthly AED treatments. The simple unweighted and unadjusted analysis reveals a marginal within-subject effect OR=1.51 95% CI=(1.03, 2.22), which disappears after MSM weighting OR=1.18 95% CI=(0.80, 1.75). Note that the weighted average effect is significantly protective OR=0.63 95% CI=(0.46, 0.85) indicating that increased treatment was associated with decreased risk of a suicide attempt. Covariate adjustment decreased the unweighted OR=1.41 95% CI=(0.97, 2.04) and weighted OR−1.10 95% CI=(0.75, 1.61) associations. These findings reveal that the benefit observed in the original MSM analysis was due in large part to between-subject effects where subjects with more AED treatment have lower suicide attempt rate. Within subjects the weighted analysis reveals no association between AED treatment and suicide attempts.

10.6.10 Stratified Cox and Random-effect Survival Models

The bipolar dataset is not well suited to analysis using a stratified Cox model because there is no obvious clustering unit besides the individual and no obvious way to partition the within subject data into episodes based on the rarity of the suicide attempt outcome. Interestingly as illustrated in the previous example, the hybrid model permits a decomposition of between and within-subject effects even without random-effects. This is unique to a time-to-event model, because it is the only model where the exposure variable can be time-varying but the outcome is not repeatedly experienced. To illustrate use of the models in the more general clustered case we turn to an example originally described by Gibbons et al. (2012a,b) on suicidal ideation and behavior data from 41 randomized longitudinal placebo-controlled clinical trials of fluoxetine and venlafaxine. Here the clustering variable is study, and study-specific variability in both the background rate and treatment effect can be included in the corresponding mixed-effects model. Given randomization, there is no possible correlation between the study-specific random-effect and exposure variable (i.e., antidepressant treatment) so concern regarding the violation of the independence assumption does not apply. For the first illustration using these data, we restrict attention to the entire adult population (37 studies and 5,821 subjects aged 18 and older), see Table 10.15. The models included terms for treatment, age, and sex on time to suicidal event. For the stratified Cox model, the treatment effect (expressed as a hazard ratio) was HR=0.66, 95% CI=(0.56, 0.77). Identical results were obtained for the mixed-effects discrete-time survival model with a random intercept HR=0.66, 95% CI=(0.56, 0.77), and similar results when the model is extended to include treatment hetero-geneity HR=0.66, 95% CI=(0.56, 0.79). The same is not true, however, when the data are restricted to young adults, ages 18-24, for which the black box warning was extended by the U.S. FDA in 2006. There were 32 studies, 378 subjects, and 44 suicidal events for this age group (see Table 10.16). Here, the stratified Cox model yielded HR=1.12, 95% CI=(0.55, 2.26), whereas the discrete-time survival model yielded HR=1.00, 95% CI=(0.54, 1.85). The fundamental difference here is that 12 of the 32 studies had zero events and therefore did not contribute to the likelihood of the stratified Cox model. When the event rate is low and the sample is limited, the random-effect approach may provide both increased statistical power and reduction in bias compared to the stratified Cox model. This is a similar result as previously shown in the comparison of fixed effect versus full-likelihood random-effect methods for meta-analysis of rare binary events in Chapter 6.

10.6.11   Conclusion

Drawing causal inference from observational data is complicated in general, but even more complicated for the study of suicide. First, suicide and suicide attempts are rare events, and their determinants are difficult to estimate precisely in all but the largest samples. Second, suicide is related to the indication for treatment (i.e., a psychiatric disorder) and is therefore difficult to disentangle from the possible effects of treatment. Third, a suicide attempt can lead to the identification of the psychiatric disorder that can in turn lead to treatment. It is not uncommon to find patients who have a suicide attempt,

TABLE 10.15: Summary of the Number of Events and Censored Values for the Adult Data (18 and older)

Study	Total	Events	Censored	% Censored
1	58	5	53	91.38
2	80	6	74	92.50
3	270	45	225	83.33
4	70	5	65	92.86
5	569	47	522	91.74
6	262	21	241	91.98
7	69	12	57	82.61
8	131	24	107	81.68
9	83	7	76	91.57
10	89	18	71	79.78
11	80	9	71	88.75
12	178	16	162	91.01
13	27	7	20	74.07
14	464	66	398	85.78
15	82	10	72	87.80
16	42	10	32	76.19
17	149	16	133	89.26
18	156	11	145	92.95
19	109	17	92	84.40
20	132	17	115	87.12
21	146	31	115	78.77
22	130	13	117	90.00
23	169	20	149	88.17
24	200	17	183	91.50
25	305	28	277	90.82
26	280	40	240	85.71
27	229	14	215	93.89
28	40	8	32	80.00
29	128	15	113	88.28
30	24	2	22	91.67
31	121	8	113	93.39
32	94	8	86	91.49
33	105	6	99	94.29
34	179	18	161	89.94
35	244	30	214	87.70
36	138	7	131	94.93
37	189	13	176	93.12
	5821	647	5174	88.89

diagnosis of depression or bipolar disorder, and initiate treatment all on the same day. While this suicide attempt is not the consequence of initiating treatment, it can inflate the rate of suicide attempts observed prior to initiation of treatment or in those patients that do not receive treatment. Fourth, the

TABLE 10.16: Summary of the Number of Events and Censored Values for the Young Adult Data (18 to 24)

Study	Total	Events	Censored	% Censored
1	4	0	4	100.00
2	7	1	6	85.71
3	21	4	17	80.95
4	2	1	1	50.00
5	38	5	33	86.84
6	24	2	22	91.67
7	7	0	7	100.00
8	5	1	4	80.00
9	7	2	5	71.43
10	12	4	8	66.67
11	3	1	2	66.67
12	15	1	14	93.33
13	6	0	6	100.00
14	1	0	1	100.00
15	9	0	9	100.00
16	7	0	7	100.00
17	11	3	8	72.73
18	2	0	2	100.00
19	8	0	8	100.00
20	5	0	5	100.00
21	7	0	7	100.00
22	16	1	15	93.75
23	15	3	12	80.00
24	12	1	11	91.67
25	9	2	7	77.78
26	8	2	6	75.00
27	8	1	7	87.50
28	52	6	46	88.46
29	25	2	23	92.00
30	13	0	13	100.00
31	12	1	11	91.67
32	7	0	7	100.00
	378	44	334	88.36

natural course of psychiatric illnesses exhibits a decrease in suicide attempts over time from diagnosis. This can make it appear that the suicide attempt rate is higher prior to treatment initiation than after, giving the false appearance of a protective effect. Fifth, patients who receive treatment often have increased severity of illness and may therefore be at increased suicidal risk to begin with.

These analyses reveal no evidence that AEDs increase risk of suicide attempts relative to patients not treated with an AED or lithium. Among patients not receiving any concomitant CNS treatment, the suicide attempt rate in AED treated patients was significantly lower than untreated patients. These analyses also reveal that there is a selection effect in that the pre-treatment suicide attempt rate is 5 times higher than the rate in untreated patients. If pre-treatment suicide attempt rates reflect severity of illness, it is the more severely impaired patients who receive treatment with an AED or lithium. Nevertheless, the post-treatment suicide attempt rate is significantly reduced relative to their elevated pre-treatment levels to the level found at or below patients not receiving treatment. This finding suggests a possible protective effect of AED treatment on suicidality. Possible exceptions are topiramate and carbamazepine which did not show significant reduction in suicide attempt rates with treatment and had post-treatment suicide attempt rates significantly higher than untreated levels. Nevertheless, even for these two AEDs, there was no evidence that they increased suicide rates.

Sensitivity analyses revealed that these findings are robust to duration of treatment, defined as duration of 30 days or more, or defined on a monthly basis. The later analysis reveals that despite the systematic decreases in suicide attempt rates over time, there remains a statistically significant decrease in suicide attempt rate for patients treated with an AED. Similar results were found for multiple attempts or a single attempt per person. Similar results were observed when monotherapy was defined for the entire year following the index episode or just until the first suicide attempt. Excluding all suicide attempts that occurred on the index episode date produced an odds ratio less than 1.0, but was no longer statistically significant. This finding suggests that some of the difference between patients treated with an AED and those not treated may be due to the identification of bipolar disorder because of the suicide attempt. Propensity score matching was used to further examine this possibility, by matching AED treated and untreated patients in terms of potential confounders and pre and post-treatment periods based on the treatment initiation day for the treated patient. Treated patients still had elevated pre-treatment suicide attempt rate, but no difference following treatment. AED treatment therefore appears to produce a larger decrease in suicide attempt rates because the patients who ultimately receive AED treatment have a higher rate of suicide attempts prior to receiving treatment. The exception to this is the case of patients who received no CNS treatment at all versus those that only received an AED, where the post AED treatment rate was significantly lower than the no treatment rate (3/1000 patient years versus 15/1000 patient years). Finally, restricting attention to those patients at highest risk for suicide attempt (i.e., those patients making a suicide attempt in the year prior to the index episode) revealed an even larger significant reduction in suicide attempt rate with AED treatment, suggesting that benefit of AED treatment may be greatest for the highest risk patients.

When we relax the requirement of AED monotherapy and include patients who might take multiple AEDs during the first six months following their index diagnosis of a new bipolar disorder, the naive analyses do suggest a positive association between treatment with an AED and suicide attempt.

Decomposing this effect into between-subject and within-subject components reveals that the protective effect is explained largely by a positive association between the proportion of time a patient receives AED treatment during the first six months following diagnosis. The within-subject association is not statistically significant, but is in the direction of increased risk during months that patients receive treatment. Marginal structural models reveal that this trend is due to dynamic confounding, which when accounted for by weighting yields an odds ratio close to 1.0. Although we generally view the between-subject effect as merely a confounder, here it suggests that if patients receive treatment with an AED, the more consistent that treatment the lower the risk of a suicide attempt.

Finally, we have also illustrated the use of a stratified Cox model and a mixed-effects discrete-time survival model for analysis of clustered survival data in a research synthesis of 37 studies of antidepressant treatment in adults. When the number of studies is large and the number of subjects within those studies is large, and when all studies record events, both approaches yield virtually identical results. However, when the number of subjects within studies is smaller and some studies have no events of interest, the stratified Cox model can exhibit bias similar to fixed-effects models used in meta-analysis of rare binary events.

10.7 Conclusion

In many ways, this chapter is the heart of this book. With the emergence and accessibility of "big data" comes the responsibility for their careful and thoughtful analysis. These are generally observational data and have no immunity to bias. Size does not insulate one from bias as shown repeatedly in this chapter. Of the various methods described here, it should be directly apparent that those methods which focus on within-subject associations are the least prone to bias. Even here, however, dynamic confounding can play a role providing the appearance of an association between two time-series which are both merely related to a third dynamic confounder, for example changes in the severity of illness. Given their wide use and generally good performance for work in drug safety, we have provided a detailed review of fixed-effects approaches for analysis of clustered and longitudinal data. These include SCCS and stratified Cox models. Both are extremely important and useful tools for high quality work in drug safety. Nevertheless we have illustrated that there are conditions in which their generally good performance is compromised in terms of limited statistical power and even bias in the presence of treatment heterogeneity. We have drawn attention to less well known alternatives based on mixed-effects regression models and ways around their sometimes restrictive assumptions which have diminished enthusiasm for their general use in this area.

11

Methods to be Avoided

"I don't use drugs, my dreams are frightening enough."
(M.C. Escher)

11.1 Introduction

As evidenced in the previous chapters, there are a great many statistical approaches to the analysis of drug safety data. Not all methods are good for all problems and as we have seen, methods which exploit dynamic exposures within individuals may well provide the greatest promise for future work in this area. Nevertheless, there are some approaches, often widely used in practice, which should be avoided as they are so prone to bias, misleading, and uninterpretable results that they are better off left alone. In this chapter, we try to highlight what these methods are and why they should be avoided and for what purposes.

11.2 Spontaneous Reports

For many years the primary tool used by pharmaceutical companies and the U.S. FDA involved the collection of spontaneous reports from patients, doctors, lawyers, ... , regarding drugs that they have taken and adverse events that they have experienced. Chapter 5 provides a detailed review of statistical approaches to the analysis of such data. While some methods are more promising than others, it is our opinion that such data are so limited that they should only be considered for very specific purposes. Problems associated with the use of spontaneous reports in drug safety include (1) confounding by indication (i.e., patients taking a particular drug may have a disease that is itself associated with a higher incidence of the AE (e.g., antidepressants, depression, and suicide)), (2) systematic underreporting, (3) questionable representativeness of patients, (4) effects of publicity in the media on numbers of reports,

(5) extreme duplication of reports, (6) attribution of the event to a single drug when patients may be exposed to multiple drugs, and (7) extensive amounts of missing data. These limitations degrade the capacity for optimal data mining and analysis (Hauben et al. 2007). Spontaneous reports are useful for the identification of very rare adverse events early in a drug's history of use which have little or anything to do with the indication for which the drug is used. For example, taking a drug and turning a bright shade of blue is a very different thing than taking a drug and feeling blue. If the drug is given to patients who are at increased risk of depression, the frequency of patients reporting that they feel blue will undoubtedly be elevated relative to other side-effects (disproportionality), but the association provides no basis for causal inference. Turning blue is a very different matter and the evidence of even a small number of cases of patients turning blue after a drug exposure is important whether it is disproportional or not. Many have taken this type of example (turning blue) as support for the in-discriminant use of such data (spontaneous reports) to draw inferences regarding examples of the latter (feeling blue). We now have much better data and methods for drawing inferences for more common adverse events (e.g., analysis of large-scale observational datasets such as medical claims data), and they should replace analysis of spontaneous reports for all but the most unusual occurrences.

11.3   Vote Counting

In chapter 6, we provide an extensive review of meta-analytic techniques for research synthesis, pointing out their various strengths and weaknesses, particularly for analysis of rare adverse events. Unfortunately, there are many cases where a simple tally of the number of positive studies is reported and taken as evidence for efficacy, safety, or the lack thereof. This is a practice that should clearly be avoided. One can easily imagine a series of small studies which are underpowered to detect an association between treatment and an adverse event such that none of the individual studies report a statistically significant association and the vote count is 0 in terms of evidence in favor of such an association. In the aggregate, however, the association may well be clinically and statistically significant given the increased statistical power of the combined analysis. The reverse can also be true. A series of biased studies can yield a high vote count in favor of an association that is an artificial byproduct of confounding. Another problem with vote-counting is that it ignores sample size, and the results of a series of small studies may provide a high or low vote count which is discordant with the greatest mass of the data which might be restricted to a few large and well controlled studies. A good example relates to the question of whether antidepressants cause birth defects. Several studies which have compared mothers who took antidepressants versus those that did not have shown increased risk of birth defects (including cardiac birth defects) in mothers who took antidepressants during the first trimester (see Alwan et al. 2007, Louik et al. 2007). However, Jimenez-Solem et al. (2012) did a similar comparison, but instead of comparing mother's who did or did not take antidepressants during pregnancy, which is confounded by depression, they compared mothers who halted antidepressant treatment during pregnancy versus those who continued taking antidepressants. Here the authors found that while children of exposed mothers had increased risk of cardiac malformations relative to unexposed mothers (OR=2.01, 95% CI=1.60, 2.53), the same difference was seen between mothers who halted their use of antidepressants during pregnancy and non-exposed mothers (OR=1.85, 95% CI=1.07, 3.20), probability value for the difference = 0.94. Vote counting would likely yield strong evidence in support of an association which may have little to do with the exposure to antidepressants and much more to do with the effects of depression on other exposures (e.g., people with depression have a higher rate of smoking) which are in turn related to birth defects.

11.4 Simple Pooling of Studies

Another bad approach to synthesizing evidence across studies is to simply pool them and perform an overall analysis on the combined data without taking the clustering of observations within studies into account. This is an all too common practice. Not only can this provide incorrect standard errors and tests of hypotheses, it can also produce biased results. For example, imagine a series of randomized controlled trials of which half used 1:1 randomization to treatment versus control and the other half used 3:1 randomization. More severely ill patients might risk enrollment in an RCT that provided three times the likelihood of receiving active treatment, but might not enroll if the chance was only 50%. If severity of illness is associated with the likelihood of the adverse event, then there would be more events in the 3:1 randomized trials, and since there are three times as many treated patients in these trials, this would give the appearance that the drug increased the risk of the adverse event. Even more dangerous would be the attribution that one can draw a causal inference from these data because the individual trials were randomized. Of course a proper meta-analysis would adjust for this imbalance and account for differences in the baseline risk between the studies in estimating the overall treatment effect.

11.5   Including Randomized and Non-randomized Trials in Meta-analysis

It is all too common to see a research synthesis which involves a mixture of randomized (Phase II or III) and non-randomized trials (Phase I). This is a similar problem to the previous example in that studies in which everyone receives treatment will often include more severely ill patients who would otherwise not enroll in a study in which they have a chance of being randomized to placebo. If severity of illness is related to adverse event of interest, the results of such an analysis will provide incorrect evidence of a relationship between the drug and the adverse event. This is true even if a proper meta-analysis is performed because in the studies without randomization there is no control condition and severity of illness will be confounded with the effect of treatment.

11.6   Multiple Comparisons and Biased Reporting of Results

While less of a factor in the peer reviewed literature, in litigation it is not uncommon to see an expert report in which hundreds or even thousands of results are reviewed and a handful of those results which are statistically significant in the desired direction are reported without discussion of disconfirming results or any information on the number of results reviewed. This is often the rule rather than the exception because in RCTs, summary results for large numbers of potential adverse events are routinely reported without any adjustment for multiplicity. While this makes sense for the purpose of regulatory review where there is greater concern of a false negative than a false positive, this can lead to biased and misleading summaries of a literature or a set of published and unpublished studies where the focus is on litigation. To make matters worse, it is often the case that results that are not statistically significant are reported in this way without regard to their confidence interval or distance of the point estimate from the null. In extreme cases, experts will attribute risk to any odds ratio or relative risk greater than 1.0 and safety to any odds ratio or relative risk less than 1.0. Of course, if the null hypothesis is true and the OR=RR=1.0, then we would expect 50% of the estimated ORs and RRs to be less than 1.0 and 50% to be greater than 1.0 by chance alone. These data which provide evidence of no association between the exposure and the adverse event of interest can therefore be used to support either a protective or harmful association depending on the prerogative of the reviewer. This type of practice is a very unfortunate consequence of our legal system.

11.7 Immortality Time Bias

Immortality time bias refers to the span of time during the observation period where the event of interest could not have occurred (Suissa 2007). The classic examples are two studies from the 1970s on the benefit of heart transplant on survival time. In the first study 15 treated patients who received a heart transplant survived an average of 111 days (including waiting time for the organ) were compared to 42 patients on the wait-list who survived an average of only 74 days (Messmer et al. 1969). In the second study survival was 200 days for the 20 patients in the transplant group versus 34 days for the 14 wait-list controls. As noted by Gail (1972) inclusion of the period of time spent waiting for transplant in the survival time of the transplanted group provides a biased upward estimate of the survival time for the transplanted group because the subjects in the transplanted group must survive until the time of transplant.

In pharmacoepidemiology, immortal time bias occurs when the time between the cohort entry and initiation of treatment is attributed to the exposure condition. If the event is not repeatable or interest is in time to the first event, the time between cohort entry and exposure is immortal since subjects who experience the event are not included and the time during which the event cannot occur is added to the exposure group only. As noted by Suissa (2007), the solution is to treat exposure as a time-dependent exposure in a time-to-event model or to classify the period prior to the first exposure as unexposed. A second example of immortal time bias occurs when the cohort is defined on the basis of having two or more exposures. The period of time between the first exposure and the second is immortal because the subject must survive until the second exposure in order to be considered. Subjects who died after the first exposure cannot be included in the exposed group; therefore, biasing their estimated survival time. A third example involves definition of the exposed group as having both a diagnosis and exposure (i.e., filled prescription) on the same day and a comparison group of subjects who were not exposed during the first year from diagnosis. Groups are then compared during a follow-up period. In order to be in the control group, the patients must survive for a year, during which the survival time for the controls is ignored. A graphical example originally presented by Lévesque et al. (2010) is presented in Figure 11.1.

Suissa (2007) demonstrated the effect of misclassified and excluded immortal time by showing effectiveness of two drug classes, inhaled beta-agonists (IBA) and gastrointestinal drugs (GID), that are not known to treat cardiovascular disease (CVD). He selected the base cohort using health insurance databases from Saskatchewan, Canada. The cohort included those patients hospitalized for primary diagnosis of CVD. To illustrate the immortal time bias arising from misclassification and exclusion, he formed two cohorts. The

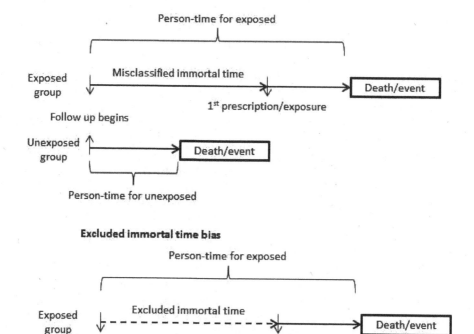

FIGURE 11.1: Examples of immortality bias.

first cohort was formed by defining cohort entry as a hospital discharge date following the CVD diagnosis, and the exposure was defined at the first prescription of IBA during the first 180 days of follow up. A total of 1542 subjects were included in the study, of whom 771 did not fill an IBA prescription during the 180-day period, i.e, unexposed. They contributed 674.6 person-years to the study and 148 deaths were observed resulting into 21.9 deaths per 100 subjects per year. Among the remaining 771 subjects who did fill an IBA prescription during the 180-day period, 114 died during follow up. The total person-time contributed by the exposed group was 713.0 person-year, of which 102.4 person-years were observed between entry and exposure. The rate of death in this group was 16 per 100 exposure years. The death rate ratio calculated from this misclassified approach showed 0.73 (0.57-0.93) times lower death rate for patients treated with IBA, even though the drug has never been associated with CVD treatment prior to this analysis. Clearly, the follow up time between hospital discharge date and dispensing of IBA prescription is immortal for the exposed group. The correctly classified analysis transfers the unexposed person-time to the denominator of the unexposed group risk. The resulting total person-time in the unexposed is increased by 102.4 person-year and decreased by the same amount in the exposed. Consequently, the correct rate of death in unexposed is 19.2 per 100 subjects per year and in exposed is 18.7 per 100 exposure per year. The resulting death rate ratio is 0.95 (0.77-1.25) and correctly shows that the IBA is not significantly effective in reducing mortality among CVD patients.

The second cohort was selected such that the immortal time is excluded from the exposure follow up. The cohort was formed by first selecting 640 subjects who received GID in the first year after discharge. The unexposed group included 640 subjects who did not receive GID in the first year after discharge. The exposed subjects were followed for 1-year after the GID exposure and unexposed subjects were followed for 1-year after the day of discharge. Of the 640 exposed subjects, 99 died during the follow up and total person-time contribution was 581.3 person-years. Of the 640 unexposed subjects, 125 died during a 1-year follow up. A total of 561.0 person-years were observed for the unexposed group. The rate ratio comparing the exposed to unexposed group was 0.78 (0.61-0.99) indicating a significant reduction in death rate among the exposed group. However, a proper accounting of 131.5 person-years that preceded exposure as unexposed person-time changed the rate ratio to 0.94 (0.73-1.20), indicating non-significant reduction in mortality rate attributable to GID treatment.

These two analyses that purposefully introduced immortal time in cohort selection highlight the danger in conducting observational studies. The immortal time bias is pervasive in the literature. Several reviews have revealed a number of studies that suffer from this bias. Suissa (2007) has listed 20 observational studies of the effects of various drugs on mortality and morbidity. Some of those studies were published in reputable journals such the Journal of the American Medical Association. Suissa and Azoulay (2012) also reviewed studies of the risk of cancer associated with metformin use and found 13 observational studies on the subject that have incurred the same bias.

Two general strategies for eliminating such bias are (a) to treat exposure as a time-dependent variable comparing rates of repeatable events within individuals or simply as a time-varying predictor in a time to a single event analysis, and (b) in a cohort defined in terms of a new diagnosis, matching control observation periods to the time after index diagnosis of the exposure for each of the treated subjects. An example of the matching is to begin the observation period for a control subject 10 days after diagnosis as a match for an exposed subject who began pharmacologic treatment 10 days after diagnosis. Of course, day 1 of the observation period would begin on day 10 following the index diagnosis for both subjects. Here the first 10 days are immortal in both exposed and unexposed subjects, thereby eliminating bias associated with the immortality. The matching strategy provides a way of eliminating immortality bias in a between-subject comparison, whereas treating exposure as a time-varying effect can be used to estimate the within-subject exposure effect using methods described in Chapter 10.

12

Summary and Conclusions

"Words are, of course, the most powerful drug used by mankind."
(Rudyard Kipling)

12.1   Final Thoughts

Drug safety is an international priority. However, all drugs have adverse effects; what ultimately matters is if the benefits of a drug outweigh the risks. To this end, a scientifically accurate characterization of risks and benefits is essential. A drug like varenicline which is the most effective anti-smoking treatment in existence has a black box warning for neuropsychiatric events and suicide risk despite the absence of a signal derived from RCTs and large-scale well controlled observational studies. The evidence in support of this association is restricted to spontaneous reports of such events. It seems unlikely that the frequency of spontaneous reports is indicative of a causal association in the absence of any signal based on higher quality randomized and observational data (Gibbons and Mann 2013). Nevertheless, the black box warning has limited use of this highly effective smoking cessation medication the consequences of which must include increased risk of lung cancer and death. There is something seriously wrong with this risk-benefit equation.

We have reviewed a wide variety of statistical approaches for the analysis of drug safety data, many of which will hopefully lead to improved future practice and increased interest by statisticians in conducting future statistical research in this important area. Drug safety is clearly an area which benefits from the availability of "big data." However, big data in and of themselves is not the solution. These data must be paired with thoughtful designs and analyses to prevent bias and false discovery. The need for rigorous statistical thinking and practice is all the more important as the size of available data streams increase. These are observational data and their perils have been well known to statisticians and epidemiologists for decades.

While we have outlined many different approaches to providing a detailed review of a putative drug adverse event association, an important direction of future research should be in the area of the use of these methods for large-scale screening of millions of possible drug adverse event interactions. We have highlighted some of these approaches but much more work in this area is needed.

As in all areas of science, we must look for coherence across findings from different perspectives using different types of studies, both randomized and observational, prior to drawing inferences. We must also look for disconfirming evidence and not simply build a research platform to support a preconceived notion. The consequences of both failing to detect a drug safety signal and falsely concluding that there is a safety concern when one does not exist are enormous in terms of the protection of public health and maximizing human capital.

Bibliography

K. Abrams and B. Sanso. Approximate Bayesian inference for random effects meta-analysis. *Statistics in Medicine*, 17(2):201–218, 1998.

A. Agresti. *Categorical Data Analysis*. John Wiley & Sons, 1990.

I. Ahmed, F. Haramburu, A. Fourrier-Réglat, F. Thiessard, C. Kreft-Jais, G. Miremont-Salamé, B. Bégaud, and P. Tubert-Bitter. Bayesian pharmacovigilance signal detection methods revisited in a multiple comparison setting. *Statistics in Medicine*, 28(13):1774–1792, 2009.

I. Ahmed, C. Dalmasso, F. Haramburu, F. Thiessard, P. Broët, and P. Tubert-Bitter. False discovery rate estimation for frequentist pharmacovigilance signal detection methods. *Biometrics*, 66(1):301–309, 2010a.

I. Ahmed, F. Thiessard, G. Miremont-Salame, B. Begaud, and P. Tubert-Bitter. Pharmacovigilance data mining with methods based on false discovery rates: a comparative simulation study. *Clinical Pharmacology & Therapeutics*, 88(4):492–498, 2010b.

I. Ahmed, F. Thiessard, G. Miremont-Salame, F. Haramburu, C. Kreft-Jais, B. Begaud, and P. Tubert-Bitter. Early detection of pharmacovigilance signals with automated methods based on false discovery rates. *Drug Safety*, 35(6):495–506, 2012.

M. A. Al-Osh and A. A. Alzaid. First order integer-valued autoregressive (inar (1)) process. *Journal of Time Series Analysis*, 8(3):261–275, 1987.

P. D. Allison. Discrete-time methods for the analysis of event histories. *Sociological Methodology*, 13(1):61–98, 1982.

P. D. Allison. *Survival Analysis Using the SAS System: A Practical Guide*. SAS Institute, 1995.

P. D. Allison. *Fixed Effects Regression Models*. Sage Los Angeles, 2009.

J. S. Almenoff, W. DuMouchel, L. A. Kindman, X. Yang, and D. Fram. Disproportionality analysis using empirical Bayes data mining: a tool for the evaluation of drug interactions in the post-marketing setting. *Pharmacoepidemiology and Drug Safety*, 12(6):517–521, 2003.

S. Alwan, J. Reefhuis, S. A. Rasmussen, R. S. Olney, and J. M. Friedman. Use of selective serotonin-reuptake inhibitors in pregnancy and the risk of birth defects. *New England Journal of Medicine*, 356(26):2684–2692, 2007.

A. Amatya, D. K. Bhaumik, S. Normand, J. Greenhouse, E. Kaizar, B. Neelon, and R. D. Gibbons. Likelihood-based random effect meta-analysis of binary events. *Journal of Biopharmaceutical Statistics*, 2014.

J. D. Angrist, G. W. Imbens, and D. B. Rubin. Identification of causal effects using instrumental variables. *Journal of the American Statistical Association*, 91(434):444–455, 1996.

P. C. Austin. Propensity-score matching in the cardiovascular surgery literature from 2004 to 2006: a systematic review and suggestions for improvement. *The Journal of Thoracic and Cardiovascular Surgery*, 134(5): 1128–1135, 2007.

A. Bate and S. J. W. Evans. Quantitative signal detection using spontaneous adr reporting. *Pharmacoepidemiology and Drug Safety*, 18(6):427–436, 2009.

A. Bate, M. Lindquist, I. R. Edwards, S. Olsson, R. Orre, A. Lansner, and R. M. De Freitas. A Bayesian neural network method for adverse drug reaction signal generation. *European Journal of Clinical Pharmacology*, 54 (4):315–321, 1998.

D. K. Bhaumik, A. Amatya, S. T. Normand, J. Greenhouse, E. Kaizar, B. Neelon, and R. D. Gibbons. Meta-analysis of rare binary adverse event data. *Journal of the American Statistical Association*, 107(498):555–567, 2012.

R. Bock. *Multilevel Analysis of Educational Data*. Academic Press, 1989.

R. D. Bock. Estimating multinomial response relations. In R. C. Bose, editor, *Contributions to Statistics and Probability*, pages 453–479. University of North Carolina Press, Chapel Hill, NC, 1970.

R. D. Bock. *Multivariate Statistical Methods in Behavioral Research*. McGraw-Hill, 1975.

R. D. Bock. The discrete Bayesian. In H. Wainer and S. Messick, editors, *Modern Advances in Psychometric Research*, pages 103–115. Erlbaum, Hillsdale, N.J., 1983a.

R. D. Bock. Within-subject experimentation in psychiatric research. In R. D. Gibbons and M. W. Dysken, editors, *Statistical and Methodological Advances in Psychiatric Research*, pages 59–90. Spectrum New York, 1983b.

D. Bohning, U. Malzahn, E. Dietz, P. Schlattmann, C. Viwatwongkasem, and A. Biggeri. Some general points in estimating heterogeneity variance with the DerSimonian and Laird estimator. *Biostatistics*, 3(4):445–457, 2002.

J. Bound, D. A. Jaeger, and R. M. Baker. Problems with instrumental variables estimation when the correlation between the instruments and the endogenous explanatory variable is weak. *Journal of the American Statistical Association*, 90(430):443–450, 1995.

P. T. Brandt, J. T. Williams, B. O. Fordham, and B. Pollins. Dynamic modeling for persistent event-count time series. *American Journal of Political Science*, pages 823–843, 2000.

A. S. Bryk and S. W. Raudenbush. *Hierarchical Linear Models: Applications and Data Analysis Methods*. Sage Publications, Inc, 1992.

W. E. Bunney, D. L. Azarnoff, B. W. Brown, R. Cancro, R. D. Gibbons, J. C. Gillin, S. Hullett, K. F. Killam, D. J. Kupfer, J. H. Krystal, et al. Report of the institute of medicine committee on the efficacy and safety of halcion. *Archives of General Psychiatry*, 56(4):349–352, 1999.

S. P. Burke, A. Baciu, K. Straton, D. Blumenthal, A. Breckenridge, A. Charo, S. Edgman-Levitan, S. Ellenberg, R. D. Gibbons, and Others. *The Future of Drug Safety: Promoting and Protecting the Health of the Public*. National Academy Press, Washington D.C., 2006.

K. Cahill, L. F. Stead, and T. Lancaster. Nicotine receptor partial agonists for smoking cessation. *The Cochrane Library*, 2008.

K. Cahill, L. Stead, and T. Lancaster. A preliminary benefit-risk assessment of varenicline in smoking cessation. *Drug Safety*, 32(2):119–135, 2009.

A. C. Cameron and P. K. Trivedi. *Regression Analysis of Count Data*. Number 53. 2013.

O. Caster. Mining the who drug safety database using lasso logistic regression. *UUDM Project Report*, 16, 2007.

O. Caster, G. N. Norén, D. Madigan, and A. Bate. Large-scale regression-based pattern discovery: The example of screening the who global drug safety database. *Statistical Analysis and Data Mining*, 3(4):197–208, 2010.

G. Chamberlain and G. Imbens. Random effects estimators with many instrumental variables. *Econometrica*, 72(1):295–306, 2004.

J. Chen and A. K. Gupta. *Parametric Statistical Change Point Analysis: with Applications to Genetics, Medicine, and Finance*. Springer, 2011.

L. Chen and D. M. Ashcroft. Risk of myocardial infarction associated with selective cox-2 inhibitors: Meta-analysis of randomised controlled trials. *Pharmacoepidemiology and Drug Safety*, 16(7):762–772, 2007.

E. M. Chi and G. C. Reinsel. Models for longitudinal data with random effects and ar (1) errors. *Journal of the American Statistical Association*, 84(406): 452–459, 1989.

W. G. Cochran. The effectiveness of adjustment by subclassification in removing bias in observational studies. *Biometrics*, pages 295–313, 1968.

M. R. Conaway. Analysis of repeated categorical measurements with conditional likelihood methods. *Journal of the American Statistical Association*, 84(405):53–62, 1989.

A. J. Cook, R. C. Tiwari, R. D. Wellman, S. R. Heckbert, L. Li, P. Heagerty, T. Marsh, and J. C. Nelson. Statistical approaches to group sequential monitoring of postmarket safety surveillance data: current state of the art for use in the mini-sentinel pilot. *Pharmacoepidemiology and Drug Safety*, 21(S1):72–81, 2012.

N. R. Cook, S. R. Cole, and C. H. Hennekens. Use of a marginal structural model to determine the effect of aspirin on cardiovascular mortality in the physicians' health study. *American Journal of Epidemiology*, 155(11):1045–1053, 2002.

D. R. Cox. Analysis of binary data, 1970. *Methuen, London*, pages 103–8, 1970.

D. R. Cox. Regression models and life-tables. *Journal of the Royal Statistical Society*, 34(2):187–220, 1972.

D. R. Cox. Partial likelihood. *Biometrika*, 62(2):269–276, 1975.

R. B. D'Agostino. Tutorial in biostatistics: propensity score methods for bias reduction in the comparison of a treatment to a non-randomized control group. *Statistics in Medicine*, 17(19):2265–2281, 1998.

R. B. D'Agostino and R. B. D'Agostino. Estimating treatment effects using observational data. *Journal of American Medical Association*, 297(3):314–316, 2007.

R. B. D'Agostino, M. Lee, A. J. Belanger, L. Cupples, K. Anderson, and W. B. Kannel. Relation of pooled logistic regression to time dependent Cox regression analysis: the Framingham Heart Study. *Statistics in Medicine*, 9 (12):1501–1515, 1990.

R. B. D'Agostino, S. Grundy, L. M. Sullivan, P. Wilson, et al. Validation of the framingham coronary heart disease prediction scores: results of a multiple ethnic groups investigation. *Journal of American Medical Association*, 286 (2):180–187, 2001.

M. J. Daniels and C. Gatsonis. Hierarchical polytomous regression models with applications to health services research. *Statistics in Medicine*, 16(20): 2311–2325, 1997.

N. M. Davies, D. Gunnell, K. H. Thomas, C. Metcalfe, F. Windmeijer, and R. M. Martin. Physicians' prescribing preferences were a potential instrument for patients' actual prescriptions of antidepressants. *Journal of Clinical Epidemiology*, 66(12):1386–1396, 2013.

J. De Leeuw and I. Kreft. Random coefficient models for multilevel analysis. *Journal of Educational and Behavioral Statistics*, 11(1):57–85, 1986.

J. C. Delaney, M. D. Daskalopoulou, S. Stella, and S. Suissa. Traditional versus marginal structural models to estimate the effectiveness of β-blocker use on mortality after myocardial infarction. *Pharmacoepidemiology and Drug Safety*, 18(1):1–6, 2009.

A. P. Dempster, D. B. Rubin, and R. K. Tsutakawa. Estimation in covariance components models. *Journal of the American Statistical Association*, 76 (374):341–353, 1981.

R. DerSimonian and R. Kacker. Random-effects model for meta-analysis of clinical trials: an update. *Contemporary Clinical Trials*, 28(2):105–114, 2007.

R. DerSimonian and N. Laird. Meta-analysis in clinical trials. *Controlled Clinical Trials*, 7(3):177–188, 1986.

P. Diggle, P. Heagerty, K. Liang, and S. Zeger. *Analysis of Longitudinal Data*. Oxford University Press, 2002.

J. G. Donahue, S. T. Weiss, M. A. Goetsch, J. M. Livingston, D. K. Greineder, and R. Piatt. Assessment of asthma using automated and full-text medical records. *Journal of Asthma*, 34(4):273–281, 1997.

W. DuMouchel. Bayesian data mining in large frequency tables, with an application to the FDA spontaneous reporting system. *The American Statistician*, 53(3):177–190, 1999.

W. DuMouchel and R. Harpaz. Regression-adjusted gps algorithm (RGPS). Technical report, Oracle Health Sciences, 2012. White paper.

W. DuMouchel and D. Pregibon. Empirical Bayes screening for multi-item associations. In *Proceedings of the Seventh ACM SIGKDD International Conference on Knowledge Discovery and Data Mining*, KDD '01, pages 67–76, New York, NY, USA, 2001. ACM.

B. Efron. Logistic regression, survival analysis, and the Kaplan-Meier curve. *Journal of the American Statistical Association*, 83(402):414–425, 1988.

T. G. Egberts. Causal or casual? *Pharmacoepidemiology and Drug Safety*, 14 (6):365–366, 2005.

R. C. Elandt-Johnson and N. L. Johnson. *Survival Distributions*. John Wiley & Sons, Inc., 1999.

V. P. Eugène, A. Egberts, E. R. Heerdink, and H. Leufkens. Detecting drug–drug interactions using a database for spontaneous adverse drug reactions: an example with diuretics and non-steroidal anti-inflammatory drugs. *European Journal of Clinical Pharmacology*, 56(9-10):733–738, 2000.

L. Evans. The effectiveness of safety belts in preventing fatalities. *Accident Analysis & Prevention*, 18(3):229–241, 1986.

S. J. Evans, P. C. Waller, and S. Davis. Use of proportional reporting ratios (PRRs) for signal generation from spontaneous adverse drug reaction reports. *Pharmacoepidemiology and Drug Safety*, 10(6):483–486, 2001.

C. P. Farrington. Relative incidence estimation from case series for vaccine safety evaluation. *Biometrics*, pages 228–235, 1995.

G. M. Fitzmaurice, N. M. Laird, and J. H. Ware. *Applied Longitudinal Data*. NJ: John Wiley & Sons, Inc., 2004.

J. L. Fleiss. Significance tests have a role in epidemiologic research: reactions to am walker. *American Journal of Public Health*, 76(5):559–560, 1986.

T. R. Fleming and D. P. Harrington. *Counting Processes and Survival Analysis*, volume 169. John Wiley & Sons, 2011.

M. H. Gail. Does cardiac transplantation prolong life? A reassessment. *Annals of Internal Medicine*, 76(5):815–817, 1972.

L. A. García Rodríguez and S. Pérez Gutthann. Use of the UK general practice research database for pharmacoepidemiology. *British Journal of Clinical Pharmacology*, 45(5):419–425, 1998.

A. Genkin, D. D. Lewis, and D. Madigan. Large-scale Bayesian logistic regression for text categorization. *Technometrics*, 49(3):291–304, 2007.

R. D. Gibbons. *Trend in Correlated Proportions*. PhD dissertation, University of Chicago, 1981.

R. D. Gibbons and R. D. Bock. Trend in correlated proportions. *Psychometrika*, 52(1):113–124, 1987.

R. D. Gibbons and J. J. Mann. Strategies for quantifying the relationship between medications and suicidal behaviour. *Drug Safety*, 34(5):375–395, 2011.

R. D. Gibbons and J. J. Mann. Varenicline, smoking cessation, and neuropsychiatric adverse events. *American Journal of Psychiatry*, 170(12):1460–1467, 2013.

R. D. Gibbons, D. Hedeker, S. C. Charles, and P. Frisch. A random-effects probit model for predicting medical malpractice claims. *Journal of the American Statistical Association*, 89(427):760–767, 1994.

R. D. Gibbons, B. Brown, D. L. Azarnoff, W. E. Bunney, R. Cancro, J. C. Gillin, S. Hullett, K. F. Killam, J. H. Krystal, D. J. Kupfer, et al. Assessment of the safety and efficacy data for the hypnotic halcion (r): Results of an analysis by an institute of medicine committee. *Journal of the American Statistical Association*, 94(448):993–1002, 1999.

R. D. Gibbons, N. Duan, D. Meltzer, A. Pope, E. D. Penhoet, N. N. Dubler, C. Francis, B. Gill, E. Guinan, M. Henderson, et al. Waiting for organ transplantation: results of an analysis by an institute of medicine committee. *Biostatistics*, 4(2):207–222, 2003.

R. D. Gibbons, K. Hur, D. K. Bhaumik, and J. J. Mann. The relationship between antidepressant medication use and rate of suicide. *Archives of General Psychiatry*, 62(2):165–172, 2005.

R. D. Gibbons, K. Hur, D. K. Bhaumik, and J. J. Mann. The relationship between antidepressant prescription rates and rate of early adolescent suicide. *American Journal of Psychiatry*, 163(11):1898–1904, 2006.

R. D. Gibbons, C. Brown, K. Hur, S. Marcus, D. Bhaumik, and J. Mann. Relationship between antidepressants and suicide attempts: an analysis of the veterans health administration data sets. *American Journal of Psychiatry*, 164(7):1044–1049, 2007.

R. D. Gibbons, E. Segawa, G. Karabatsos, A. Amatya, D. K. Bhaumik, H. Brown, K. Kapur, S. M. Marcus, K. Hur, and J. J. Mann. Adaptive centering with random effects: An alternative to the fixed effects model for studying time-varying treatments in school settings. *Statistics in Medicine*, 27(11):1814–1833, 2008.

R. D. Gibbons, K. Hur, C. H. Brown, and J. J. Mann. Relationship between antiepileptic drugs and suicide attempts in patients with bipolar disorder. *Archives of General Psychiatry*, 66(12):1354–1360, 2009.

R. D. Gibbons, C. H. Brown, K. Hur, J. M. Davis, and J. J. Mann. Suicidal thoughts and behavior with antidepressant treatment: reanalysis of the randomized placebo-controlled studies of fluoxetine and venlafaxine. *Archives of General Psychiatry*, 69(6):580–587, 2012a.

R. D. Gibbons, K. Hur, C. H. Brown, J. M. Davis, and J. J. Mann. Benefits from antidepressants: synthesis of 6-week patient-level outcomes from double-blind placebo-controlled randomized trials of fluoxetine and venlafaxine. *Archives of General Psychiatry*, 69(6):572–579, 2012b.

R. D. Gibbons, M. Coca Perraillon, K. Hur, R. M. Conti, R. J. Valuck, and D. A. Brent. Antidepressant treatment and suicide attempts and self-inflicted injury in children and adolescents. *Pharmacoepidemiology and Drug Safety*, 2014.

S. K. Goldsmith, T. C. Pellmar, A. M. Kleinman, and W. E. Bunney. *Reducing suicide: A National Imperative*. National Academies Press, 2002.

H. Goldstein. *Multilevel Statistical Models*, volume 922. John Wiley & Sons, 2011.

X. S. Gu and P. R. Rosenbaum. Comparison of multivariate matching methods: Structures, distances, and algorithms. *Journal of Computational and Graphical Statistics*, 2(4):405–420, 1993.

T.A. Hammad. Review and evaluation of clinical data., 2004. URL http://www.fda.gov/ohrms/dockets/ac/04/briefing/ 2004-4065b1-10-TAB08-Hammads-Review.pdf.

D. J. Hand. Data mining: Statistics and more? *The American Statistician*, 52(2):112–118, 1998.

B. B. Hansen. Full matching in an observational study of coaching for the sat. *Journal of the American Statistical Association*, 99(467):609–618, 2004.

R. J. Hardy and S. G. Thompson. A likelihood approach to meta-analysis with random effects. *Statistics in Medicine*, 15:619–629, 1996.

L. R. Harrold, K. G. Saag, R. A. Yood, T. R. Mikuls, S. E. Andrade, H. Fouayzi, J. Davis, K. A. Chan, M. A. Raebel, and W. A. Von. Validity of gout diagnoses in administrative data. *Arthritis Care & Research*, 57(1):103–108, 2007.

J. Hartzel, A. Agresti, and B. Caffo. Multinomial logit random effects models. *Statistical Modelling*, 1(2):81–102, 2001.

T. Hastie, R. Tibshirani, and J. Friedman. *The Elements of Statistical Learning*. Springer, New York, 2001.

M. Hauben and X. Zhou. Quantitative methods in pharmacovigilance. *Drug Safety*, 26(3):159–186, 2003.

M. Hauben, S. Horn, and L. Reich. Potential use of data-mining algorithms for the detection of surpriseadverse drug reactions. *Drug Safety*, 30(2):143–155, 2007.

D. Hedeker. *Random Regression Models with Autocorrelated Errors*. PhD dissertation, University of Chicago, Department of Psychology, 1989.

D. Hedeker. A mixed-effects multinomial logistic regression model. *Statistics in Medicine*, 22(9):1433–1446, 2003.

D. Hedeker and R. D. Gibbons. A random-effects ordinal regression model for multilevel analysis. *Biometrics*, pages 933–944, 1994.

D. Hedeker and R. D. Gibbons. *Longitudinal Data Analysis*, volume 451. John Wiley & Sons, 2006.

D. Hedeker and R. D. Gibbons. A comparison of fixed-effect and random-effect models for survival analysis. Technical report, University of Chicago, Center for Health Statistics, 2015.

D. Hedeker, R. D. Gibbons, C. Waternaux, and J. M. Davis. Investigating drug plasma levels and clinical response using random regression models. *Psychopharmacology Bulletin*, 25(2):227–231, 1988.

D. Hedeker, O. Siddiqui, and F. B. Hu. Random-effects regression analysis of correlated grouped-time survival data. *Statistical Methods in Medical Research*, 9(2):161–179, 2000.

L. Held, M. Höhle, and M. Hofmann. A statistical framework for the analysis of multivariate infectious disease surveillance counts. *Statistical Modeling*, 5(3):187–199, 2005.

S. Hennessy, C. E. Leonard, C. P. Freeman, R. Deo, C. Newcomb, S. E. Kimmel, B. L. Strom, and W. B. Bilker. Validation of diagnostic codes for outpatient-originating sudden cardiac death and ventricular arrhythmia in medicaid and medicare claims data. *Pharmacoepidemiology and Drug Safety*, 19(6):555–562, 2010.

P. T. Higgins and S. G. Thompson. Quantifying heterogeneity in a meta-analysis. *Statistics in Medicine*, 21(11):1539–1558, 2002.

P. W. Holland. Statistics and causal inference. *Journal of the American Statistical Association*, 81(396):945–960, 1986.

D. Hosmer, S. Lemeshow, and S. May. *Applied Survival Analysis*. NJ, Wiley, 2008.

P. J. Huber. The behavior of maximum likelihood estimates under nonstandard conditions. In *Proceedings of the Fifth Berkeley Symposium on Mathematical Statistics and Probability*, volume 1, pages 221–233, 1967.

S. L. Hui and J. O. Berger. Empirical Bayes estimation of rates in longitudinal studies. *Journal of the American Statistical Association*, 78(384):753–760, 1983.

E. Jimenez-Solem, J. T. Andersen, M. Petersen, K. Broedbaek, J. K. Jensen, S. Afzal, G. H. Gislason, C. Torp-Pedersen, and H. E. Poulsen. Exposure to selective serotonin reuptake inhibitors and the risk of congenital malformations: a nationwide cohort study. *British Medical Journal*, 2(3), 2012.

J. D. Kalbfleisch and R. L. Prentice. *The Statistical Analysis of Failure Time Data*, volume 360. John Wiley & Sons, 2011.

G. King. Variance specification in event count models: From restrictive assumptions to a generalized estimator. *American Journal of Political Science*, pages 762–784, 1989.

I. Kirsch, B. J. Deacon, T. B. Huedo-Medina, A. Scoboria, T. J. Moore, and B. T. Johnson. Initial severity and antidepressant benefits: a meta-analysis of data submitted to the food and drug administration. *PLoS medicine*, 5 (2):e45, 2008.

M. Kulldorff, R. L. Davis, M. Kolczakar, E. Lewis, T. Lieu, and R. Platt. A maximized sequential probability ratio test for drug and vaccine safety surveillance. *Sequential Analysis*, 30(1):58–78, 2011.

N. M. Laird. Missing data in longitudinal studies. *Statistics in Medicine*, 7 (1-2):305–315, 1988.

N. M. Laird and J. H. Ware. Random-effects models for longitudinal data. *Biometrics*, pages 963–974, 1982.

K. K. Gordon Lan and D. L. DeMets. Discrete sequential boundaries for clinical trials. *Biometrika*, 70(3):659–663, 1983.

D. S. Lee, L. Donovan, P. C. Austin, Y. Gong, P. P. Liu, J. L. Rouleau, and J. V. Tu. Comparison of coding of heart failure and comorbidities in administrative and clinical data for use in outcomes research. *Medical Care*, 43(2):182–188, 2005.

A. C. Leon and D. Hedeker. Quintile stratification based on a misspecified propensity score in longitudinal treatment effectiveness analyses of ordinal doses. *Computational Statistics and Data Analysis*, 51(12):6114–6122, 2007.

C. E. Leonard, K. Haynes, A. R. Localio, S. Hennessy, J. Tjia, A. Cohen, S. E. Kimmel, H. I. Feldman, and J. P. Metlay. Diagnostic e-codes for commonly used, narrow therapeutic index medications poorly predict adverse drug events. *Journal of Clinical Epidemiology*, 61(6):561–571, 2008.

L. E. Lévesque, J. A. Hanley, A. Kezouh, and S. Suissa. Problem of immortal time bias in cohort studies: example using statins for preventing progression of diabetes. *British Medical Journal*, 340, 2010.

J. D. Lewis, R. Schinnar, W. B. Bilker, X. Wang, and B. L. Strom. Validation studies of the health improvement network (thin) database for pharmacoepidemiology research. *Pharmacoepidemiology and Drug Safety*, 16(4): 393–401, 2007.

L. Li. A conditional sequential sampling procedure for drug safety surveillance. *Statistics in Medicine*, 28(25):3124–3138, 2009.

K. Liang and S. L. Zeger. Longitudinal data analysis using generalized linear models. *Biometrika*, 73(1):13–22, 1986.

R. Little and D. B. Rubin. *Statistical Analysis With Missing Data.* Wiley, 2002.

R. J. Little. Modeling the drop-out mechanism in repeated-measures studies. *Journal of the American Statistical Association*, 90(431):1112–1121, 1995.

D. Liu, R. Y. Liu, and M. Xie. Exact meta-analysis approach for discrete data and its application to 2× 2 tables with rare events. *Journal of the American Statistical Association*, 2014.

N. T. Longford. A fast-scoring algorithm for maximum likelihood estimation in unbalanced mixed models with nested random effects. *Biometrika*, 74 (4):817–827, 1987.

N. T. Longford. *Random Coefficient Models.* Springer, 1995.

C. Louik, A. E. Lin, M. M. Werler, S. Hernández-Díaz, and A. A. Mitchell. First-trimester use of selective serotonin-reuptake inhibitors and the risk of birth defects. *New England Journal of Medicine*, 356(26):2675–2683, 2007.

J. Ludwig and D. E. Marcotte. Anti-depressants, suicide, and drug regulation. *Journal of Policy Analysis and Management*, 24(2):249–272, 2005.

D. G. Luenberger. *Introduction to Linear and Nonlinear Programming.* Addison-Wesley, Reading, MA, second edition, 1984.

M. Maclure. The case-crossover design: a method for studying transient effects on the risk of acute events. *American Journal of Epidemiology*, 133(2):144–153, 1991.

G. S. Maddala. *Limited-dependent and Qualitative Variables in Econometrics.* Number 3. Cambridge University Press, 1983.

D. Madigan, P. E. Stang, J. A. Berlin, M. Schuemie, J. M. Overhage, M. A. Suchard, W. Dumouchel, A. G. Hartzema, and P. B. Ryan. A systematic statistical approach to evaluating evidence from observational studies. *Annual Review of Statistics and Its Application*, 1:11–39, 2014.

J. R. Magnus and H. Neudecker. *Matrix Differential Calculus with Applications in Statistics and Econometrics.* John Wiley & Sons, 1995.

R. J. Månsson, M. Marshall, W. Sun, and S. Hennessy. On the estimation and use of propensity scores in case-control and case-cohort studies. *American Journal of Epidemiology*, 166(3):332–339, 2007.

N. Mantel and W. Haenszel. Statistical aspects of the analysis of data from retrospective studies of disease. *Journal of National Cancer Institute*, 22 (4):719–748, 1959.

P. McCullagh. Regression models for ordinal data. *Journal of the Royal Statistical Society. Series B (Methodological)*, pages 109–142, 1980.

P. McCullagh and J. A. Nelder. *Generalized Linear Models*. Chapman and Hall, London, England, 1989.

B. J. Messmer, R. D. Leachman, J. J. Nora, and D. A. Cooley. Survival-times after cardiac allografts. *The Lancet*, 293(7602):954–956, 1969.

T. E. Meyer, L. G. Taylor, S. Xie, D. J. Graham, A. D. Mosholder, J. R. Williams, D. Moeny, R. P. Ouellet-Hellstrom, and T. S. Coster. Neuropsychiatric events in varenicline and nicotine replacement patch users in the military health system. *Addiction*, 108(1):203–210, 2013.

D. R. Miller, S. A. Oliveria, D. R. Berlowitz, B. G. Fincke, P. Stang, and D. E. Lillienfeld. Angioedema incidence in US veterans initiating angiotensin-converting enzyme inhibitors. *Hypertension*, 51(6):1624–1630, 2008.

E. Miller, P. Farrington, M. Goldacre, S. Pugh, A. Colville, A. Flower, J. Nash, L. MacFarlane, and R. Tettmar. Risk of aseptic meningitis after measles, mumps, and rubella vaccine in UK children. *The Lancet*, 341 (8851):979–982, 1993.

J. E. Miller, M. Z. Molnar, C. P. Kovesdy, J. J. Zaritsky, E. Streja, I. Salusky, O. A. Arah, and K. Kalantar-Zadeh. Administered paricalcitol dose and survival in hemodialysis patients: a marginal structural model analysis. *Pharmacoepidemiology and Drug Safety*, 21(11):1232–1239, 2012.

R. G. Miller. *Survival analysis*, volume 66. John Wiley & Sons, 2011.

K. Ming and P. R. Rosenbaum. Substantial gains in bias reduction from matching with a variable number of controls. *Biometrics*, 56(1):118–124, 2000.

N. Moore, G. Hall, M. Sturkenboom, R. Mann, R. Lagnaoui, and B. Begaud. Biases affecting the proportional reporting ratio (prr) in spontaneous reports pharmacovigilance databases: the example of sertindole. *Pharmacoepidemiology and Drug Safety*, 12(4):271–281, 2003.

N. Moore, F. Thiessard, and B. Begaud. The history of disproportionality measures (reporting odds ratio, proportional reporting rates) in spontaneous reporting of adverse drug reactions. *Pharmacoepidemiology and Drug Safety*, 14(4):285–286, 2005.

H. Morgenstern. Ecologic studies in epidemiology: concepts, principles, and methods. *Annual Review of Public Health*, 16(1):61–81, 1995.

M. Nerlove and S. J. Press. *Univariate and Multivariate Log-linear and Logistic Models*, volume 1306. Rand Corporation, Santa Monica, CA, 1973.

J. M. Neuhaus and J. D. Kalbfleisch. Between-and within-cluster covariate effects in the analysis of clustered data. *Biometrics*, pages 638–645, 1998.

J. M. Neuhaus and C. E. McCulloch. Separating between-and within-cluster covariate effects by using conditional and partitioning methods. *Journal of the Royal Statistical Society: Series B (Statistical Methodology)*, 68(5): 859–872, 2006.

J. M. Neuhaus, J. D. Kalbfleisch, and W. W. Hauck. A comparison of cluster-specific and population-averaged approaches for analyzing correlated binary data. *International Statistical Review/Revue Internationale de Statistique*, pages 25–35, 1991.

G. N. Norén, R. Sundberg, A. Bate, and I. R. Edwards. A statistical methodology for drug–drug interaction surveillance. *Statistics in Medicine*, 27(16): 3057–3070, 2008.

P. C. O'Brien and T. R. Fleming. A multiple testing procedure for clinical trials. *Biometrics*, pages 549–556, 1979.

Institute of Medicine. *Organ Procurement and Transplantation: Assessing Current Policies and the Potential Impact of the DHHS Final Rule.* National Academy Press, Washington D.C., 1999.

M. Olfson and S. C. Marcus. National patterns in antidepressant medication treatment. *Archives of General Psychiatry*, 66(8):848–856, 2009.

R. Orre, A. Lansner, A. Bate, and M. Lindquist. Bayesian neural networks with confidence estimations applied to data mining. *Computational Statistics and Data Analysis*, 34(4):473–493, 2000.

R. C. Paule and J. Mandel. Consensus values and weighting factors. *Journal of Research of the National Bureau of Standards*, 87(5):377–385, 1982.

L. J. Paulozzi, D. S. Budnitz, and Y. Xi. Increasing deaths from opioid analgesics in the United States. *Pharmacoepidemiology and Drug Safety*, 15(9): 618–627, 2006.

Y. Pawitan. Change-point problem with biostatistical applications. In *Wiley StatsRef: Statistics Reference Online.* Wiley Online Library, 2014.

M. B. Perry, J. J. Pignatiello, and J. R. Simpson. Estimating the change point of a poisson rate parameter with a linear trend disturbance. *Quality and Reliability Engineering International*, 22(4):371–384, 2006.

R. L. Plackett. *The Analysis of Categorical Data.* Griffin, London, 1974.

M. Pladevall, D. C. Goff, M. Z. Nichaman, F. Chan, D. Ramsey, C. Ortiz, and D. R. Labarthe. An assessment of the validity of ICD code 410 to identify hospital admissions for myocardial infarction: The corpus christi heart project. *International Journal of Epidemiology*, 25(5):948–952, 1996.

S. J. Pocock. Interim analyses for randomized clinical trials: the group sequential approach. *Biometrics*, pages 153–162, 1982.

R. F. Potthoff and S. N. Roy. A generalized multivariate analysis of variance model useful especially for growth curve problems. *Biometrika*, 51(3-4): 313–326, 1964.

R. L. Prentice and L. A. Gloeckler. Regression analysis of grouped survival data with application to breast cancer data. *Biometrics*, pages 57–67, 1978.

Y. Qian, X. Ye, W. Du, J. Ren, Y. Sun, H. Wang, B. Luo, Q. Gao, M. Wu, and J. He. A computerized system for detecting signals due to drug–drug interactions in spontaneous reporting systems. *British Journal of Clinical Pharmacology*, 69(1):67–73, 2010.

S. W. Raudenbush. Adaptive centering with random effects: An alternative to the fixed effects model for studying time-varying treatments in school settings. *Education*, 4(4):468–491, 2009.

S. W. Raudenbush and A. S. Bryk. *Hierarchical Linear models: Applications and Data Analysis Methods*, volume 1. Sage, 2002.

M. D. Rawlins. Postmarketing surveillance of adverse reactions to drugs. *British Medical Journal (Clinical Research ed.)*, 288(6421):879, 1984.

D. Revelt and K. Train. Mixed logit with repeated choices: households' choices of appliance efficiency level. *Review of Economics and Statistics*, 80(4):647–657, 1998.

J. M. Robins, M. A. Hernan, and B. Brumback. Marginal structural models and causal inference in epidemiology. *Epidemiology*, 11(5):550–560, 2000.

P. R. Rosenbaum. A characterization of optimal designs for observational studies. *Journal of the Royal Statistical Society. Series B (Methodological)*, pages 597–610, 1991.

P. R. Rosenbaum. Quantiles in nonrandom samples and observational studies. *Journal of the American Statistical Association*, 90(432):1424–1431, 1995.

P. R. Rosenbaum. *Observational Studies*. Springer, second edition, 2002.

P. R. Rosenbaum. Differential effects and generic biases in observational studies. *Biometrika*, 93(3):573–586, 2006.

P. R. Rosenbaum and D. B. Rubin. The central role of the propensity score in observational studies for causal effects. *Biometrika*, 70(1):41–55, 1983.

P. R. Rosenbaum and D. B. Rubin. Reducing bias in observational studies using subclassification on the propensity score. *Journal of the American Statistical Association*, 79(387):516–524, 1984.

P. R. Rosenbaum and D. B. Rubin. The bias due to incomplete matching. *Biometrics*, pages 103–116, 1985.

P. R. Rosenbaum, R. N. Ross, and J. H. Silber. Minimum distance matched sampling with fine balance in an observational study of treatment for ovarian cancer. *Journal of the American Statistical Association*, 102(477):75–83, 2007.

K. J. Rothman, S. Greenland, and T. L. Lash. *Modern Epidemiology*. Lippincott Williams & Wilkins, 2008.

D. B. Rubin. Inference and missing data. *Biometrika*, 63(3):581–592, 1976.

D. B. Rubin. Bayesian inference for causal effects: The role of randomization. *The Annals of Statistics*, pages 34–58, 1978.

D. B. Rubin. Estimating causal effects from large data sets using propensity scores. *Annals of Internal Medicine*, 127(8_Part_2):757–763, 1997.

D. B. Rubin. On principles for modeling propensity scores in medical research. *Pharmacoepidemiology and Drug Safety*, 13(12):855–857, 2004.

G. Rucker, G. Schwarzer, J. Carpenter, and M. Schumacher. Undue reliance on I^2 in assessing heterogeneity may mislead. *BMC Medical Research Methodology*, 8(1):79, 2008.

S. Schneeweiss. A basic study design for expedited safety signal evaluation based on electronic healthcare data. *Pharmacoepidemiology and Drug Safety*, 19(8):858–868, 2010.

A. Schömig, J. Mehilli, A. de Waha, M. Seyfarth, J. Pache, and A. Kastrati. A meta-analysis of 17 randomized trials of a percutaneous coronary intervention-based strategy in patients with stable coronary artery disease. *Journal of the American College of Cardiology*, 52(11):894–904, 2008.

G. Schwarz. Estimating the dimension of a model. *The Annals of Statistics*, 6(2):461–464, 1978.

T. Schweder and N. Hjort. Confidence and likelihood. *Scandinavian Journal of Statistics*, 29(2):309–332, 2002.

J. J. Shuster. Empirical vs natural weighting in random effects meta-analysis. *Statistics in Medicine*, 29(12):1259–1265, 2010.

K. Sidik and J. N. Jonkman. Simple heterogeneity variance estimation for meta-analysis. *Journal of the Royal Statistical Society: Series C (Applied Statistics)*, 54(2):367–384, 2005.

J. D. Singer and J. B. Willett. Its about time: Using discrete-time survival analysis to study duration and the timing of events. *Journal of Educational and Behavioral Statistics*, 18(2):155–195, 1993.

J. D. Singer and J. B. Willett. *Applied Longitudinal Data Analysis: Modeling Change and Event Occurrence.* Oxford University Press, 2003.

K. Singh, M. Xie, and W. E. Strawderman. Combining information from independent sources through confidence distributions. *The Annals of Statistics,* 33(1):159–183, 2005.

A. Sjölander, P. Lichtenstein, H. Larsson, and Y. Pawitan. Between–within models for survival analysis. *Statistics in Medicine,* 32(18):3067–3076, 2013.

L. So, D. Evans, and H. Quan. ICD-10 coding algorithms for defining comorbidities of acute myocardial infarction. *BMC Health Services Research,* 6 (1):161, 2006.

P. E. Stang, P. B. Ryan, J. A. Racoosin, J. Overhage, A. G. Hartzema, C. Reich, E. Welebob, T. Scarnecchia, and J. Woodcock. Advancing the science for active surveillance: rationale and design for the observational medical outcomes partnership. *Annals of Internal Medicine,* 153(9):600–606, 2010.

R. Stiratelli, N. Laird, and J. H. Ware. Random-effects models for serial observations with binary response. *Biometrics,* pages 961–971, 1984.

J. F. Strenio, H. I. Weisberg, and A. S. Bryk. Empirical Bayes estimation of individual growth-curve parameters and their relationship to covariates. *Biometrics,* pages 71–86, 1983.

B. L. Strom. Data validity issues in using claims data. *Pharmacoepidemiology and Drug Safety,* 10(5):389–392, 2001.

B. L. Strom. *Pharmacoepidemiology.* John Wiley & Sons, 2006.

A. H. Stroud and D. Secrest. *Gaussian Quadrature Formulas.* Prentice Hall, 1966.

S. Suissa. Immortal time bias in observational studies of drug effects. *Pharmacoepidemiology and Drug Safety,* 16(3):241–249, 2007.

S. Suissa and L. Azoulay. Metformin and the risk of cancer time-related biases in observational studies. *Diabetes Care,* 35(12):2665–2673, 2012.

A. Szarfman, S. G. Machado, and R. T. ONeill. Use of screening algorithms and computer systems to efficiently signal higher-than-expected combinations of drugs and events in the US FDA'S spontaneous reports database. *Drug Safety,* 25(6):381–392, 2002.

P. L. Thomas. U.S. Food and Drug Administration clinical review relationship between antidepressant drugs and suicidality in adults, 2006. URL http://www.fda.gov/ohrms/dockets/ac/06/briefing/2006-4272b1-01-FDA.pdf. [accessed on 22 July 2007].

L. Tian, T. Cai, M. A. Pfeffer, N. Piankov, P. Cremieux, and L. J. Wei. Exact and efficient inference procedure for meta-analysis and its application to the analysis of independent 2×2 tables with all available data but without artificial continuity correction. *Biostatistics*, 10(2):275–281, 2009.

S. Toh and J. E. Manson. An analytic framework for aligning observational and randomized trial data: application to postmenopausal hormone therapy and coronary heart disease. *Statistics in Biosciences*, 5(2):344–360, 2013.

E. A. Torkamani, S. Niaki, M. Aminnayeri, and M. Davoodi. Estimating the change point of correlated poisson count processes. *Quality Engineering*, 26 (2), 2014.

H. Tunstall-Pedoe. Validity of ICD code 410 to identify hospital admission for myocardial infarction. *International Journal of Epidemiology*, 26(2): 461–462, 1997.

E. H. Turner, A. M. Matthews, E. Linardatos, R. A. Tell, and R. Rosenthal. Selective publication of antidepressant trials and its influence on apparent efficacy. *New England Journal of Medicine*, 358(3):252–260, 2008.

M. Valenstein, H. M. Kim, D. Ganoczy, D. Eisenberg, P. N. Pfeiffer, K. Downing, K. Hoggatt, M. Ilgen, K. L. Austin, K. Zivin, et al. Antidepressant agents and suicide death among us department of veterans affairs patients in depression treatment. *Journal of Clinical Psychopharmacology*, 32(3): 346, 2012.

C. Varas-Lorenzo, J. Castellsague, M. R. Stang, L. Tomas, J. Aguado, and S. Perez-Gutthann. Positive predictive value of ICD-9 codes 410 and 411 in the identification of cases of acute coronary syndromes in the Saskatchewan Hospital automated database. *Pharmacoepidemiology and Drug Safety*, 17 (8):842–852, 2008.

G. R. Venning. Identification of adverse reactions to new drugs. II - how were 18 important adverse reactions discovered and with what delays? *British Medical Journal (Clinical Research ed.)*, 286(6361):289, 1983.

G. Verbeke and G. Molenberghs. *Linear Mixed Models for Longitudinal Data.* Springer, 2000.

W. Viechtbauer. Confidence intervals for the amount of heterogeneity in meta-analysis. *Statistics in Medicine*, 26(1):37–52, 2007.

J. Villerd, Y. Toussaint, and A. Lillo-Le Louët. Adverse drug reaction mining in pharmacovigilance data using formal concept analysis. In *Machine Learning and Knowledge Discovery in Databases*, pages 386–401. 2010.

P. M. Wahl, K. Rodgers, S. Schneeweiss, B. F. Gage, J. Butler, C. Wilmer,

M. Nash, G. Esper, N. Gitlin, and N. Osborn. Validation of claims-based diagnostic and procedure codes for cardiovascular and gastrointestinal serious adverse events in a commercially-insured population. *Pharmacoepidemiology and Drug Safety*, 19(6):596–603, 2010.

D. E. Warn, S. G. Thompson, and D. J. Spiegelhalter. Bayesian random effects meta-analysis of trials with binary outcomes: methods for the absolute risk difference and relative risk scales. *Statistics in Medicine*, 21(11):1601–1623, 2002.

J. P. Weber. Epidemiology of adverse reactions to nonsteroidal antiinflammatory drugs. *Advances in Inflammation Research*, 1984.

C. H. Weiss. Detecting mean increases in poisson INAR(1) processes with EWMA control charts. *Journal of Applied Statistics*, 38(2):383–398, 2011.

C. H. Weiss and M. C. Testik. CUSUM monitoring of first-order integer-valued autoregressive processes of poisson counts. *Journal of Quality Technology*, 41(4):389–400, 2009.

H. White. A heteroskedasticity-consistent covariance matrix estimator and a direct test for heteroskedasticity. *Econometrica: Journal of the Econometric Society*, pages 817–838, 1980.

H. White. Maximum likelihood estimation of misspecified models. *Econometrica: Journal of the Econometric Society*, pages 1–25, 1982.

M. Wilchesky, R. M. Tamblyn, and A. Huang. Validation of diagnostic codes within medical services claims. *Journal of Clinical Epidemiology*, 57(2): 131–141, 2004.

R. Wolfinger. Laplace's approximation for nonlinear mixed models. *Biometrika*, 80(4):791–795, 1993.

G. Y. Wong and W. M. Mason. The hierarchical logistic regression model for multilevel analysis. *Journal of the American Statistical Association*, 80 (391):513–524, 1985.

X. Wu, D. Barbará, and Y. Ye. Screening and interpreting multi-item associations based on log-linear modeling. In *Proceedings of the ninth ACM SIGKDD International Conference on Knowledge Discovery and Data Mining*, pages 276–285, 2003.

M. Xie, K. Singh, and W. E. Strawderman. Confidence distributions and a unifying framework for meta-analysis. *Journal of the American Statistical Association*, 106(493), 2011.

W. Yang and M. M. Joffe. Subtle issues in model specification and estimation of marginal structural models. *Pharmacoepidemiology and Drug Safety*, 21 (3):241–245, 2012.

S. L. Zeger. A regression model for time series of counts. *Biometrika*, 75(4): 621–629, 1988.

S. L. Zeger and K. Liang. Longitudinal data analysis for discrete and continuous outcomes. *Biometrics*, pages 121–130, 1986.

S. L. Zeger and B. Qaqish. Markov regression models for time series: a quasi-likelihood approach. *Biometrics*, pages 1019–1031, 1988.

S. L. Zeger, K. Liang, and P. S. Albert. Models for longitudinal data: a generalized estimating equation approach. *Biometrics*, pages 1049–1060, 1988.

T. Zhang and F. J. Oles. Text categorization based on regularized linear classification methods. *Information Retrieval*, 4(1):5–31, 2001.

Index